T0198194

Cavus Foot Deformity

Editor

HARRY JOHN VISSER

CLINICS IN PODIATRIC MEDICINE AND SURGERY

www.podiatric.theclinics.com

Consulting Editor
THOMAS J. CHANG

July 2021 • Volume 38 • Number 3

ELSEVIER

1600 John F. Kennedy Boulevard • Suite 1800 • Philadelphia, Pennsylvania, 19103-2899

http://www.theclinics.com

CLINICS IN PODIATRIC MEDICINE AND SURGERY Volume 38, Number 3
July 2021 ISSN 0891-8422, ISBN-13: 978-0-323-79595-1

Editor: Lauren Boyle
Developmental Editor: Diana Grace Ang

© **2021 Elsevier Inc. All rights reserved.**

This periodical and the individual contributions contained in it are protected under copyright by Elsevier, and the following terms and conditions apply to their use:

Photocopying
Single photocopies of single articles may be made for personal use as allowed by national copyright laws. Permission of the Publisher and payment of a fee is required for all other photocopying, including multiple or systematic copying, copying for advertising or promotional purposes, resale, and all forms of document delivery. Special rates are available for educational institutions that wish to make photocopies for non-profit educational classroom use. For information on how to seek permission visit www.elsevier.com/permissions or call: (+44) 1865 843830 (UK)/(+1) 215 239 3804 (USA).

Derivative Works
Subscribers may reproduce tables of contents or prepare lists of articles including abstracts for internal circulation within their institutions. Permission of the Publisher is required for resale or distribution outside the institution. Permission of the Publisher is required for all other derivative works, including compilations and translations (please consult www.elsevier.com/permissions).

Electronic Storage or Usage
Permission of the Publisher is required to store or use electronically any material contained in this periodical, including any article or part of an article (please consult www.elsevier.com/permissions). Except as outlined above, no part of this publication may be reproduced, stored in a retrieval system or transmitted in any form or by any means, electronic, mechanical, photocopying, recording or otherwise, without prior written permission of the Publisher.

Notice
No responsibility is assumed by the Publisher for any injury and/or damage to persons or property as a matter of products liability, negligence or otherwise, or from any use or operation of any methods, products, instructions or ideas contained in the material herein. Because of rapid advances in the medical sciences, in particular, independent verification of diagnoses and drug dosages should be made.

Although all advertising material is expected to conform to ethical (medical) standards, inclusion in this publication does not constitute a guarantee or endorsement of the quality or value of such product or of the claims made of it by its manufacturer.

Clinics in Podiatric Medicine and Surgery (ISSN 0891-8422) is published quarterly by Elsevier Inc., 360 Park Avenue South, New York, NY 10010-1710. Months of issue are January, April, July, and October. Business and Editorial Offices: 1600 John F. Kennedy Blvd., Ste. 1800, Philadelphia, PA 19103-2899. Customer Service Office: 3251 Riverport Lane, Maryland Heights, MO 63043. Periodicals postage paid at New York, NY and additional mailing offices. Subscription prices are $310.00 per year for US individuals, $750.00 per year for US institutions, $100.00 per year for US students and residents, $382.00 per year for Canadian individuals, $776.00 for Canadian institutions, $462.00 for international individuals, $776.00 per year for international institutions, $100.00 per year for Canadian students/residents, and $220.00 per year for foreign students/residents. To receive student/resident rate, orders must be accompanied by name of affiliated institution, date of term, and the *signature* of program/residency coordinator on institution letterhead. Orders will be billed at individual rate until proof of status is received. Foreign air speed delivery is included in all *Clinics* subscription prices. All prices are subject to change without notice. POSTMASTER: Send address changes to *Clinics in Podiatric Medicine and Surgery*, Elsevier Health Sciences Division, Subscription Customer Service, 3251 Riverport Lane, Maryland Heights, MO 63043. **Customer Service: 1-800-654-2452 (US). From outside of the US, call 314-447-8871. Fax: 314-447-8029. E-mail: JournalsCustomerService-usa@elsevier.com (for print support); JournalsOnlineSupport-usa@elsevier.com (for online support).**

Reprints. For copies of 100 or more of articles in this publication, please contact the Commercial Reprints Department, Elsevier Inc., 360 Park Avenue South, New York, NY 10010-1710. Tel.: 212-633-3874; Fax: 212-633-3820; E-mail: reprints@elsevier.com.

Clinics in Podiatric Medicine and Surgery is covered in *MEDLINE/PubMed (Index Medicus)* and *EMBASE/Excerpta Medica.*

Printed in the United States of America.

Contributors

CONSULTING EDITOR

THOMAS J. CHANG, DPM
Clinical Professor and Past Chairman, Department of Podiatric Surgery, California College of Podiatric Medicine, Faculty, The Podiatry Institute, Redwood Orthopedic Surgery Associates, Santa Rosa, California, USA

EDITOR

HARRY JOHN VISSER, DPM, FACFAS
Director of Residency Training in Foot and Ankle Surgery, SSM DePaul Health Center, Bridgeton, Missouri, USA

AUTHORS

SHARIF ABDELFATTAH, DPM, PGY III
Resident, East Liverpool City Hospital, East Liverpool, Ohio, USA

RAUL AVILES, DPM
Resident, Foot and Ankle Surgery Residency, SSM Health DePaul Hospital, Bridgeton, Missouri, USA

JOELAKI CARTMAN, DPM, PGY II
Resident, East Liverpool City Hospital, East Liverpool, Ohio, USA

DAVID CHAN, DPM, PGY III
Resident, East Liverpool City Hospital, East Liverpool, Ohio, USA

AUSTIN CHINN, DPM
Podiatric Medicine and Surgery Residency Program PGY2, Advocate Christ Medical Center, Oak Lawn, Illinois, USA

CLARE CORMIER, DPM
Podiatric Medicine and Surgery Residency Program PGY2, Advocate Christ Medical Center, Oak Lawn, Illinois, USA

LAWRENCE A. DIDOMENICO, DPM, FACFAS
Residency Director, East Liverpool City Hospital, East Liverpool, Ohio, USA; Director of Fellowship Training, NOMS Ankle and Foot Care Centers, Section Chief, St. Elizabeth Hospital, Youngstown, Ohio, USA

ROBERT K. DUDDY, DPM, FACFAS
Attending Physician, SSM Health DePaul Hospital, Foot and Ankle Surgery Residency, St Louis, Missouri, USA

LAWRENCE M. FALLAT, DPM, FACFAS
Director, Beaumont Health Wayne Podiatric Foot and Ankle Surgical Residency,
Beaumont Hospital Wayne, Wayne, Michigan, USA

JOHN F. GRADY, DPM, FASPS, FAAPSM, FACFAS, FACFAOM, FRCPS(G)
Director, Podiatric Residencies, Advocate Christ Medical Center and Advocate Children's
Hospital, Foot and Ankle Institute of Illinois, Foot and Ankle Institute for Research (FAIR),
Oak Lawn, Illinois, USA; Professor of Surgery and Applied Biomechanics, Rosalind
Franklin University (Adjunct Track), North Chicago, Illinois, USA

ALLEN MARK JACOBS, DPM, FACFAS
Attending, Foot and Ankle Surgery Residency, SSM Health DePaul Hospital, St Louis,
Missouri, USA

DAVID E. KARGES, DO
Professor, Department of Orthopaedic Surgery, Chief of Foot and Ankle Surgery, St. Louis
University School of Medicine, St Louis, Missouri, USA

EMILY KEETER, DPM
Fellow, American Foundation of Lower Extremity Surgery and Research, Alamogordo,
New Mexico, USA

REKHA KOURI, DPM
Resident, Foot and Ankle Surgery Residency, SSM Health DePaul Hospital, St Louis,
Missouri, USA

KATHRYN LAVIOLETTE, DPM
Podiatric Medicine and Surgery Residency Program Graduate, Advocate Christ Medical
Center, Oak Lawn, Illinois, USA

TYLER D. MCKEE, DPM, AACFAS
Fellow, American Health Network Foot and Ankle Reconstructive Surgery Fellowship,
Carmel, Indiana, USA

JAY J. MORADIA, DPM
Attending Physician, SSM Health DePaul Hospital, Foot and Ankle Surgery Residency,
St Louis, Missouri, USA

KALLI E. MORTENSON, DPM
Resident, Submitted During Postgraduate Year 2, Beaumont Health Wayne Podiatric Foot
and Ankle Surgical Residency, Beaumont Hospital Wayne, Wayne, Michigan, USA

MELINDA NICHOLES, DPM
Second-Year Resident, SSM Health DePaul Hospital, Foot and Ankle Surgery Residency,
St Louis, Missouri, USA; SSM Health DePaul Hospital, Bridgeton, Missouri, USA

LAWRENCE OSHER, DPM
Professor, Radiology, Division of Podiatric and General Medicine, Kent State University
College of Podiatric Medicine, Independence, Ohio, USA

THORSTEN Q. RANDT, MD, MBA
Consultant, Department of Foot Surgery, Clinics of Traumatology and Orthopedics,
St. George Hospital, Hamburg, Germany

ZACHARY RASOR, DPM, AACFAS
Assistant Director, Professional Education and Research Institute, Roanoke,
Virginia, USA

JACOB RIZKALLA, DPM, PGYII
Resident, East Liverpool City Hospital, East Liverpool, Ohio, USA

BLAKE T. SAVAGE, DPM
Resident, SSM Health DePaul Hospital, Foot and Ankle Surgery Residency, St Louis, Missouri, USA

BENJAMIN SAVASKY, DPM, AACFAS
Fellow, Professional Education and Research Institute, Roanoke, Virginia, USA

JACLYN SCHUMANN, DPM
Podiatric Medicine and Surgery Residency Program PGY3, Advocate Christ Medical Center, Oak Lawn, Illinois, USA

JEFFREY E. SHOOK, DPM
Adjunct Faculty, St. Vincent Charity Medical Center, Cleveland, Ohio, USA

CLAY SHUMWAY, DPM, PGY III
Resident, East Liverpool City Hospital, East Liverpool, Ohio, USA

BRITTANY R. STAPLES, DPM
Attending Physician, Foot and Ankle Surgery Residency, SSM Health DePaul Hospital, St Louis, Missouri, USA

NICHOLAS J. STAUB, DPM
Third-Year Resident, Foot and Ankle Surgery Residency, SSM Health DePaul Hospital, St Louis, Missouri, USA

JORDAN TACKTILL, DPM, FACFAS
Attending Physician, Kaiser Permanente Midatlantic, Washington Hospital Center Residency, Upper Marlboro, Maryland, USA; Fellow, Professional Education and Research Institute, Roanoke, Virginia, USA

HARRY JOHN VISSER, DPM, FACFAS
Director of Residency Training in Foot and Ankle Surgery, SSM DePaul Health Center, Bridgeton, Missouri, USA

JARED J. VISSER, DPM, FACFAS
Attending Physician, Foot and Ankle Surgery Residency, SSM Health DePaul Hospital, St Louis, Missouri, USA

JESSE R. WOLFE, DPM, AACFAS
Foot and Ankle Surgeon, Northwest Iowa Bone, Joint, & Sports Surgeons, Spencer, Iowa, USA

JOSHUA WOLFE, DPM, MHA
Chief Resident, Foot and Ankle Surgery Residency, SSM Health DePaul Hospital, St Louis, Missouri, USA

HANNAN H. ZAHID, DPM
Second-Year Resident, Foot and Ankle Surgery Residency, SSM Health DePaul Hospital, St Louis, Missouri, USA

CHARLES M. ZELEN, DPM, FACFAS
Fellowship Director, Professional Education and Research Institute, Roanoke, Virginia, USA

Contents

Foreword: Cavus Issue   xiii

Thomas J. Chang

Preface: A Comprehensive Evaluation of the Cavus Foot Deformity   xv

Harry John Visser

**Pes Cavus Deformity: Anatomic, Functional Considerations, and Surgical
Implications**   291

Allen Mark Jacobs

Pes cavus is a complicated, multiplanar deformity that requires a thorough understanding in order to provide the appropriate level of care. The foot and ankle surgeon should perform a comprehensive examination, including a neurologic evaluation, in the workup of this patient population. Understanding the cause of the patient's deformity is a critical step in predicting the disease course as well as the most acceptable form of treatment. The surgical correlation with the patient's pathologic anatomy requires an in-depth clinical evaluation, in addition to the radiographic findings, as the radiographic findings do not necessarily correlate with the patient's discomfort.

Imaging of the Pes Cavus Deformity   303

Lawrence Osher and Jeffrey E. Shook

Direct-type cavus foot deformities are most commonly encountered and are primarily sagittal plane deformities. Direct deformities should be delineated from rarer triplane pes cavovarus deformities. The lateral weight-bearing radiograph is the cornerstone of imaging evaluation of direct pes cavus foot deformity. The apex of Meary talo-first metatarsal angle on the lateral radiograph represents the pinnacle of the cavus deformity and assists in subclassification of the deformity. With routine application, ancillary radiographic imaging techniques, such as the modified Saltzman view or the modified Coleman block test, can give valuable insight into deformity assessment and surgical planning.

Neurologic Conditions Associated with Cavus Foot Deformity   323

Harry John Visser, Joshua Wolfe, Rekha Kouri, and Raul Aviles

The cavus foot deformity is an often less understood deformity within the spectrum of foot and ankle conditions. The hallmark concern is the possibility of an underlying neurologic or neuromuscular disorder. Although a proportion of these deformities are idiopathic, a significant majority do correlate with an underlying disorder. The appropriate evaluation of this deformity, in coordination within the multidisciplinary scope of health care, allows for a timely diagnosis and understanding of the patient's condition. We provide an abbreviated survey of possible underlying etiologies for the patient with the cavus foot deformity as a reference to the foot and ankle surgeon.

Hallux and Lesser Digits Deformities Associated with Cavus Foot   343

Lawrence A. DiDomenico, Jacob Rizkalla, Joelaki Cartman, and Sharif Abdelfattah

It is important to identify the level of the deformity or deformities. It is important to get the limb as close to anatomic alignment as possible. Many levels and multiple procedures may be involved with this reconstruction.

The Subtle Cavovarus Foot Deformity: The Nonneurologic Form of Cavus Foot Deformity   361

Harry John Visser, Hannan H. Zahid, Jared J. Visser, Brittany R. Staples, and Nicholas J. Staub

Conditions of ankle instability, peroneal tendon tears, and stress fractures of the lateral metatarsals are commonly encountered in a clinical foot and ankle practice. Evaluation of the supporting foot structure is critical to prevent failure of index procedures. The prominence of the subtle cavus foot is now a recognized entity and must be properly diagnosed and addressed surgically.

Use of Calcaneal Osteotomies in the Correction of Inframalleolar Cavovarus Deformity   379

Jesse R. Wolfe, Tyler D. McKee, and Melinda Nicholes

Cavovarus deformity is a complicated condition most commonly resulting from neurologic, posttraumatic, or iatrogenic pathologic conditions. Careful evaluation of the cavovarus patient is necessary in determining appropriate treatment course. Weight-bearing radiographs are necessary, and advances in computed tomographic technology can be beneficial in identifying level of involvement. In the case of operative treatment of inframalleolar deformity, assessment of the subtalar joint position and relation of calcaneocuboid joint can be of assistance. Multiple osteotomies have been described providing uniplanar, biplanar, and triplanar correction and in the appropriate setting can prove beneficial to the surgeon in treating hind-foot cavovarus deformity.

Management of Midfoot Cavus   391

John F. Grady, Jaclyn Schumann, Clare Cormier, Kathryn LaViolette, and Austin Chinn

There is a deficiency in publications on the topic of midfoot cavus. The limited research available does not have a standard definition for the diagnosis of this deformity and lacks a reliable algorithm for its surgical management. The authors performed an extensive review of the literature that found a majority of patients are satisfied with the Cole osteotomy and the dorsiflexory first metatarsal osteotomy for treatment of this condition. High patient satisfaction has been observed with lateralizing calcaneal osteotomies in the setting of midfoot cavus with a secondary rigid rearfoot deformity. Further research on this topic is encouraged.

Principles of Triple Arthrodesis and Limited Arthrodesis in the Cavus Foot   411

Kalli E. Mortenson and Lawrence M. Fallat

Cavus foot is a complex podiatric deformity that requires precise and in-depth work-up through an objective, physical, and radiographic examination. The goal of surgical treatment is to eliminate pain while establishing a plantigrade foot structure. Triple arthrodesis has proven to be an effective surgical procedure for treatment of moderate to severe rearfoot deformity with or without the presence of rearfoot arthritic changes. The foot and ankle surgeon must always be aware that no two cavus deformity cases are alike, therefore one may require additional surgical procedures including soft tissue balancing, joint-sparing osteotomies, and/or supplementary arthrodesing procedures.

Tendon Transfers and Their Role in Cavus Foot Deformity   427

Thorsten Q. Randt, Joshua Wolfe, Emily Keeter, and Harry John Visser

Management of the cavus foot is a difficult task for the foot and ankle surgeon. Tendon transfers have been a longstanding accepted treatment for the flexible cavus foot. Performing tendon transfers requires an in-depth understanding of the patient's medical history, factors leading to the development of deformity, as well as the deforming forces contributing to the deformity. Evaluation of the patient for rigid, progressive, and/or spastic deformities is critical to avoid postoperative complications. Educating the patient on postoperative rehabilitation, potential complications, and postoperative expectations is essential to ensure appropriate surgical outcomes.

The Role of Peroneal Tendinopathy and the Cavovarus Foot and Ankle   445

Harry John Visser, Blake T. Savage, Jay J. Moradia, and Robert K. Duddy

Peroneal tendon pathology is often an overlooked and underdiagnosed condition. It is often confused with chronic ankle instability. It is important when surgically managed to assess the condition of the tendons, muscle viability and strength, and associated cavovarus deformity. Complex reconstruction may be needed, including 2-stage procedures with a silicone rod and tendon transfer.

The Cavovarus Ankle: Approaches to Ankle Instability and Inframalleolar Deformity   461

Lawrence A. DiDomenico, Sharif Abdelfattah, David Chan, and Clay Shumway

Pathologic affects from a cavus foot deformity range from flexible subtle to rigid severe deformities and are related to many pathologic conditions of the foot and ankle. Understanding the underlying deformity and the deforming force is essential in treating the cavus ankle and foot. Every deformity is different and unique to a given patient; therefore, surgical plans should be modified to each patient.

Ankle and Pantalar Arthrodesis: End-Stage Salvage in Cavus Foot   483

David E. Karges, Joshua Wolfe, and Raul Aviles

Bony alignment is the primary goal in foot and ankle reconstruction of the cavovarus foot. This condition presents as a malalignment causing a medial overload of the ankle articular surface and lateral overload of the hindfoot, midfoot, and forefoot. A painful gait associated with articular degeneration of the numerous joints can lead to a chronic and rigid arthrosis of joints, warranting arthrodesis of the affected joints accordingly.

Consideration for Total Ankle Replacement in the Varus Ankle and Cavovarus Foot Type   497

Jordan Tacktill, Zachary Rasor, Benjamin Savasky, and Charles M. Zelen

The varus ankle and cavus foot pose challenges in surgical correction with regard to total ankle replacement surgery. Etiology of cavus foot type and varus ankle must be evaluated and confirmed. Pesccavus is increased height of the arch with metatarsus adductus and increased calcaneal inclination angle. There often is intrinsic musculature irregularity leading to imbalance of the foot. Although not all cavus foot types and varus ankle deformities are sequelae of neuromuscular disorder, neurologic etiology must be considered. Attaining neutral alignment of ankle joint articular surface is paramount to longevity and functionality of ankle joint replacement implant.

CLINICS IN PODIATRIC MEDICINE AND SURGERY

FORTHCOMING ISSUES

October 2021
Podiatric Dermatology
Tracey C. Vlahovic, *Editor*

January 2022
Pediatric Orthopedics
Mark E. Solomon, *Editor*

April 2022
The Legacy and Impact of Podiatric FellowshipTraining
Thomas Zgonis and Christopher Hyer, *Editors*

RECENT ISSUES

April 2021
Posterior and Plantar Heel Pain
Eric A. Barp, *Editor*

January 2021
OrthoplasticTechniques for Lower Extremity Reconstruction - Part II
Edgardo R. Rodriguez-Collazo and Suhail Masadeh, *Editors*

October 2020
OrthoplasticTechniques for Lower Extremity Reconstruction - Part I
Edgardo R. Rodriguez-Collazo and Suhail Masadeh, *Editors*

SERIES OF RELATED INTEREST

Orthopedic Clinics
https://www.orthopedic.theclinics.com/
Clinics in Sports Medicine
https://www.sportsmed.theclinics.com/
Foot and Ankle Clinics
https://www.foot.theclinics.com/
Physical Medicine and Rehabilitation Clinics
https://www.pmr.theclinics.com/

THE CLINICS ARE AVAILABLE ONLINE!
Access your subscription at:
www.theclinics.com

Foreword

Cavus Issue

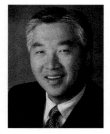

Thomas J. Chang, DPM
Consulting Editor

Over the past 20 to 30 years, there has been an incredible amount of research, debate, and scientific publications on the topic of the adult acquired flatfoot deformity. Every foot and ankle meeting has included a track on the flatfoot deformity, and the presentations and discussions have brought our level of experience with this common presentation to the highest level. I feel the opposite is true for the cavus foot deformity.

During medical school, I remember one lecture on the cavus foot, while 4 to 5 lectures were dedicated to the flatfoot topics. We recognize there is often a neuromuscular contribution to the cavus foot. We are aware of isolated anatomic regions of the foot where cavus deformities can present. We understand the cavus foot is predominantly a sagittal plane deformity, but really is triplanar in its development. Due to this topic being somewhat of a "neglected stepchild," I wanted to devote an issue on the current "state-of-the-art" discussion on all topics relevant to this area.

Dr Visser has been a longtime educator on the local and national level, working in residency training for over 35 years in the St. Louis area. I applaud his approach to this issue, with an extremely complete list of topics covering medical and surgical articles on the cavus deformity. He has also invited some international and allopathic medical authors to participate in this issue, providing more depth and shared experiences from several disciplines.

I hope this will prove to be a comprehensive mini textbook on this often-forgotten topic. I am looking forward to it.

Thomas J. Chang, DPM
Redwood Orthopedic Surgery Associates
208 Concourse Boulevard
Santa Rosa, CA 95403, USA

E-mail address:
thomaschang14@comcast.net

Clin Podiatr Med Surg 38 (2021) xiii
https://doi.org/10.1016/j.cpm.2021.04.002
0891-8422/21/© 2021 Published by Elsevier Inc.

podiatric.theclinics.com

Preface

A Comprehensive Evaluation of the Cavus Foot Deformity

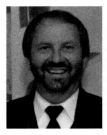

Harry John Visser, DPM, FACFAS
Editor

This issue of *Clinics in Podiatric Medicine and Surgery* presents the extensive topic of cavus foot deformity. The cavus foot represents a pergola of unique and complex conditions. Although when initially considered it represents an entanglement of complex neurologic conditions, it also may be part of a more subtle nonneurologic condition. This issue serves to wade through these extensive topics. It is my hope that this issue, serving a peony of topics, will serve as a "textbook" to students and practitioners.

I would like to personally thank all my authors, who are all well known in their own right. They are all philomaths of a great profession. It is quite obvious the time they have spent constructing these articles. They represent the nuance of dramaturgy within our profession. As Lyndon B. Johnson said to his principle speech writer, Richard Goodwin, "Put the music to it, Dick,"…and they have. I would also like to offer special acknowledgment to the residency program at SSM DePaul St. Louis, Missouri and its contributing residents. It is a distinct honor to be a part of this program and its very supportive administration.

Finally, I would like to personally thank Dr Thomas Chang for allowing me to edit this issue. It is a very distinct honor. Also, I offer my eternal gratitude to Dr Allen Jacobs. As my residency director, he has instilled a thirst for learning that has remained immutable into my older age.

Harry John Visser, DPM, FACFAS
SSM DePaul Health Center
12255 Depaul Drive, Suite 705
Bridgeton, MO 63044, USA

E-mail address:
tsarhjv@aol.com

Clin Podiatr Med Surg 38 (2021) xv
https://doi.org/10.1016/j.cpm.2021.04.001
0891-8422/21/© 2021 Published by Elsevier Inc.

podiatric.theclinics.com

Pes Cavus Deformity
Anatomic, Functional Considerations, and Surgical Implications

Allen Mark Jacobs, DPM*

KEYWORDS

- Cavus foot deformity • Anatomy • Cavus correction

KEY POINTS

- In many cases, cavus foot deformity is associated with an underlying neurologic cause.
- A complete neuromuscular examination is required as part of the evaluation of cavus foot deformity, particularly when surgical intervention is contemplated.
- Structural deformity in cavus foot may be the result of functional disorders, which must be addressed for successful management.
- Varus heel deformity does not necessarily mandate calcaneal osteotomy and may be the result of factors extrinsic to the calcaneus, such as first ray plantar flexion or neuromuscular imbalance.
- In many cases, arthrodesis procedures must include concurrent tendon lengthenings, transfers, or recessions in order to reduce the incidence of recurrent deformity.

INTRODUCTION

Also we can affirm, without fear of being taxed for exaggeration, that it is in the school of anatomy, particularly in topographic anatomy, that the best surgeons are formed.

Testut and Jacob[1]

The term cavus foot (pes cavus) is used to characterize a broad spectrum of abnormalities generally intended to describe a foot with a higher-than-normal arch structure.[2] Cavus foot deformities may be supple to presentation or may represent advanced and significant disease. These deformities may be flexible or rigid. They may be progressive or nonprogressive. The deformity may manifest in the pediatric, adolescent, or adult patient. The deformities encompassing the term cavus foot may include deformity of the distal tibia, ankle, calcaneus, subtalar joint, midtarsal

Foot and Ankle Surgery Residency, SSM Health DePaul Hospital, St Louis, MO 63117, USA
* Dr. Allen M. Jacobs and Associates, Ltd., P.C., 6400 Clayton Road, Suite 402, St Louis, MO 63117.
E-mail address: allenthepod@sbcglobal.net

Clin Podiatr Med Surg 38 (2021) 291–302
https://doi.org/10.1016/j.cpm.2020.12.012
0891-8422/21/© 2021 Elsevier Inc. All rights reserved.

joint, metatarsus, and metatarsals. In addition, digital deformities are not infrequently associated with cavus foot deformity. Careful analysis of the patient with a cavus foot deformity, including detailed history, gait analysis, neurologic examination, musculoskeletal evaluation, and appropriate bone and joint imaging, is required in each case to best determine appropriate nonoperative or operative intervention.[3] Clinical manifestations may include metatarsalgia, pain associated with hammertoes, sesamoid pain, osteoarthritis of the midfoot, lateral ankle joint instability, peroneal tendon pathologic condition, plantar fasciitis, osteoarthritis of the ankle, subtalar joint, or midfoot. Postural symptoms, such as chronic low back pain, osteoarthritis of the hips, knees, or ankle joints, may be exacerbated in the patient with a cavus foot deformity, particularly deformities that are rigid. Rigid pes cavus deformities are associated with decreased shock absorption and may contribute to postural or arthritic deformities of the back, hips, and knees.[4]

There are no universal presentations to the anatomic components of cavus foot deformity. Triplanar morbidly is common. In addition, in planning surgical intervention for the correction of cavus foot deformity, a clear understanding of functional versus structural deformity is essential. For example, varus deformity of the calcaneus is a frequent component of cavus foot deformity. The calcaneus and subtalar joint may have the ability to undergo eversion; however, the positioning of the calcaneus may be influenced by excessive plantarflexion of the first metatarsal/first ray with compensatory varus positioning of the heel.[5] In such a circumstance, elevation of the first metatarsal with additional other indicated surgical interventions may result in reduction of heel varus without the necessity for calcaneal osteotomy. Alternatively, the first ray may be excessively plantarflexed secondary to overactivity of the peroneus longus, dominance of the extensor or flexor hallucis muscles, or the presence of a hallux hammertoe. Again, although anatomic evaluation would indicate abnormal plantarflexion positioning of the first ray, procedures other than osteotomy or arthrodesis of the first ray may be indicated. Therefore, the key to understanding surgical planning for the correction of cavus foot deformity is to understand that *anatomic (morphologic) findings do not necessarily indicate the cause of any particular component of cavus foot.*[6] Weakness of the gastrocnemius and soleus muscles, such as seen in lower motor neuron disorders, will result in increased calcaneal inclination on clinical and radiographic evaluation. Under such circumstances, osteotomy of the calcaneus to reduce calcaneal inclination may not be preferable to alternative procedures, such as tendon transfers, to increase the strength of the posterior musculature.

CAUSE OF PES CAVUS

It is generally accepted that greater than 50% of cavus foot deformities are the result of neuromuscular imbalance and resultant progressive or nonprogressive deformity.[7] Particularly in the presence of more advanced cavus foot deformity, occult neuromuscular disorders must be considered, as the presence and type of neuromuscular disorder are significant factors in determining the appropriate surgical management of cavus foot deformity. Neuromuscular disorders associated with cavus foot deformity include hereditary sensory-motor neuropathies, the most common of which is likely presentations of Charcot-Marie-Tooth disease.[8] It has been suggested that in the presence of bilateral cavus foot deformity, the probability that the patient has Charcot-Marie-Tooth disease or some neurologic disorder is between 62% and 75%.[9] Although commonly associated with hereditary sensory motor neuropathies, cavus foot deformity may be associated with lower motor neuron disorders (classical disorders, such as poliomyelitis or peripheral nerve injury), primary myopathies (for example, muscular dystrophy), upper motor neuron disorders (such as stroke, cerebral palsy), spinocerebellar ataxias (such as Friedreich ataxia, Roussy-Levy syndrome).[10] Cavus foot deformity may also occur following peripheral nerve injury, such as injury to the superficial peroneal nerve, resulting in weakness of the pronator muscles and gradual progressive deformity secondary to dominance of the supinator muscles. In the pediatric and adolescent patient, evaluation for undiagnosed spinal cord disorders is important in seeking the cause of the deformity.[11]

Cavus foot deformity may also occur lacking the presence of a definitive and definable neurologic disorder, with abnormalities in neurologic testing, such as electrodiagnostic studies or epidermal nerve fiber density testing, or clinical evaluation.

Cavus foot may occur following trauma or peripheral nerve injury or may be idiopathic.[12]

In the presence of peripheral nerve injury or neuromuscular disorders, the nature and extent of such disorders must be appreciated before undertaking surgical correction of a cavus foot deformity. For example, in the presence of upper motor neuron disease (spastic deformities), split-tendon transfers, or tendon recession surgery, may be preferable to whole-tendon motor transfer secondary to the risk of overcorrection in the presence of spasticity. Furthermore, when neurologic disease is progressive in nature, osteotomy or arthrodesis may provide only temporary realignment, with recurrence of deformity secondary to continuation of muscle imbalance. As an example, in the presence of Charcot-Marie-Tooth disease, there may be less disease involvement of the supinator muscles than the pronator muscles and less involvement of the dorsiflexion muscles than the plantarflexion muscles. Arthrodesis of the subtalar joint, or triple arthrodesis, may be followed by progressive medial subluxation of the ankle joint, secondary to the fact that the neuromuscular imbalance has not been addressed. Although some neurologic disorders may be considered nonprogressive in nature, for example, a stroke, the resulting muscle imbalance will result in progressive deformity of the foot and ankle, although the primary neurologic deficit itself is not progressive. Injury to the deep peroneal nerve may result in weakening of the anterior tibial muscle. Although the nerve injury is not progressive, the imbalance created between the weakened anterior tibial muscle and the peroneus longus may result in a progressive plantar flexion deformity of the first metatarsal.

Idiopathic cavus foot deformity may occur lacking any neuromuscular disorder. Such deformity may be unilateral or bilateral. Subtle forms of pes cavus may also occur. As noted earlier, posttraumatic pes cavus and pes cavus associated with tarsal coalition may occur.

Anatomic Considerations in Pes Cavus

Hindfoot/ankle

Components of deformity in pes cavus deformity involving the hindfoot and ankle may include tibia varum, ankle varus, and varus of the calcaneus/subtalar joint. Most commonly, varus deformity of the calcaneus is present when a hindfoot varus deformity exists. It is however important to assess the distal tibia and ankle joint for the presence of significant varus deformity, which may require reduction by appropriate osteotomy or soft tissue procedures.

The calcaneus may be malaligned primarily in the frontal and sagittal planes. Increased calcaneal inclination may be present and require reduction by osteotomy. Similarly, increased varus of the calcaneus may be present and require reduction. A variety of osteotomies, generally variants of the classic Dwyer calcaneal osteotomy, are used to reduce the frontal plane deformity alone (varus reducing osteotomy), the sagittal plane deformity alone, or the combined deformities. For example, if preoperative imaging studies do not demonstrate a true varus deformity within the calcaneus itself, but rather varus positioning of the calcaneus together with increased calcaneal inclination, a linear osteotomy may be performed allowing dorsiflexion and frontal plane rotation of the calcaneus. If a true varus deformity exists within the calcaneus itself, shortening of the lateral wall of the calcaneus by utilization of cuneiform, wedge, or trapezoidal osteotomy will allow reduction of varus, and if needed, reduction of calcaneal inclination. Generally, a computed tomographic (CT) scan examined in transverse plane sectioning allows an appreciation of any true deformity within the calcaneus itself. In performing an osteotomy of the calcaneus to reduce varus, it should be recalled that varus is a frontal plane deformity. Therefore, ideally, reduction of a frontal plane deformity would require an osteotomy parallel to the body of the calcaneus. The more horizontally oriented the osteotomy through the calcaneus, the more frontal plane rotation occurs, but rather, the posterior portion of the calcaneus is transposed in a lateral direction, providing transverse plane but reduced frontal plane correction. Thus, the more obliquely oriented the calcaneal osteotomy, the greater the resultant frontal plane correction. Alternatively, the medial cortex can be osteotomized, allowing frontal plane correction together with shortening of the lateral portion of the calcaneus, and if necessary, proximal positioning of the calcaneus to reduce increased calcaneal inclination.

The Achilles tendon inserts into the posterior aspect of the calcaneus. In the presence of a significant varus deformity of the calcaneus, the tendon will contract maintaining the excessive supination position of the hindfoot. Calcaneal osteotomy for correction of a pes cavus deformity allows repositioning of the insertion of the gastrocnemius and soleus muscles (Achilles tendon), which will reduce the supination, maintaining position of the tendon, and may provide a neutralizing or pronation, encouraging positioning of the tendon. Repositioning of the calcaneus also serves to correct the center of gravity at heel contact and midstance.[2]

Not infrequently, pes cavus is associated with a relative plantar flexion of the forefoot on the hindfoot. As a result, increased range of motion of the ankle joint is required in order to obtain adequate dorsiflexion of the forefoot relative to the hindfoot and ankle.[13] The increased demand for dorsiflexion at the ankle joint resulting from the plantar-flexed forefoot positioning may result in a functional limitation of ankle joint dorsiflexion, or pseudoequinus. Dorsal displacement of a calcaneal osteotomy may result in a functional lengthening of the gastrocnemius and soleus muscles. Gastrocnemius recession or lengthening of the Achilles tendon may be required in some circumstances.

In the presence of lower motor neuron disorders, decreased strength of the gastrocnemius and soleus muscles results in decreased plantar flexion force on the calcaneus itself and may result in increased calcaneal inclination. Under such circumstances, assessment of available motor units available for transfer to provide increased plantar flexor strength to the Achilles tendon may be considered. Appropriate muscles may include the peroneal muscles, or the long flexor muscles to the digits. However, appropriate evaluation of the motor units to be transferred with regard to the strength and probability of involvement in any existing neuromuscular disorder, or the tendon transfers, will result in surgical failure or future surgical failure over time.

Varus heel positioning may be functional. With the patient in a prone position, the ability to evert the calcaneus should be determined. If the calcaneus can be easily everted beyond neutral, osteotomy of the calcaneus is probably not indicated, and a cause for functional varus positioning of the calcaneus should be sought. The

Coleman block test has been classically suggested as a means by which a plantarflexion of the first ray inducing heel varus may be assessed.[14,15]

Plantar Fascia and Intrinsic Musculature

In the presence of a cavus foot deformity, the plantar fascia is not infrequently thickened and contracted. Shortening of the length of the foot results in contracture of the plantar fascia and a persistence of the deformity, increased deformity rigidity, and frequently requires release in order to allow reduction of the deformity at the time of surgery. Because the contracture involves all components of the plantar release, open surgical release is typically used. Inflammatory changes of the plantar fascia at the insertion, with eventual scarring of the plantar fascia, may result in plantar fasciitis. In addition to the loss of fascia plasticity, decreased shock absorption at heel contact results in repetitive mechanical trauma to the plantar fascia. Secondary to the contracture of the plantar fascia, abnormalities in the normal Windlass function of the plantar fascia contribute to the cause and persistence of hammertoe deformities typical of pes cavus deformity.[16]

Contracture and overpull of the intrinsic muscles of the foot in pes cavus deformity will contribute to progressive digital deformity, forefoot plantar flexion relative to the hindfoot, and resistance to correction. Similarly, atrophy and weakness of the intrinsic foot muscular has been identified as a factor in cavus foot deformity. As a result, release of the intrinsic musculature may be required concurrently with release of the plantar fascia in order to affect a cavus foot structural correction. Classically, such a release consists of a classic or variation of the Steindler stripping procedure. In many neurologic disorders, the intrinsic muscles of the foot appear to be less affected than the extrinsic muscles, resulting in an imbalance and resultant deformities of the forefoot. Occasionally, denervation of the intrinsic musculature, as performed in procedures such as the Garceau-Brahms procedure, may be indicated.[17]

The First Ray and Great Toe

The first ray consists of the first metatarsal, first cuneiform, navicular, and talus with their intervening joints. Not infrequently, excessive plantarflexion of the first ray represents 1 anatomic component of pes cavus deformity. Typically, isolated plantarflexion deformity of the first ray is a component of a more complex pes cavus deformity. Clinical and radiographic evaluation of the first ray deformity, primarily in the sagittal plane, must determine the level at which the deformity occurs. Typically, the plantarflexion deformity occurs at the level of the metatarsal cuneiform joint, or the navicular cuneiform joint. Arthrodesis of the indicated metatarsal cuneiform joint or intertarsal joints may be appropriate rather than osteotomy of the first metatarsal, of which bone is seldom deformed in isolation, accounting for plantarflexion prominence of the first ray.

Plantarflexion of the first ray may also be the result of neuromuscular imbalance. Not infrequently, the neuromuscular imbalance affecting the first ray is characterized by a hallux hammertoe. Hallux hammertoe deformity is most commonly the result of the imbalance between the flexor and extensor muscles to the great toe, resulting in buckling or elevation of the great toe and secondary first ray plantar flexion. Arthrodesis of the hallux Interphalangeal joint together with appropriate tendon transfers or the flexor or extensor muscles to the great toe, when the plantarflexion deformity is flexible, is a frequently indicated further correction of a plantarflexion deformity of the first ray, in addition to osteotomy or arthrodesis.

Plantarflexion deformity of the first ray may also be secondary to overactivity of the peroneus longus muscle as a result of hypertonicity, spasticity, or antagonist weakness. When this clinical scenario is present, plantarflexion deformity of the first ray is addressed by appropriate peroneal tendon lengthening or peroneus longus to brevis tendon transfers, as indicated.[18,19]

The Lesser Metatarsals

Most commonly, metatarsus adductus is present together with plantarflexion deformity of the forefoot, resulting in increased forefoot weight-bearing. Ankle, hindfoot, or midfoot varus deformity results in secondary frontal plane deformity of the lesser metatarsals, increasing weight-bearing to the lateral aspect of the foot with resultant pain or callus formation. Metatarsalgia and pressure callus formation may be present at the base of the fifth metatarsal, or plantar lateral to the fifth metatarsal head. Forefoot equinus associated with metatarsal-tarsal plantarflexion deformity is typically rigid and not reducible. Forefoot equinus, with prominent lesser metatarsals, may be the result of midtarsal joint plantarflexion, which is initially reducible on examination. The distinction between a Lisfranc level and Chopart level plantarflexion deformity is of significant clinical relevance. The former deformity may dictate the need for distal osteotomies or arthrodesis, whereas the latter may be addressed by arthrodesis or tendon transfers or other muscle tendon balancing techniques.[20,21]

The Lesser Digits

Some degree of digital deformity, typically hammertoe deformities in the sagittal plane, is characteristic of pes cavus deformity. Less commonly, transverse plane deformity with adduction of the digits may occur. Etiologic factors include imbalance between the flexor, extensor, and intrinsic muscles inserting into the digits secondary to underlying neuromuscular disease. In the presence of flexible forefoot, contracted and inelastic plantar fascia with associated abnormal Windlass mechanism may contribute to the persistence of digital deformities. Flexible forefoot equinus may be addressed, when appropriate, by proximal transfer of extensor tendons classically illustrated by the Hibbs tenosuspension and its variations. Flexor tendon transfers may be appropriate when the flexor tendons to the lesser digits are determined to be a primary etiologic factor. Care must be exercised in patients with upper motor neuron (spastic) disorders. Arthrodesis of the digital interphalangeal joints is frequently required together with appropriate tendon transfers.[22–24]

Anatomic Classification of Cavus Foot Deformity

Cavus foot deformity is a complex deformity occurring in the frontal, sagittal, and transverse planes. The apex of the deformity should be appreciated, as it does assist in operative planning for correction.[25]

In the sagittal plane, anatomic classification of cavus foot deformity may include increased calcaneal inclination, deformity apex at the mid tarsal joint, deformity apex within the mid tarsal bones, or plantar flexion deformity of the first ray. First-ray plantar flexion deformity may occur at the first metatarsal cuneiform joint, the navicular cuneiform joints, or the talonavicular joint. Relative plantar flexion of the forefoot relative to the hindfoot may be present. Such deformities may be initially flexible, typically becoming more rigid over time. Anatomic classification in the sagittal plane does not account for the contribution of neuromuscular disease and soft tissue balance, and therefore, surgical decision making should not be based solely on lateral radiographs and clinical examination to determine the sagittal plane apex of deformity.

Transverse plane deformity in the cavus foot may typically occur as a metatarsus adductus or deformity at the midtarsal joint.

Frontal plane deformity in the form of forefoot valgus or supination deformity of the midfoot and hindfoot or ankle is frequently present.

As a result, the anatomic classification of pes cavus is a nosology based on the components of each deformity. In the presence of posterior muscle weakness and increased calcaneal inclination, the term calcaneocavus is appropriate. If a significant midfoot varus deformity is present, the term calcaneocavovarus is appropriate. Plantar flexion of the forefoot relative to the hindfoot is anatomically classified as a forefoot equinus, which may be flexible or rigid. Significant transverse plane deformity together with varus and sagittal plane deformity is anatomically a cavoadductovarus deformity. Plantar flexion of the first ray driving a compensatory hindfoot varus deformity represents an anatomic forefoot valgus. However, such morphologic classifications do not address the etiologic neuromuscular factors, which must also be considered and addressed at the time of surgical correction.[4]

Radiographic Anatomy

Appropriate bone and joint imaging is helpful in elucidating the osseous and articular components of cavus foot deformity. Imaging may be used to define the frontal, transverse, and sagittal plane components of each deformity, the level at which the deformity is occurring, individual components of the cavus foot deformity, and any articular or osseous adaptive changes. However, although bone and joint imaging is helpful in determining appropriate osteotomy or arthrodesis procedures, if the correction has cavus deformity, it must always be recalled that in many circumstances the cause of cavus foot deformity is the result of adaptive soft tissue contractures, as well as progressive or nonprogressive neuromuscular disorders. Therefore, when planning surgical intervention for the correction of cavus foot deformity, it must always be recalled that bone and joint imaging represents a static representation of the deformity, which may progress, or recur, or remain subtotally corrected, with a failure to address the dynamic nature of the associated soft tissue adaptive changes and neuromuscular imbalance, which may be progressive or result in slowly progressive deformity, following seemingly successful surgical correction. Although important in the evaluation of cavus foot deformity, decision making regarding the appropriate surgical intervention in any particular case must be determined by a global examination and consideration of multiple factors, and not determined solely on the basis of imaging.[26]

Typically, at a minimum, weight-bearing radiographs are obtained in dorsal plantar, lateral, and oblique projections of the foot as well as weight-bearing calcaneal axial views. Radiographs of the ankle joint and distal leg structures, or the use of a long leg posterior leg, ankle, or heel projection, are useful in determining any component of tibial deformity, or ankle deformity, contributing to the pes cavus.

On occasion, advanced imaging, such as CT scanning, with weight-bearing or 3-dimensional reconstruction, may provide additional information for operative planning.

The lateral weight-bearing radiograph provides information regarding sagittal plane deformity in the cavus foot. Standard angular relationships measured include calcaneal inclination, greater than 30°. Hibb angle, representing the angle between the long axis of the calcaneus and first metatarsal, is considered abnormal when greater than 45°. Meary angle, the angle between the long axis of the talus and first metatarsal, is considered abnormal when greater than 5° of plantar flexion. The lateral radiograph also allows an evaluation or external rotation of the leg, a frequent coexisting abnormality in pes cavus deformity. External rotation is evident by posterior positioning of the fibula relative to the tibia and a lateral radiograph and presentation of the sinus tarsi as being more spherical to presentation, or "bulletlike." Relative plantarflexion of the first ray as well as the presence of hammertoe deformities, frequently associated with cavus deformity, may also be appreciated on the lateral weight-bearing radiograph. The tibiotalar ankle is considered abnormal on lateral radiograph when greater than 105°, in addition to which the talus may appear to be "flattened" in pes cavus deformity. The tibial-talar angle may also be appreciated on a lateral radiograph. In a cavus foot deformity, this ankle is decreased from a normal angle of 150°. The tibial calcaneal angle may also be used for the evaluation of the cavus foot deformity. The normal tibiocalcaneal angle is less than 80°. This angular relationship is increased in the presence of a cavus foot deformity. Finally, the angular relationship between the inferior border of the calcaneus and fifth metatarsal will be less than 150° on the lateral radiograph in a cavus foot deformity.[27–29]

Weight-bearing dorsal plantar radiographs are useful to appreciate the extent of transverse plane deformity in pes cavus and are helpful in determining the nature and orientation of an osteotomy or arthrodesis to be performed. For example, when a significant midfoot medial transverse plane deformity is present, osteotomies or arthrodesis procedures, which allow lateral rotation of the midfoot, such as a Cole procedure or a midfoot dome osteotomy, might be considered appropriate to allow reduction of adduction, as opposed to other osteotomies, such as a Japas procedure, which also allows sagittal plane correction but minimal correction in the transverse plane.

Narrowing of the normal talocalcaneal angle, with less than 25° medial orientation of the midtarsal joint with medial subluxation of the talonavicular and calcaneocuboid joints, and metatarsus adductus deformity, may be appreciated on standard weight-bearing dorsal plantar radiographs.

Radiographs of the heel in axial projection, or posterior long leg projection, are of importance in the evaluation of cavus deformity. Heel varus represents a significant component of many pes cavus deformities. Although readily appreciated on radiographs, it should be recalled that heel varus may be fixed or functional, for example, the results of a plantarflexion performed to the first metatarsal, overactivity of the peroneal musculature, or relative overpowering of the posterior tibial muscle. Therefore, although a quantitative assessment of the degree of heel varus may be determined on axial or posterior long leg views, the reducibility of the varus deformity cannot be appreciated on radiograph. As a result, the presence of heel varus, and the need for varus reducing osteotomy of the calcaneus, or varus reducing subtalar joint arthrodesis, should not be determined solely on the presence of calcaneal varus on radiographs. Although less common in cavus foot deformity, calcaneal position may be neutral or even slightly valgus.

Radiographic evaluation of the ankle and distal leg is similarly important when reconstruction of the foot or reduction of a pes cavus deformity is considered. Ankle varus, or distal tibia varus deformities, may be present in an individual demonstrating a pes cavus deformity. Both ankle varus and distal tibial varum deformities may be primary or secondary and may require reduction at the time of surgical correction.

Weight-bearing CT scans of the foot and ankle may provide additional information for the evaluation of pes cavus deformity in selected patients. Complex deformities, such as pes cavus deformity, may be better understood, and surgical planning improved, with the use of weight-bearing CT scanning. Three-dimensional reconstruction of the cavus foot using CT scanning may also provide additional insight into reconstruction of the foot in any given patient.

Additional considerations in the radiographic evaluation of cavus foot deformity include the presence of osteoarthritis, in which case arthrodesis procedures may be required. Although uncommon, tarsal coalition may be associated with pes cavus deformity. Therefore, observation for primary or secondary signs of tarsal coalition should be undertaken as a matter of routine in the clinical and radiographic evaluation of pes cavus deformity.

Gait Abnormality in Pes Cavus

The term pes cavus (cavus foot) represents a continuum of presentations generally characterized as having a higher arch than normal. The gait abnormality associated with cavus foot depends on the nature of the underlying neuromuscular disease, the extent of the disease presentation, and the extent of resultant deformity that is present.

Lesser degrees of the deformity may be associated with progressive and painful hammertoes, increased weight-bearing to the lesser metatarsals with associated metatarsalgia, or pressure callus formation. Increased varus components may result in ankle instability or recurring ankle injury, pain, or pressure callus of the fifth metatarsal head and/or fifth metatarsal base. Plantar fasciitis/fasciopathy may result from decreased shock absorption during the contact phase of gait.

Significant cavus foot deformities are associated with external rotation of the leg, which may be observed by gait analysis. Increased lateral weight-bearing may be noted in the presence of varus positioning of the heel. Increased strike force during heel contact may be noted on gait analysis. A more rigid gait pattern with persistence of high arch through late contact and midstance phases of gait may be appreciated. Some degree of clinical drop-foot deformity may be noted in those patients in whom the disease process, such as Charcot-Marie-Tooth disease, weakens the anterior leg musculature.

SUMMARY

Cavus foot is a complex deformity. It is frequently a manifestation of diagnosed or occult neuromuscular disorders. Neurologic evaluation is important in any evaluation of cavus foot deformity. Surgical decision making is based on age, anatomic presentation, and underlying neurologic cause. Complete and family history, detailed clinical examination, appropriate radiographic studies, and gait analysis are typically required in order to determine the most appropriate operative or nonoperative management in each case.

Pathoanatomic and Pathophysiologic Surgical Correlates

Contracture and deformity of the plantar fascia
   Open plantar fasciotomy
   Percutaneous plantar fasciotomy
   Overactivity/overpull of the intrinsic musculature
   Release of the intrinsic musculature and plantar fascia (Steindler stripping)
   Innervation of the intrinsic foot musculature (Garceau and Brahms)
   Weakness of the peroneus brevis muscle
   Overactivity of the peroneus longus muscle
   Peroneus longus to brevis transfer
   Peroneus longus recession or lengthening
   Ankle equinus deformity
   Gastrocnemius recession
   Lengthening of the Achilles tendon (open, percutaneous)
   Nonreducible heel varus
   Varus reducing calcaneal osteotomy (Dwyer type)
   Planar calcaneal osteotomy with valgus rotation of the posterior fragment

Reducible heel varus
Dorsiflexion osteotomy of the first metatarsal
Dorsiflexion arthrodesis first metatarsal-cuneiform joint
Peroneus longus to brevis transfer
Peroneus longus recession
Peroneus longus lengthening
Excessive calcaneal inclination
Dorsal sliding linear osteotomy of the calcaneus
Peroneal or digital flexor transfer to the Achilles tendon
Excessive calcaneal inclination with shortening of the hindfoot
Oblique, posterior-superior displacement osteotomy of the calcaneus (Mitchell type)
Forefoot equinus, nonreducible
Multiple lesser metatarsal dorsiflexion osteotomies
Lisfranc joint arthrodesis (truncated wedge)
Forefoot equinus, reducible (flexible)
Transfer of the long extensor muscles to the lesser metatarsals proximally
Anterior transfer of the posterior tibial tendon
Plantarflexion deformity secondary to weakness of the anterior leg musculature
Anterior transfer of the posterior tibial muscle/tendon
Transfer of the long extensor tendons into the cuneiform bones (Cole procedure)
Reduction of midfoot deformity at the apex of the deformity
Pan-tarsal metatarsal arthrodesis
Midtarsal dorsal wedge osteotomy (Cole type)
Midtarsal dorsiflexor osteotomy (Japas type)
Percutaneous osteotomy with gradual correction using external fixation
Reduction of adduction deformity
Modified Cole procedure with truncated wedge/trapezoid configuration
Calcaneocuboid arthrodesis
Percutaneous osteotomy with gradual correction using external fixation
Release of the abductor hallucis
Hammertoe/claw toe deformities
Transfer of the long extensor tendons to the metatarsals (Hibbs procedure) or its variants
Arthrodesis of the digital interphalangeal joints
Flexor digitorum longus dorsal digital tendon transfer (Girdlestone-Taylor type)
Reducible plantarflexion of the first ray
Transfer of the extensor hallucis longus into the first metatarsal neck (Jones suspension)
Arthrodesis of the hallux interphalangeal joint
Arthrodesis of the first metatarsal-cuneiform joint
Arthrodesis of the navicular-cuneiform joints
Nonreducible plantarflexion of the first ray
Dorsiflexory osteotomy of the first metatarsal
Dorsiflexory first metatarsal-cuneiform arthrodesis
Complex multiplanar deformity ± osteoarthritis
Triple arthrodesis
Percutaneous osteotomy with distraction using external fixation
Distal tibia varus deformity
Corrective osteotomy of the distal tibial metaphysis
Percutaneous osteotomy with gradual correction using external fixation
Ankle varus

Lateral ligament reconstruction
Arthrodesis of the ankle
Deltoid ligament release

CLINICS CARE POINTS

- Accurate and timely diagnosis of the cause related to the patient's cavus deformity is critical to effectively treat this patient population and promote patient outcomes, particularly in the pediatric population.

- Physical evaluation of cavus deformities should take into consideration soft tissue deforming forces as well as osseous deformities and their planar malalignment.

- Effective treatment of the pes cavus patient should include identification of the apex or center of rotation of angulation of the deformity.

- It is important to avoid pitfalls with regards to cavus, as anatomic (morphologic) findings do not necessarily indicate the cause of any particular component of cavus foot.

DISCLOSURE

Dr A.M. Jacobs has nothing to disclose regarding this topic.

REFERENCES

1. Testut L, Jacob O. Traite d'anatomie topographique avec applications1. Paris, Doin: Medico-Chirugicales; 1909. p. p3.
2. Aminian A, Sangeorzan BJ. The anatomy of cavus foot deformity. Foot Ankle Clin 2008;13:191–8.
3. Rosenbum AJ, Lisella J, Patel N. The cavus foot. Med Clin North Am 2014;98: 301–12.
4. Maynou C, Szymanski C, Thiounn A. The adult cavus foot. EFORT Open Rev 2017;2(5):221–9.
5. Holmes JR, Hansen ST. Foot and ankle manifestations of Charcot-Marie-Tooth disease. Foot Ankle 1993;14(8):14–476.
6. Ganley J. Lectures in orthopedics. Pennsylvania College of Podiatric Medicine, 1972 (personal notes).
7. Brewerton DA, Sandifer PH, Sweetman D. Idiopathic pes cavus: an investigation of its etiology. Br Med J 1963;2(5358):358–659.
8. McClusky WP, Lovell WW, Cummings RJ. The cavovarus foot deformity. Etiology and management. Clin Orthop Relat Res 1989;247:24.
9. Nagel MK, Chan G, Guille GT, et al. Prevalence of Charcot-Marie-Tooth disease in patients who have bilateral cavovarus feet. J Pediatr Orthop 2006;26(4):438–43.
10. Heron JR. Neurological syndromes associated with pes cavus. Proc R Soc Med 1969;62:270.
11. Winter RB, Haven JJ, Moe JH, et al. Diastematomyelia and congenital spine deformities. J Bone Joint Surg Am 1974;56-A:27.
12. Bigos SJ, Coleman SS. Foot deformity secondary to gluteal injection in infancy. J Pediatr Orthop 1984;4:560.
13. Ortiz C, Wagner E, Keller A. Cavovarus foot reconstruction. Foot Ankle Clin 2009; 14(3):471–87.
14. Coleman SS, Chestnut WJ. A simple test for hindfoot flexibility in the cavovarus foot. Clin Orthop Relat Res 1997;123:60–2.

15. Price BD, Price CT. A simple demonstration of hindfoot flexibility in the cavovarus foot. J Pediatr Orthop 1997;17:18.
16. Thometz JG, Gould JS. Cavus deformity. In: Drennan J, editor. The child's foot and ankle. P343. New York (NY): Raven Press; 1992.
17. Levitt RI, Canale ST, Cooke AJ, et al. The role of foot surgery in progressive neuro-muscular disorders in children. J Bone Joint Surg Am 1973;55-A:1396.
18. Bentzon PG. Pes cavus and the m. peroneus longus. Acta Orthop Scand 1933; 4:50.
19. Kim BS. Reconstruction of the cavus foot: a review. Open Orthop J 2017;11: 651–9.
20. Jahss MH. Evaluation of the cavus foot for orthopedic treatment. Clin Orthop 1983;181:52.
21. Jahss M. Tarsal metatarsal truncated-wedge arthrodesis for pes cavus and equinovarus deformity of the fore part of the foot. J Bone Joint Surg Am 1980; 62-A:713.
22. Grambart ST. Hibbs tenosuspension. Clin Podiatr Med Surg 2016;33(1):63–9.
23. Lauwerens JWK. Operative treatment algorithm for foot deformities in Charcot-Marie-Tooth disease. Oper Orthop Traumatol 2018;30(2):130–46.
24. Taylor RG. The treatment of claw toes by multiple transfer of flexors into extensor tendons. J Bone Joint Surg Am 1951;33-B:539.
25. Oganesyan OV, Is Istomina, Kuzmin VI. Treatment of equinovarus deformity in adults with the use of hinged distraction apparatus. J Bone Joint Surg Am 1996;78(4):546–56.
26. Perera A, Guha A. Clinical and radiographic evaluation of the cavus foot: surgical implications. Foot Ankle Clin 2013;18(4):619–28.
27. Samilson RL, Dillon W. Cavus, cavovarus, and calcaneocavus. An update. Clin Orthop Relat Res 1983;177:125.
28. Hibbs RA. An operation for "clawfoot". JAMA 1919;73:1573.
29. Meary R. Symposium: Le Pied Creux Essential. Rev Chir Orthop 1967;53:385.

Imaging of the Pes Cavus Deformity

Lawrence Osher, DPM[a],*, Jeffrey E. Shook, DPM[b,1]

KEYWORDS

- Direct pes cavus deformity • Sagittal plane deformity • Meary angle
- Calcaneal inclination angle • Cavovarus deformity • Modified Coleman block test
- Modified Saltzman view

KEY POINTS

- Direct-type cavus foot deformities are most commonly encountered and are primarily sagittal plane deformities. Direct deformities should be delineated from rarer triplane pes cavovarus deformities.
- The lateral weight-bearing radiograph is the cornerstone of imaging evaluation of direct pes cavus foot deformity.
- The apex of Meary talo-first metatarsal angle on the lateral radiograph represents the pinnacle of the cavus deformity and assists in subclassification of the deformity.
- With routine application, ancillary radiographic imaging techniques, such as the modified Saltzman view or the modified Coleman block test, can give valuable insight into deformity assessment and surgical planning.
- Advanced multiplanar computed tomographic (CT) imaging techniques along with 3-dimensional reconstructions promise to improve on precision and accuracy in delineating the presence and extent of intraosseous and interosseous deformity. In addition, weight-bearing CT can facilitate hindfoot alignment and compensatory motions in pes cavus deformity.

IMAGING OF PES CAVUS

Pes cavus is commonly perceived as a pedal deformity with grossly apparent elevation of the medial and lateral longitudinal foot arches imparting an overall hollow or cave-like appearance to the foot. The direct type of pes cavus (direct pes cavus) is most common, and is defined primarily as a sagittal plane deformity.[1] Although the distinction is often ignored, direct pes cavus should not be equated with the rarer

There are no financial or commercial conflicts of interest as it pertains to this topic. There are no sources of funding for this article.
[a] Radiology, Division of Podiatric and General Medicine, Kent State University College of Podiatric Medicine, 6000 Rockside Woods Blvd. N, Independence, OH 44131, USA; [b] Adjunct Faculty, St. Vincent Charity Medical Center, Cleveland, OH, USA
[1] Present address: 447 13th Avenue, Huntington, WV 25701.
* Corresponding author.
E-mail address: Losher@kent.edu

Clin Podiatr Med Surg 38 (2021) 303–321
https://doi.org/10.1016/j.cpm.2021.03.004
0891-8422/21/© 2021 Elsevier Inc. All rights reserved.

podiatric.theclinics.com

triplane cavovarus deformity (eg, associated CMT disease, clubfoot). In contradistinction from the uniplanar (sagittal plane) direct pes cavus deformity, cavovarus deformity entails rotation of the foot and calcaneus on the distal tibial-fibular articulation as a unit (calcaneopedal unit) via the subtalar joint, minus the talus.[1,2] Consequentially, cavovarus deformity typically results in compensatory supination of the calcaneopedal unit, eventual development of calcaneal varus with external rotation of talo-tibfibular unit, forefoot/metatarsal equinus, and forefoot-midfoot adduction.

Although advanced imaging modalities, such as weight-bearing (WB) computed tomographic (CT) scanning, show promise as potential future adjuncts in the evaluation of pes cavus deformity, plain radiographs currently comprise the cornerstone of imaging in the evaluation of this deformity. Plain radiographs, along with modified specialized views, are key in helping to (a) confirm the clinical diagnosis, (b) classify the deformity, and (c) aid in surgical planning. Standard WB plain radiographic imaging typically includes WB pedal anteroposterior (AP), lateral, and calcaneal axial views. In addition, standard ankle studies are recommended to assess for associated extrapedal causes and associations such as ankle/tibia plafond varus deformities or significant rotational malalignments.

Pedal Radiographs

Anteroposterior weight-bearing radiographic assessment
AP foot radiographs provide essential insight into transverse plane malalignments in cavus foot deformities, perhaps with the greatest benefit in the evaluation of cavovarus deformities.

AP foot radiographs can provide insight into the degree of (a) metatarsus adduction, (b) forefoot adduction (or displacement in clubfoot), (c) degree of midfoot and subtalar joint supination (talocalcaneal [TC] and talonavicular), (d) overlap of midfoot and rearfoot bones, or (e) parallelism of the talus and calcaneus (marked decrease of TC angle <5°; normal values 25°–30°) most notably in a triplanar cavus foot deformity associated with a clubfoot or incompletely treated clubfoot. In these instances, the longitudinal talar axis is directed through the lateral rays (eg, fourth and fifth metatarsals) as opposed to normal alignment through (or slightly medial to) the first metatarsal bone. A more detailed discussion of the pes cavus associated with clubfoot/residual clubfoot deformity is beyond the scope of the section.

Lateral weight-bearing plain radiographic assessment
Whether for helping to confirm the clinical diagnosis, classifying the deformity, or planning for surgical correction, the lateral WB radiograph is integral to the evaluative process of the sagittal plane deformity seen in direct pes cavus. As the mainstay for imaging direct pes cavus, the lateral radiograph is also essential in assessing the sagittal plane component of the triplanar cavovarus deformity. In this latter instance, multiplanar CT scanning incorporating 3-dimensional (3D) reconstruction of the foot and ankle appear better suited for preoperative and postoperative evaluation of cavovarus deformity.[3]

A. Primary WB lateral radiographic determinations.[1,4–6] The following comprise the main measurements and/or determinations in pes cavus deformity (**Figs. 1** and **2**):
   1. Calcaneal inclination angle (CIA, also known as calcaneal "pitch" angle). The angle is formed by a tangent to the inferior calcaneal surface and the WB reference line. Normal values are 25° ± 5°. Values greater than 30° are indicative of moderate pes cavus/increase in pitch. Severe cavus deformity often demonstrates excessive CIAs of 40° or greater. It is not uncommon for neurologic cavus foot deformities to radiographically present with CIAs in this range.

2. Talo-first metatarsal (Meary) angle.[7] The angle is formed by the intersection of the longitudinal axis of the talus and the first metatarsal. Normal values range from 0° to 5°. Normal (rectus) foot alignment generally demonstrates a colinear relationship of the talar and first metatarsal axes. As first metatarsal declination increases, Meary angle generally increases. Values greater than 15° to 18° are typically encountered in pes cavus.

3. Sagittal apex of pes cavus deformity. Deformity is determined by where the apex of the Meary talo-first metatarsal angle is positioned. The apex is a key guideline used in helping to subclassify pes cavus deformities.

4. Calcaneal-first metatarsal (Hibbs) angle. The angle is formed by the intersection of the longitudinal axes (center, bisections) of the calcaneus and first metatarsal bones. Hibb angles less than 150° are indicative of pes cavus. Severe pes cavus deformities may demonstrate decreased angles approaching 90°. The usefulness of this angle has been questioned in that it does not aid in the determination of the apex of the deformity.

5. Lateral TC angle. The angle is formed the by the intersection of the calcaneal and talar longitudinal axes. Normal values are 35° to 50°. Geometrically equal to the sum of the calcaneal inclination and talar declination angles, the lateral talocalcaneal angle tends to increase with pronation and decrease with supination. Classically used to evaluate clubfoot correction, this angle can be an aid in the subclassification of the pes cavus deformity. Marked decreases in the lateral talocalcaneal angle can be encountered with pes cavus deformities.

6. First metatarsal declination angle. The angle formed by the longitudinal axis of the first metatarsal and the WB reference line (formed between the most posteroinferior points of the os calcis and inferior-most point of the fifth metatarsal head). Normal values range from 15° to 23°. First metatarsal declination angles commonly increase beyond 25° in cavus deformity (eg, anterior cavus).

7. Tibiotalar angle. The angle is formed by the longitudinal axes of the talus and tibia. Normal values are 110°. The angle decreases with cavus deformity associated with ankle joint dorsiflexion and vice versa.

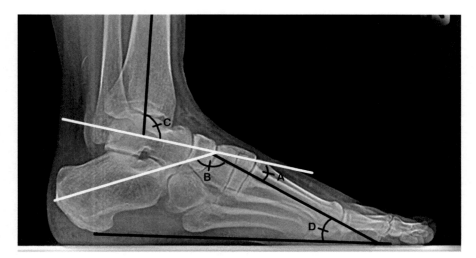

Fig. 1. Angle A: Meary talo-first metatarsal angle. Angle B: Hibbs calcaneo-first metatarsal angle. Angle C: tibiotalar angle. Angle D: first metatarsal declination angle.

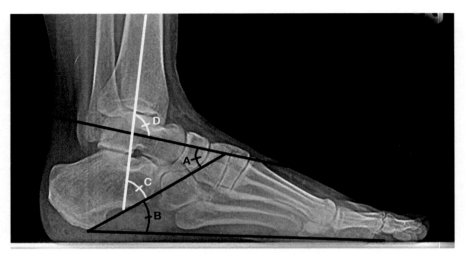

Fig. 2. Angle A: lateral TC angle. Angle B: CIA. Angle C: tibiocalcaneal angle. Angle D: tibiotalar angle.

8. Tibiocalcaneal angle. The angle formed by a tangent to the inferior calcaneal surface and the longitudinal axis of the tibia. Normal pediatric angle range is 60° to 90°. Increased angles generally associated with ankle and/or rearfoot equinus. This angle tends to decrease with increasing values of calcaneal pitch/CIA and/or with ankle dorsiflexion (calcaneus position).

B. Secondary WB lateral radiographic findings. The following are largely qualitative observations associated with alterations in bony positions, overlaps, and/or shapes associated with pes cavus deformity (**Fig. 3**):
   a. Horizontal orientation of the talus
   b. Posterior displacement of distal fibula
   c. Double overlap talar dome
   d. "Bullet-hole" sinus tarsi
   e. Posterior cyma line
   f. "Bell-shaped" cuboid
   g. Markedly decreased posterior facet declination angle (normal 30°–40°)

Radiography of cavus foot classifications: anterior, posterior, or combined

Primarily based on the lateral/sagittal plane determination of the apex of the deformity, pes cavus deformities are generally classified as either forefoot/anterior cavus (anterior equinus) deformity, hindfoot/rearfoot deformity, or combined rearfoot + forefoot deformity.[1,3–8]

I. Anterior cavus ("forefoot driven hindfoot varus"): Anterior cavus is primarily a sagittal plane deformity associated with excessive plantarflexion of either the first ray or the forefoot equinus, although eversion of the entire forefoot may be present (**Fig. 4**). CMT (and other hereditary sensory motor neuropathies) is one of the more frequent conditions associated with forefoot-driven hindfoot varus, typically presenting with relative weakness of the peroneus brevis (PB) and anterior tibial muscles and sparing of the peroneus longus and tibialis posterior.[3]

General radiographic findings, anterior cavus deformity (**Fig. 5**): Increased declination angles of the metatarsal bones. For local first ray deformity, first metatarsal

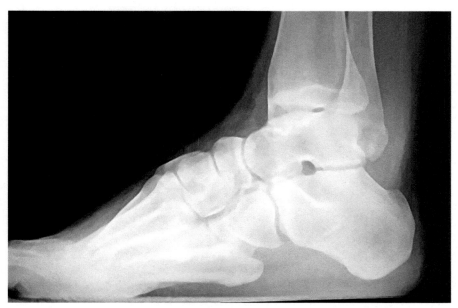

Fig. 3. Secondary pes cavus findings; virtually all listed findings present. Note horizontal orientation of the talus, double overlap of talar dome, posterior displacement of distal fibula, conspicuous "bullet hole" sinus tarsi, posterior cyma line, and so-called bell-shaped cuboid. In addition, marked decrease in posterior facet declination angle is apparent.

declination angles commonly increase into ranges of 25° to 35°. CIA less than 30, Meary greater than 10. The Meary (Tomeno) line is disrupted. The apex of the Meary angle is at the level of either the cuneiforms or the cuneiform-metatarsal (first metatarsal/Lisfranc) joints. The tibiotalar angle decreases with global anterior cavus deformity secondary to compensatory ankle joint dorsiflexion.

It is perhaps best to think of these deformities as involving either sagittal plane depression of the medial forefoot column or pillar, or both the medial and the lateral pillars of the forefoot. Depression of the medial foot pillar may be either a sagittal plane depression of the entire medial pillar or a local plantarflexed first ray. As noted by DiGiovanni and Smith,[9] both deformities create a frontal plane valgus relationship of the forefoot to the rearfoot that is compensated at the subtalar joint by supination. Therefore, compensation would predictably result in a decreased lateral TC angle and a high normal CIA. In the event of depression of both medial and lateral forefoot pillars, that is, total forefoot equinus deformity, compensation primarily occurs by dorsiflexion of the ankle joint and not the subtalar joint. In this case, the talus and calcaneus act as a unit and are suggested by the radiographic findings of increased CIA with a normal lateral TC angle. Finally, in the event of forefoot valgus combined with depression of the lateral forefoot pillar, compensation would result in both decreased lateral TC angle and increased CIA.[9]

II. Posterior (hindfoot) cavus deformity (**Fig. 6**): Posterior cavus deformities are typically associated with weakness of the gastrocnemius ("equinocavus foot") or triceps surae muscles, or varus deformities of the distal tibia (eg, secondary to malunion of pilon fracture). Clinically, there is a lack of adequate dorsiflexion of

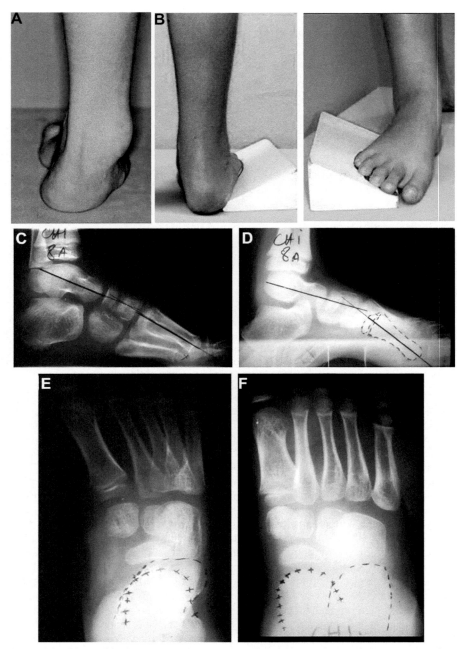

Fig. 4. (*A*) Oblique block test. A posterior view of the foot with significant inversion/heel varus. (*B*). Oblique block test. The oblique block corrects the heel varus. (*C–F*) Lateral radiograph without (*C*) and with (*D*) the oblique block: the oblique block corrects the abnormalities in the transverse plane, allowing appropriate measurement of Meary angle. Dorsoplantar radiograph without (*E*) and with (*F*) the oblique block: note the restoration of TC divergence. (*From* Wicart P. Cavus foot, from neonates to adolescents. Orthop Traumatol Surg Res. 2012 Nov;98(7):813-28. https://doi.org/10.1016/j.otsr.2012.09.003. Epub 2012 Oct 23. PMID: 23098772.)

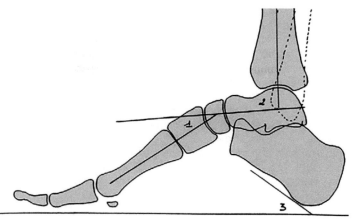

Fig. 5. Direct anterior pes cavus demonstrating increased Meary angle, increased CIA, and decreased tibiotalar angle (normal 110°). (*From* Wicart P. Cavus foot, from neonates to adolescents. Orthop Traumatol Surg Res. 2012 Nov;98(7):813-28. https://doi.org/10.1016/j.otsr. 2012.09.003. Epub 2012 Oct 23. PMID: 23098772.)

the ankle. Radiographically, the common presentation is a deformity of the hindfoot associated with an isolated increase in the CIA and compensatory plantarflexion/equinus of the ankle. In the event of varus plafond/tibial varus deformities (eg, malunited pilon fracture), if the subtalar joint has sufficient motion in the direction of eversion, it may compensate for the extrinsic varus, and the hindfoot can assume a relatively normal position. When sufficient motion does not exist at the subtalar joint, the hindfoot will reflect the varus ankle/varus plafond and also assume the varus position.[3,5] Other associations include rigid rearfoot varus, calcaneovarus secondary to compensatory motions owing to forefoot deformities, such as rigid plantarflexed first ray, and occasionally, tarsal coalition.

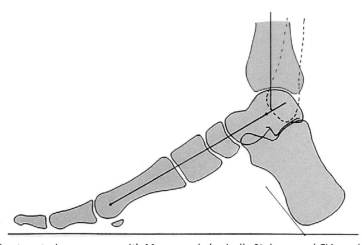

Fig. 6. Direct posterior pes cavus with Meary angle basically 0°, increased CIA, and increased tibiotalar angle. (*From* Wicart P. Cavus foot, from neonates to adolescents. Orthop Traumatol Surg Res. 2012 Nov;98(7):813-28. https://doi.org/10.1016/j.otsr.2012.09.003. Epub 2012 Oct 23. PMID: 23098772.)

Radiographic findings: CIA greater than 30, Meary less than 10. The apex/vertex of the Meary angle is typically proximal to the Chopart joint. The tibiotalar angle is typically increased in posterior cavus deformity. The lateral TC angle can show paradoxic ("reversed") increases in value in the presence of normal talar declination secondary to markedly increased CIAs.

III. Combined (mixed) cavus deformity (primary posterior; **Fig. 7**): Increased Meary angle and increased CIA greater than 30° are generally associated with high normal or mild (but not dramatic) increases in the tibiotalar angle. The apex of the Meary angle typically intersects somewhere in between the Chopart and Lisfranc joint, with the more anterior apex generally reflective of the degree or magnitude of increased metatarsal declination associated with the anterior component of the deformity. The tibiocalcaneal can be useful in delineating combined findings associated with compensated forefoot (global) equinus (**Fig. 8**). Subclassifications, such as combined primary anterior or combined primary posterior, are beyond the scope of this discussion.

Ancillary plain radiographic imaging

Ancillary radiographic views of cavus deformities include AP leg studies, ankle charger, and WB hindfoot alignment studies. There have been several studies regarding WB hindfoot alignment views, which can be quite useful in capturing coronal plane varus and valgus malalignments of the leg and foot. With respect to pes cavus deformities, varus malalignments of the ankle joint are of greatest interest. Originally proposed by Cobey,[10] the modified version of the view by Saltzman and el-Khoury[11,12] is most widely used. The specialized orthoposer along with subject positioning is shown in **Fig. 9A**. The inclination angle of the beam is 20° to the WB surface, with a long leg-plate image receptor angled 20° from the vertical, which allows for the central ray/beam to be approximately perpendicular to the center plane of the image receptor.

The view is designed to estimate the moment arm between the WB axis of the leg and the contact point of the heel. Coronal plane tibiocalcaneal alignment was defined by measuring the horizontal distance between a line representing the anatomic axis of

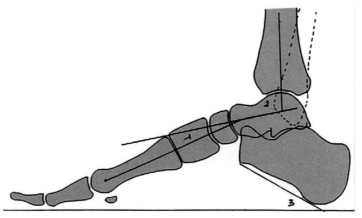

Fig. 7. Combined/mixed direct pes cavus with increased Meary angle, increased CIA, and no change in the tibiotalar angle. (*From* Wicart P. Cavus foot, from neonates to adolescents. Orthop Traumatol Surg Res. 2012 Nov;98(7):813-28. https://doi.org/10.1016/j.otsr.2012.09.003. Epub 2012 Oct 23. PMID: 23098772.)

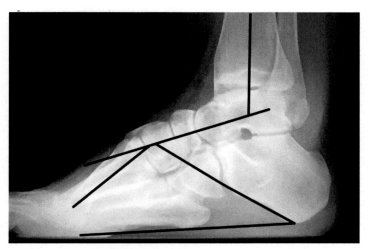

Fig. 8. Angle values (measured digitally): Lat TC = 49°; tibiotalar 109°; CIA = 34°; first met declination = 38.1; Meary = 22.7°; apex mid first cuneiform bone; tibiocalcaneal = 61.8. Interpretation: The lateral TC angle is relatively normal to slightly increased lateral along with marked increases in metatarsal declination and Meary angle, with the crossing apex at tarsometatarsal joint. These findings suggest combined/mixed cavus foot deformity. However, the low normal value of the tibiocalcaneal angle indicates the ankle has been dorsi-flexed. Therefore, in concert with the significant elevation of the CIA and only mildly elevated lateral TC angle, underlying compensated forefoot equinus should be considered.

the tibia and the most inferior aspect of the calcaneus (**Fig. 9**B). The mean moment arm placed the most inferior aspect of the calcaneus medial to the tibial bisection; this suggests that the most inferior aspect of the heel was slightly inverted to the tibial bisection or the tibial bisection is in slight external rotation compared with the inferior-most point of the calcaneus. In the Saltzman and el-Khoury study, the line of the tibia fell within 8 mm of the lowest calcaneal point in 80% of subjects and within 15 mm of the lowest calcaneal point in 95% of subjects. Johnson and colleagues[13] noted that these hindfoot studies assessing the coronal plane alignment of the calcaneus relative to the tibia do not yield an angular difference and do not demonstrate true calcaneal frontal plane alignment for several reasons. These reasons include leg rotation, unnatural subject posture (changing hindfoot alignment), and obliquity of the x-ray beam. The investigators proposed a modified technique allowing the patient to assume a natural WB posture that captures the relative angle and base between both feet. A method using multiple ellipses was used, centered over the "condensation" of the posterior calcaneal tuberosity. The angle formed between the axes of the ellipse and tibia defined coronal hindfoot alignment. The investigators conclude that their method more accurately and reliably determined the coronal axis of the posterior calcaneus (**Fig. 10**).

Reilingh and colleagues[14] subsequently compared the reliabilities of the hindfoot alignment with the so-called long axial radiographic view described by Lamm and colleagues.[15] The long axial view is modified from traditional calcaneal axial studies in that the subject stands on (over with digital radiography) the image cassette as the x-ray beam enters the posterior ankle joint area angled 45° to the image receptor plane, with the patient extending/dorsiflexing the angle by 10°. The Reilingh and colleagues study concluded that the long axial view was more reliable than the hindfoot

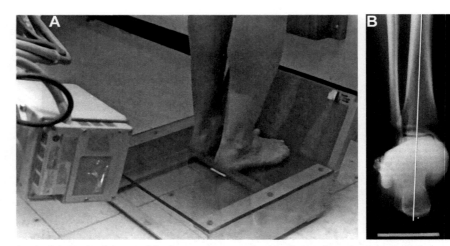

Fig. 9. (*A*) Method for positioning patient on the hindfoot alignment view platform. Patients stand on the platform facing the film with the medial border of their feet parallel and their knees in extension. A lead strip is placed tangent to the most posterior aspect of the heel, oriented perpendicular to the longitudinal axis of the foot. (*B*) Hindfoot alignment view. The apparent moment arm is determined by measuring the perpendicular distance between the longitudinal midaxis of the tibia and the lowest point on the calcaneus.

alignment view, and that the unilateral WB stance does not lead to greater measurement reliability.

Irrespective of which posterior radiographic imaging technique is used to assess the frontal plane position of the heel with respect to the leg, the accuracy of frontal plane assessment is questionable because of inconsistencies of osseous morphology and differing joint compensatory capacity between individuals. Further investigations using WB CT along with 3D CT predictably provide more accurate preoperative determination of frontal plane osseous position. As noted in the following section, WB CT scanning has more recently been used to evaluate hindfoot alignment as well as evaluate the morphology of the posterior facet.

Computed tomographic scanning/weight-bearing computed tomographic scanning
Several simulated foot loading CT scans have focused on the previously mentioned hindfoot alignment. With the advent of true physiologic loading using dedicated standing/WB multiplanar CT scanners, hindfoot alignment has been evaluated with a greater accuracy and reliability. Hirschmann and colleagues[16] found significant changes in hindfoot alignment between non-WB and "upright" WB CT scan images. Using standard radiographs and WB, Burssens and colleagues[17] evaluated 60 hindfoot malalignments with subjects divided in 2 groups of 30, one with valgus and one with varus hindfoot alignments. Standard angles were measured along with a novel method to determine the hindfoot angle by combining the anatomic axis and the coronal plane TC inclination angle.

WB CT rationally should provide for more detailed analyses of pes cavus deformity, such as identifying differences in types of pes cavus, evaluating compensatory rearfoot motions and positions, and analyses of rotational movements of foot and ankle bones. Kim and colleagues[18] retrospectively evaluated WB CT and plain radiographs of 52 normal ankles and 96 ankles with varus osteoarthritis, which were further divided

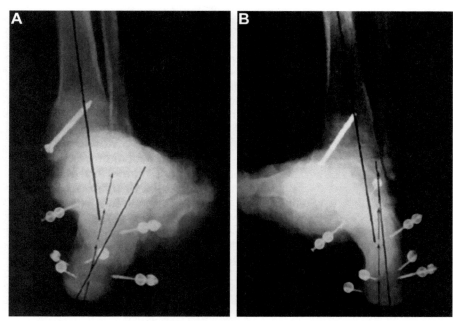

Fig. 10. (A) Coronal view of both the foot and the distal leg (cadaveric) with markers placed on the cortical "condensation" of the posterior calcaneal tuberosity. Note that the outline of the markers form an elliptical, "egg-shaped" configuration. (B) The series of ellipses are placed over the "egg" of the tuberosity to determine the coronal axis of the calcaneus as represented by the semi-major axis of the overlaid ellipse. (*From* Johnson JE, Lamdan R, Granberry WF, Harris GF, Carrera GF. Hindfoot Coronal Alignment: A Modified Radiographic Method. Foot & Ankle International. 1999;20(12):818-825, with permission.)

into moderate (50) and severe (46) osteoarthritic subgroups. Rotation of the talus in the transverse (axial) plane was evaluated via the development of a new radiographic parameter WB CT, the talus rotation ratio. The study ultimately demonstrated that abnormal internal rotation of the talus occurs in patients with varus ankle osteoarthritis and is more frequently noted in severe than in moderate varus ankle osteoarthritis.

To date, although validated studies are sparce regarding classifying pes cavus as anterior, posterior, or mixed deformities, the reliability of WB CT in evaluating pes cavus has been affirmed.[19] In general, 3D CT reconstructions of the foot can be quite useful in preoperative planning of complex triplanar cavovarus foot deformities, as well as in identifying occult osteoarthritic joints or tarsal coalition or coalitions. Most recently, Bernasconi and colleagues[20] retrospectively compared CMT cavovarus foot deformities with idiopathic (so-called subtle pes cavovarus) cavovarus feet. Using 3D WB CT analyses, CMT feet demonstrated increased forefoot supination and hindfoot malalignment compared with idiopathic forms.

WB CT research has also focused on the configuration of the posterior subtalar joint facet and its potential association with ankle joint alignment and/or osteoarthritis. Krähenbühl and colleagues[21,22] retrospectively evaluated 60 ankle radiographs (20 controls, 40 with osteoarthritis) in order to determine if an association exists between the coronal plane posterior facet/subtalar joint orientation (assessed by the subtalar joint vertical axis) and osteoarthritis of the ankle. In their cohort, varus osteoarthritis of the ankle joint occurred with varus orientation of the subtalar joint in about 50%

of subjects, with a greater percentage of subjects (70%) with valgus osteoarthritis associated with valgus subtalar joint orientation. The investigators conclude that the subtalar joint vertical axis provides a reliable and consistent method to assess the varus/valgus configuration of the subtalar joint posterior facet. No significant difference of the subtalar joint alignment was evident when comparing different stages of ankle osteoarthritis. In a 2019 retrospective study of 88 patients with symptomatic ankle joint osteoarthritis, Krähenbühl and colleagues further noted a correlation with increased valgus subtalar joint alignment in patients with varus ankle osteoarthritis and conclude that varus ankles compensate in the subtalar joint for deformities above the ankle joint.

Imaging of pes cavus with tarsal coalition
Commonly associated with pes planus, tarsal coalitions are encountered in the pes cavus foot. The frequency is unclear, but certainly not rare. In light of the decreased overlap of osseous structures and improved visualization of the subtalar joint facets on the lateral pedal radiographs, the accuracy of typical findings and the conspicuity of tarsal coalitions are improved in patients with high-arch morphologies. The 2 most commonly encountered tarsal coalitions are calcaneonavicular (CN) followed by middle facet subtalar joint. Other coalitions involving the midfoot, such as talonavicular, naviculocuboid, or calcaneocuboid bones/joints, are uncommon, and an underlying syndrome should be ruled out. In the latter case, AP ankle views should be acquired to rule-out ball-and-socket ankle joint deformity.

Classic lateral radiographic findings: tarsal coalition
a. Anteater nose sign: Hypertrophic enlargement of the anterior calcaneal process is indicative of CN coalition; alteration of the normally triangular or rounded shape to plateau (for incomplete bars) or poorly defined (for complete bars).
b. Inconspicuous/absent middle facet sign (**Fig. 11**): A loss of conspicuity of the middle facet of the subtalar joint. As a general rule, the middle facet is apparent in all but the most severe flatfoot (eg, "rocker bottom") deformities. In the absence of a severe flatfoot, loss of visualization of the middle facet is a sin qua non for a middle facet coalition, especially in cavus-type architecture.
c. C-sign: An apparent continuity of structure between the talus and the calcaneus where a continuous line can be traced from the medial talar dome to the posteroinferior margin of the sustentaculum tali (see **Fig. 11**).
d. Lateral talar process blunting: A dysmorphic rounding of the normally "V-shaped" lateral talar process, effectively becoming "U-shaped."
e. Talar neck "beaking": A dorsal talar neck osseous "spur" that not uncommonly spans the entire width of the neck between anterior ankle and talonavicular joints.

Medial oblique radiographic imaging: tarsal coalition. High-angle medial oblique views are the imaging view of choice to demonstrate and confirm diagnosis of CN coalitions (also known as "bars"). A direct synostosis may be noted, although the term anteater nose sign is also applied to the appearance of a hypertrophic anterior calcaneal process in the case of incomplete CN coalitions. In this instance, the appearance of an articulation or articulating facet between the calcaneus and navicular is suspect. High-angle medial oblique views can also be quite useful in demonstrating other rarer midfoot intertarsal coalitions as well as imaging of the anterior facet of the subtalar joint.

Harris (Harris-Beath) view: tarsal coalition. Normally, Harris views are quite useful in the coronal plane imaging of the posterior and middle subtalar joint facets along

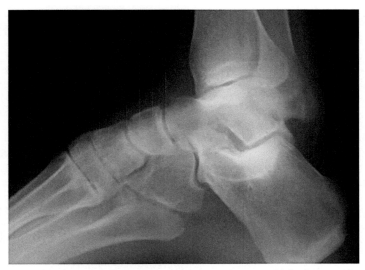

Fig. 11. Severe pes cavus deformity with poorly conspicuous middle facet and continuous (unbroken) C-sign. With the cavus morphology, these findings are strongly indicative of subtalar joint tarsal coalition.

with the morphology of the sustentaculum tali. However, because of the horizontal orientations (markedly decreased declination angles) of both the posterior and the middle subtalar joint facets with high-arched/cavus feet, Harris views cannot reliably image these subtalar joint features in subjects with pes cavus deformity. Therefore, CT scanning becomes the primary imaging modality demonstrating typical coronal plane features in subtalar joint coalition. Typical findings include dysmorphic (hypoplastic or aplastic) sustentaculum tali, altered middle facet angulation ("drunken waiter" sign), presence of incorporated os sustentacula, and the degree of posterior facet involvement in the coalition.

Adult acquired pes cavus

One of the most common, acute musculoskeletal injuries of the body is the plantar flexion/inversion injury of the ankle or the "common" ankle sprain. Although most of these injuries occur in athletically active individuals, up to half of the estimated 2 million annual ankle sprains in the United States occurred in the absence of a sporting activity.[23] An epidemiologic review of ankle sprains done by Herzog and colleagues[24] revealed an incidence ranging from 2.15 per 1000 person-years up to 26.0 per 1000 person-years. More impressive is the fact that these incidence numbers most likely represent an underestimation of ankle sprains, as Kemler and colleagues[25] estimated that the true incidence of ankle sprains is 5.5 times higher than the number of ankle sprains registered in emergency departments.

A multitude of soft tissue and osteoarticular injuries can occur either in conjunction or concurrently with an acute plantarflexion inversion lateral ankle sprain. These injuries can include (1) common peroneal nerve injuries, (2) superficial peroneal nerve injuries, (3) fifth metatarsal base fractures, (4) extensor digitorum brevis avulsion fractures of the calcaneus, (5) calcaneal anterior process "beak" fractures, (6) osteoarticular injuries to the dorsal lateral/lateral calcaneocuboid joint, (7) osteochondral injuries of the talus, (8) capsular/ligamentous damage to the dorsal/dorsolateral talonavicular joint, (9) lateral talar process fractures, (10) posterolateral process fractures of the talus, (11) ligamentous/capsular damage lateral and/or interosseous area of the subtalar joint, and (12) peroneal tendon pathologic condition.[26]

Typically, patients who sustain other injuries to the leg, ankle, and rearfoot complex associated with a lateral ankle sprain experience higher impact/force when sustaining the initial trauma. Because of this, these secondary or concomitant injuries are often overlooked and/or incompletely treated, leading to morbidity and disability. It is not uncommon for a patient to seek initial medical treatment on a delayed timeframe for the associated injury not the primary ankle sprain.

Notwithstanding the cause, one of the primary problems in a cavus foot deformity is the resultant muscle imbalance secondary to weakness or complete loss of the PB musculotendinous unit. With respect to acute injuries, the PB tendon is either (a) indirectly injured because of traction forces on the common peroneal nerve associated with plantar flexion, or (b) injured by direct mechanical trauma to the tendon. Indirect PB injury/dysfunction is rare with weakness the result of deficit at the neuromuscular junction. Direct PB injury is more common and results from mechanical tendon trauma along the course of the tendon from the musculotendinous junction to the insertion at the fifth metatarsal base. Although acute complete PB (transverse) ruptures have been reported, loss of tendon function is more commonly associated with significant tendon deformations, such as attenuated "splaying" or overt longitudinal "split" tears (**Fig. 12**). The damaged PB tendon can undergo progressive attrition secondary to multiple factors and therefore not heal. These injuries not uncommonly include (a) progressive longitudinal full-split PB tendon ruptures secondary to the tendon being compressed by the overlying peroneus longus tendon against the posterior fibula within the posterolateral ankle fibroosseous tunnel, (b) repetitive inversion ankle injuries (ankle instability), or (c) persistent peroneal tendon subluxation with superior peroneal retinacular injury. In instances of progressive deterioration of PB function, the tibialis posterior eventually, and essentially, functions unopposed, and the adult-acquired pes cavus deformity develops. Imaging the adult acquired pes cavus deformity secondary to chronic sequelae of an acute PB injury begins with WB, plain film imaging of the foot and ankle, AP and lateral of the foot, axial views of the calcaneus/tibia, and AP mortise and lateral of the ankle. However, the imaging "workhorse" in these patients is MRI. Not only does MRI image the integrity of lateral and medial ankle ligamentous structures, but it can also confirm and identify underlying peroneal tendon pathologic condition and concomitant pathologic condition (commonly occult) and assists in evaluation of extent of peroneal tendon disease. A discussion of MR evaluation of ligaments and tendons is beyond the scope of this article, but it is worth noting the caveat of magic angle artifact. The effect occurs with ordered collagen within tendons or ligaments, as they change their orientation to 55° with respect to the direction of the main MRI magnetic field. As the peroneal tendons change direction from leg to foot around the distal tip of the fibula, short echo time images (eg, T1-weighted) can demonstrate increased intratendinous signal or signals leading to an erroneous false positive interpretation of tendon rupture or ruptures. Ankle MRI is therefore best accomplished routinely with the patient placed in a prone position and the ankle plantarflexed by about 20°. In this way, the peroneal (and other ankle) tendons approximate a straighter course around the distal tip of the fibula/malleoli.

MRI in pes cavus

Apart from the aforementioned evaluation of tendon and ligament integrity/involvement in pes cavus deformity, the role of MRI of the foot and ankle is not clearly defined. The sectional and 3D imaging capabilities of MRI have not supplanted standard and

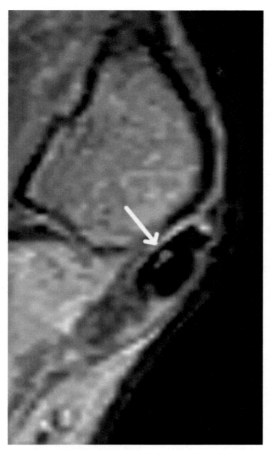

Fig. 12. Proton density MR axial lateral ankle image in a patient with adult-acquired pes cavus. Attenuation with mild splaying of PB tendon is noted. Arrow indicates area of partial split tendon rupture.

WB multiplanar and 3D CT scanning for pretreatment/preoperative reconstruction in pes cavus and cavovarus deformities. MRI is, however, an area of evolving application. With the ability to evaluate skeletal muscle, MRI has been used to assess and monitor the magnitude and progression of neuropathic disease in disorders such as CMT disease,[27–29] and also in the assessment of idiopathic clubfoot deformity.[30] In chronic neurologic denervation, involved skeletal muscle atrophies and is progressively replaced by fat. Fatty replacement is conspicuous with T1-weighted images (**Fig. 13**). Gaeta and colleagues[31] used MRI to describe patterns of disease distribution, and muscle fat fraction calculation in a family of 5 patients with CMT type 2F disease. A proximal to distal bilateral lower-extremity gradient of increasing muscle involvement was noted in the male subjects, with proximal sparing noted in all patients. Using MRI, Chung and colleagues[32] studied 62 consecutive CMT1A and CMT2A patients that had not undergone prior surgery. CMT1A patients showed selective fatty infiltration with a preference for anterior and lateral compartment muscles, whereas CMT2A patients showed a preference for superficial posterior compartment muscles (especially soleus). Early-onset CMT2A patients showed more severe leg fatty atrophy than late-onset CMT2A.

In the evaluation of progressive skeletal muscle wasting, MRI has moved to quantitative evaluation of textural changes, diameter/volume, and muscle fat fraction grading of fatty axonal denervation atrophy of both extrinsic leg muscles and intrinsic foot muscles.[33–39] Recently, Franettovich-Smith and colleagues[40] have indicated that 7 T (vs 3 T) MRIs provide superior resolution in the evaluation of intrinsic foot muscles (especially forefoot) in the assessment of segmentation of individual muscles, muscle volumes, and fat infiltration (see **Fig. 13**).

Beyond the assessment of intrinsic skeletal muscle, MRI has been used to evaluate foot and ankle deformities in cavovarus deformity. Richards and Dempsey[41] used MRI to study congenital clubfoot deformity in 10 infants preconservative and postconservative Ponsetti method therapy. MRI proved a useful tool in chronicling the alignment of the pediatric cartilaginous anlage of pediatric skeletal structures, along with chondroosseous anatomy and joint relationships over time. Peden and colleagues[42] used 3D CT and MRI in 72 subjects (36 pes cavus, 36 control) to determine whether the fibula was truly posterior or if this appearance was just an artifact. In the cavus group, the average fibula was 72% more posterior than the average fibula in the control group.

With altered WB (lateral) patterns in pes cavus/cavovarus deformity, MRI can demonstrate altered patterns of bone marrow edema, predilection for lateral stress reaction/fracture,[43] and also the potential development of arthritic changes in pes

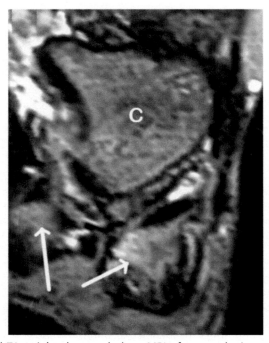

Fig. 13. Magnified T1-weighted coronal plane MRI of a neurologic pes cavus patient. Arrows indicate fatty denervation atrophy of intrinsic muscles (from medial to lateral, flexor digitorum brevis, and abductor digiti minimi). On cross-section, approximately 50% of normally isointense muscle has been replaced by high signal fat. The calcaneus is indicated by the letter "C".

cavus. In the latter instance, Krause and colleagues[44] used high-resolution T2* relaxation time mapping of ankle joint cartilage in 18 normal and 25 total pes cavus feet. The pes cavus group comprises 13 symptomatic and 12 asymptomatic/mildly symptomatic ankle joints. The study found that mean global T2* relaxation times were significantly higher (indicating arthrosis) in the symptomatic versus other groups. Ankle arthrosis (noted on plain radiographs and with American Orthopaedic Foot and Ankle Society scoring) correlated significantly with T2* values in the medial (not lateral) ankle compartment of the symptomatic group.

CLINICS CARE POINTS

- Pes cavus deformity is classified into either the sagittal, direct deformity or the more complex triplanar cavovarus (medial cavus) deformity.
- Whereas lateral weightbearing radiographs are relatively accurate in the assessment of the direct cavus deformities along with subclassifications based upon the apex of the deformity (eg. Meary's angle for anterior cavus), this is not the case for the complex triplanar deformity.
- Complex cavovarus deformities, which are almost always associated a underlying neurologic condition, require imaging the foot in multiple planes. Radiographic hindfoot alignment views can be quite useful in assessing the coronal plane deformity, although weightbearing 3D CT scans are an emerging imaging technology.
- Acquired pes cavus is generally associated with trauma (eg. lateral ankle injuries) where resultant muscle imbalance secondary to insufficiency of the peroneus brevis musculotendinous unit. Magnetic resonance imaging (MRI) can be useful in assessment of tendon rupture (eg. split rupture) or tendon subluxation/dislocation.
- MRI has been shown to be a useful tool in chronicling the alignment of the pediatric cartilaginous structures in conditions such as clubfoot. Most recently, MRI has been used in the quantitative evaluation of skeletal muscle textural changes, diameter/volume, and muscle fat fraction grading as fatty axonal denervation atrophy of both extrinsic leg muscles and intrinsic foot muscles occurs.

ACKNOWLEDGMENTS

The authors wish to gratefully acknowledge the time and efforts of Joshua Wolfe, DPM in advancing this section.

REFERENCES

1. Wicart P. Cavus foot, from neonates to adolescence. Orthopedics Traumatol Surg Res 2012;98:813–28.
2. Seringe R, Wicart P. The French Society of Orthopedics (SOFOP). The talonavicular and subtalar joints: The "calcaneopedal unit" concept. Orthopaedics & Traumatology: Surgery & Research 2013;99:S345–55.
3. Apostle KL, Sangeorzan BJ. Anatomy of the varus foot and ankle. Foot Ankle Clin N Am 2012;17:1–11.
4. Akoh CC, Phisitkul P. Clinical examination and radiographic assessment of the cavus foot. Foot Ankle Clin N Am 2019;24:183–93.
5. Krähenbühl N, Weinberg MW. Anatomy and biomechanics of cavovarus deformity. Foot Ankle Clin N Am 2019;24:173–81.

6. Herring JA. Tachdjian's pediatric orthopedics. 5th edition. Saunders; 2013. p. 834–47.

7. Meary R. On the measurement of the angle between the talus and the first metatarsal. Symposium: Le Pied Creux Essential. Rev Chir Orthop 1967;53:389.

8. Southerland JT, Boberg JS, Downey MS, et al. McGlamry's comprehensive textbook of foot and ankle surgery. 4th edition. Philadelphia: Wolters Kluwer Health/Lippincott Williams & Wilkens. pps; 2013. p. 898–9.

9. DiGiovanni JE, Smith SD. Normal biomechanics of the adult rearfoot. A radiographic analysis. J Am Podiatry Assoc. Nov. 1976;66(11):812–24.

10. Cobey JC. Posterior roentgenogram of the foot. Clin Orthop 1976;118:202–7.

11. Cobey JC, Sella E. Standardizing methods of measuring foot shape by including the effects of subtalar rotation. Foot Ankle 1981;2:30–6.

12. Saltzman CL, el-Khoury GY. The hindfoot alignment view. Foot Ankle Int 1995;16:572–6.

13. Johnson JE, Lamdan R, Granberry WF, et al. Hindfoot coronal alignment: a modified radiographic method. Foot Ankle Int 1999;20(12):818–25.

14. Reilingh ML, Beimers L, Tuijthof GJM, et al. Measuring hindfoot alignment radiographically: the long axial view is more reliable than the hindfoot alignment view. Skeletal Radiol 2010;39:1103–8.

15. Lamm BM, Mendicino RW, Catanzariti AR, et al. Static rearfoot alignment: a comparison of clinical and radiographic measures. J Am Podiatr Med Assoc 2005;95:26–33.

16. Hirschmann A, Pfirrmann CW, Klammer G, et al. Upright cone CT of the hindfoot: comparison of the non-weight-bearing with the upright weight-bearing position. Eur Radiol 2014;24(3):553–8.

17. Burssens A, Peeters J, Buedts K, et al. Measuring hindfoot alignment in weight bearing CT: a novel clinical relevant measurement method. Foot Ankle Surg 2016;22(4):233–8.

18. Kim JB, Young Y, Kim JY, et al. Weight-bearing computed tomography findings in varus ankle osteoarthritis: abnormal internal rotation of the talus in the axial plane. Skeletal Radiol 2017;46(8):1071–80.

19. Bernasconi A, Cooper L, Lyle S, et al. Intraobserver and interobserver reliability of cone beam weightbearing semi-automatic three-dimensional measurements in symptomatic pes cavovarus. Foot Ankle Surg 2019;26(5):564–72.

20. Bernasconi A, Cooper L, Lyle S, et al. Pes cavovarus in Charcot-Marie-Tooth compared to the idiopathic cavovarus foot: a preliminary weightbearing CT analysis. Foot Ankle Surg 2020;27(2):186–95.

21. Krähenbühl N, Tschuck M, Bolliger L, et al. Measurement and reliability using weightbearing CT scans of the orientation of the subtalar joint. Foot Ankle Int 2016;37(1):109–14.

22. Krähenbühl N, Siegler L, Deforth M, et al. Subtalar joint alignment in ankle osteoarthritis. Foot Ankle Surg 2019;25(2):143–9.

23. Waterman BR, Owens BD, Davey S, et al. The epidemiology of ankle sprains in the United States. J Bone Joint Surg Am 2010;92(13):2279–84.

24. Herzog MM, Kerr ZY, Marshall SW, et al. Epidemiology of ankle sprains and chronic ankle instability. J Athl Train 2019;54(6):603–10.

25. Kemler E, van de Port I, Valkenberg H, et al. Ankle injuries in The Netherlands: trends over 10–25 years. Scand J Med Sci Sports 2015;25(3):331–7.

26. Yu GV, Shook JE. Differential diagnosis of ankle sprains. In: Scurran BL, editor. Foot and ankle trauma. 2nd edition. New York: Churchill Livingstone; 1996. p. 701–29. Chapter 27.

27. Gallardo E, Garci A, Combarros O, et al. Charcot-Marie-Tooth disease type IA duplication. Spectrum of clinical and magnetic resonance imaging features in leg and foot muscles. Brain 2006;129:426–37.
28. Mercuri E, Pichiecchio A, Allsop J, et al. Muscle MRI in inherited neuromuscular disorders: past, present, and future. J Magn Reson Imaging 2007;25:433–40.
29. Wattjes MP, Kley RA, Fischer D. Neuromuscular imaging in inherited muscle diseases. Eur Radiol 2010;20:2447–60.
30. Duce SL, D'Alessandro M, Du Y, et al. 3D MRI analysis of the lower legs of treated idiopathic congenital talipes equinovarus (clubfoot). PLoS One 2013;8(1): e54100.
31. Gaeta M, Mileto A, Mazzeo A, et al. MRI findings, patterns of disease distribution, and muscle fat fraction calculation in five patients with Charcot-Marie-Tooth type 2 F disease. Skeletal Radiol 2012;41(5):515–24.
32. Chung KW, Suh BC, Shy ME, et al. Different clinical and magnetic resonance imaging features between Charcot-Marie-Tooth disease type 1A and 2A. Neuromuscul Disord 2008;18(8):610–8.
33. Burakiewicz J, Sinclair CDJ, Fischer D, et al. Quantifying fat replacement of muscle by quantitative MRI in muscular dystrophy. J Neurol 2017;264:2053–67.
34. Forbes SC, Willcocks RJ, Rooney WD, et al. MRI quantifies neuromuscular disease progression. Lancet Neurol 2016;15(1):26–8.
35. Willcocks RJ, Rooney WD, Triplett WT, et al. Multicenter prospective longitudinal study of magnetic resonance biomarkers in a large Duchenne muscular dystrophy cohort. Ann Neurol 2016;79:535–47.
36. Willis TA, Hollingsworth KG, Coombs A, et al. Quantitative magnetic resonance imaging in limb-girdle muscular dystrophy 2I: a multinational cross-sectional study. PLoS One 2014;9:e90377.
37. Gaeta M, Messina S, Mileto A, et al. Muscle fat-fraction and mapping in Duchenne muscular dystrophy: evaluation of disease distribution and correlation with clinical assessments. Preliminary experience. Skeletal Radiol 2012;41: 955–61.
38. Lee JH, Yoon YC, Kim SH, et al. Texture analysis using T1-weighted images for muscles in Charcot-Marie-Tooth disease in patients and volunteers. Eur Radiol 2020. https://doi.org/10.1007/s00330-020-07435-y.
39. Kim HS, Yoon YC, Choi BO, et al. Muscle fat quantification using magnetic resonance imaging: case-control study of Charcot-Marie-Tooth disease patients and volunteers. J Cachexia Sarcopenia Muscle 2019;10(3):574–85.
40. Franettovich Smith MM, Elliott JM, Al-Najjar A, et al. New insights into intrinsic foot muscle morphology and composition using ultrahigh-field (7-Tesla) magnetic resonance imaging. BMC Musculoskelet Disord 2021;22:97.
41. Richards BS, Dempsey M. Clubfoot treated with the French functional (physical therapy). Method J Pediatr Orthop 2007;27:214–9.
42. Peden SC, Tanner JC, Manoli A. Posterior fibula of pes cavus: real or artifact? Answer based on cross-sectional imaging. J Surg Orthop Adv 2018;27(4): 255–60.
43. Bluth B, Eagan M, Otsuka NY. Stress fractures of the lateral rays in the cavovarus foot: indication for surgical intervention. Orthopedics 2011;34(10):e696–9.
44. Krause FG, Klammer G, Benneker LM, et al. Biochemical T2* MR quantification of ankle arthrosis in pes cavovarus. J Orthop Res Dec. 2010;28:1562–8.

Neurologic Conditions Associated with Cavus Foot Deformity

Harry John Visser, DPM, Joshua Wolfe, DPM, MHA*,
Rekha Kouri, DPM, Raul Aviles, DPM

KEYWORDS

- Cavus foot deformity • Cerebrovascular accident • Muscular dystrophy
- Charcot Marie tooth • Post polio syndrome • Neuromuscular disorders
- Foot and ankle disorders

KEY POINTS

- A wide variety of conditions contribute to the development of a cavus foot deformity, many of which may stem from a neuromuscular or neurologic etiology; an appropriate evaluation must be performed.
- Neurologic and neuromuscular disorders in the cavus patient may present similarly and a thorough evaluation of the patient in conjunction with a neurologist or pediatric neurologist should be performed.
- Progressive and spastic disorders provide a unique hurdle for the correction of a patient's foot and ankle deformity.
- Understanding the nature of the deformity as well as the likelihood of progression or spasticity must be determined before any surgical intervention.

INTRODUCTION

Cavus and cavovarus foot deformities are commonly associated with neurologic disorders. These patients may present to the office undiagnosed with lower extremity complaints. These deformities can represent an early sign of a more subtle, underlying neurologic condition. Appropriate and timely diagnosis of these conditions is critical in the evaluation of the patient with cavus foot deformity. This diagnosis can significantly affect the course and the appropriate treatment plan for the patient.

Understanding and recognizing the neurologic condition allows for proper management of the patient. Evaluation of these complex patients should include a team approach. This process includes consultations with neurology, orthopedists, and genetic specialists. In the instance of talipes equinovarus, recognition may be as early as

Foot and Ankle Surgery Residency, SSM Health DePaul Hospital, 12303 DePaul Drive, Suite 701, St Louis, MO 63044, USA
* Corresponding author.
E-mail address: joshua.wolfe.dpm@gmail.com

Clin Podiatr Med Surg 38 (2021) 323–342
https://doi.org/10.1016/j.cpm.2021.03.001
0891-8422/21/© 2021 Elsevier Inc. All rights reserved.

determined by fetal ultrasound examination.[1] Most important, this diagnosis must be established before any treatment intervention.

The evaluation and workup of the patient with suspected neuromuscular disease should include baseline laboratory values, nerve conduction studies, and electromyography. These tests may be performed in the interim before evaluation by the neurologist or neuropediatrician. Baseline laboratory tests should include creatinine kinase (CK), which are primarily present in the myocardium and skeletal muscle. The presence of CK 3 times greater than normal (or more) proposes a congenital muscular dystrophy or early onset of spinal muscular atrophy.[1,2] Dystromyopathy or Becker muscular dystrophy should be ruled out in instances where plasma CK levels are more than 50 times the uppermost normal level.[1,2] Second, nerve conduction studies and electromyography should be performed to evaluate for possible peripheral neuropathic conditions, radiculopathy, and/or entrapment neuropathy. This information helps to identify the location as well as loss of muscle and sensory response owing to motor and sensory nerve impairment. In addition to nerve conduction studies and electromyography, another diagnostic tool is MRI involving the brain, spine, or both. Muscle biopsy and genetic testing can serve as a last step in determining the disease etiology. The decision to proceed with this line of testing and evaluation should be determined by the diagnostic condition based on clinical grounds. The biopsy should be performed at a specialty center in coordination with neurology.

NEUROLOGIC AND NEUROMUSCULAR CONDITIONS AND CAVUS

The etiology of cavus and cavovarus foot deformity can be derived from a variety of factors. Understanding the underlying causes is an important step in the management of this patient population. The types of neurologic and neuromuscular conditions affecting patients are immense. It is important to understand the possible and likely conditions that specifically affect the orthopedic and podiatric patient populations. The purpose of this article is not to provide an absolute or comprehensive description of these conditions, but rather to highlight some of the potential causes.

CLASSIFICATION

The classification of the patient's symptomatology is important as far as understanding the disease process and the likelihood of progression. Neurologic conditions are classified based on the anatomic location of the disorder and the hereditary manifestations, as well as the nonprogressive or progressive nature of the condition. Understanding the pathophysiology and disease course is critical for ensuring optimal patient outcomes given the complexity of these patients.

Dyck Classification

The classification of the hereditary sensorimotor neuropathies (HMSN) commonly falls within the Dyck classification. The Dyck classification has been historically used and was originally developed in 1968. HMSNs were classified from I through VII; however, only classes I through III were used with any regularity.[3] HMSN I is considered as demyelinating neuropathies with concomitant diminished nerve conduction velocity (NCV), normally seen as a median conduction velocity of less than 38 m/s.[3] HMSN II consists of axonal neuropathy with motor nerve conduction velocities that are typically normal. HMSN III refers to Dejerine–Sottas disease, which presents with severe demyelination and typically starts early on as an infant and also demonstrates a median nerve motor conduction velocity of less than 10 m/s.[3] HMSN IV refers to Refsum's syndrome. HMSN V refers to spastic paraplegia, HMSN VI refers to optic atrophy, and

HMSN VII is defined as the presence of retinitis pigmentosa. As previously stated, HMSN IV through VII are not used commonly and are rare in presentation. HMSN classifications I and II, based on their presentation, have become commonly known as CMT1 and CMT2, respectively. HMSN III has become generally accepted as Dejerine–Sottas disease. The classification of the HMSNs based on the clinical and electrophysiologic presentation alone, although helpful for understanding at a baseline, is not enough. The classification of these conditions should allow for a more thorough evaluation and understanding of the condition, including genetic causes.

STABLE AND PROGRESSIVE CAVOVARUS DEFORMITIES

A thorough understanding of whether the condition is stable or progressive lends credence to the neurologic condition contributing to the cavus deformity. This knowledge then allows for appropriate conservative and or surgical treatment plans for the patient.

LESIONS OF THE SPINAL CORD

One of the differential neurologic categories that should be considered as part of the cause of cavovarus deformity are lesions involving the spinal cord. Patients with these lesions often present with unilateral cavus deformity, but bilaterality also can occur. Lesions involving the spinal cord may not be uniform in presentation and are due to a range of causes.

Diastomatomyelia

Diastematomyelia is a rare congenital spine disorder characterized by a sagittal division of the spinal cord or cauda equina at 1 or more vertebral levels, most commonly seen within the lumbar and thoracic levels.[4] Diastematomyelia is included as a subset within the split cord malformations and is quite rare in presentation. Split cord malformations represent 1 in 5499 live births (0.02%), affecting females more often than males (1.3:1).[5,6] It has been noted to be 4 times more common in females than males.[7] Diastematomyelia with split cord malformation occurs 47% of the time between L1 and L4 and 25% at T7 and T12.[8] The type II (L3–L5) variant may present minimally with leg weakness, low back pain, scoliosis, and unilateral cavus foot. Clinically, some of the musculoskeletal manifestations include asymmetry of the peripheral extremities, pes cavus, scoliosis, and spinal dysraphism.[9] Additional clinical symptoms may include hairy patches, dimples, hemangiomas, lipomas, and sinus tracts overlying the area of involvement.[9] Although the exact mechanism for lower extremity symptoms may be multifactorial, it is derived from the changes associated with the split cord malformation. In the pediatric patient, this manifestation is seen as the vertebral column grows in length. The split is caused by an osseous, cartilaginous, or sinus septum within the spinal cord and the longitudinal division stems from patient growth.[4] This split leads to lower extremity symptomatology associated with patient growth. There are varying degrees of neurologic deficit, which depend on the level of involvement.

Diastematomyelia is commonly represented as an asymmetric or unilateral deformity. Diastematomyelia can also be present as a progressive or nonprogressive condition. However, it seems that the progressive neurologic manifestation is usually a part of the natural history of diastematomyelia.[10] In addition, surgical interventions involving the spinal deformity may help to prevent a split spinal cord. A study conducted by Miller and colleagues[10] reported that surgical intervention should be considered if a patient presents with progressive neurologic manifestations and patients who do not have progressive neurologic manifestations should be observed. Therefore, diastematomyelia should be included as a differential in a child that presents with a cavovarus deformity.

Hydromyelia

Hydromyelia is a condition in which the central spinal cord and canal is widened. Hydromyelia is usually congenital and results from the increased pressure of cerebrospinal fluid (CSF) in the fourth ventricle.[11] In addition, it is often associated with a Chiari malformation. Hydromyelia tends to mainly occur in infants and children; however, a similar condition, syringomyelia, tends to occur primarily in adults. Owing to the similarity between the 2 conditions, it is difficult for hydromyelia and syringomyelia to be distinguished from each other through imaging and the term hydrosyringomyelia may be used to encompass both conditions.[12]

The clinical picture for both of these is similar, although there may be some variation. The symptoms develop as the condition progresses including sensory loss, which presents as compromised pain and temperature sensation. Additionally, this sensory disturbance presents as a cape-like distribution over the arms and trunk[13] and often involves the lateral spinothalamic tracts. However, vibratory and proprioception sensations remain intact, which indicates preserved posterior column function. Along with sensory loss, muscle weakness involving the legs and feet is present, which may present with a unilateral cavovarus foot deformity. Like diastematomyelia, the exact changes in the lower extremity are mixed and nonspecific. Early consideration of hydromyelia can potentially provide the child with a better outcome.

Poliomyelitis

Poliomyelitis is a highly infectious viral disease that is caused by the polio picornavirus.[11] The average age of onset is around 11 months, but can affect any age group. Polio virus exists in 3 subtypes, types 1, 2, and 3. However, type 2 was eradicated in 1999 and type 3 has not been identified since 2012 in Nigeria. Types 2 and 3 have been certified as eradicated, whereas type 1 is still present in Pakistan and Afghanistan as of 2020.[14] The mode of transmission is typically through the fecal–oral route or, less commonly, through a single source such as a contaminated water or food source.[14] The virus multiplies in the alimentary tract and lymph nodes before hematogenous spread to the central nervous system.[11] The greatest effect of the disease involves the anterior horn cells of the spinal cord and/or the cranial nerve motor nuclei in the gray matter of the spinal cord or brainstem.[15] The course of the disease is divided into 3 phases.

The first phase is known as the acute phase and generally lasts from 9 to 10 days. During this phase, there is a loss of elasticity and contraction involving the tendons, fascia, and ligaments.[16] This loss leads to acute contractures of the Achilles tendon and plantar fascia. During this phase, it is important to apply appropriate bracing to maintain the patient's foot and ankle in neutral position. In the second phase, or the convalescent phase, conservative treatment care should be continued to prevent the development of an unnecessary deformity. Adequate mobilization and passive range of motion is required during this period to prevent fixed equinus, cavus, or flat foot deformities. During the final phase or the chronic phase, there may be a need for a correction of soft tissue contractures and bony deformity owing to the long-term consequences of muscle imbalance.[16] Any corresponding foot deformity depends on the population of affected anterior horn cells of the spinal cord. The different deformities of the foot and ankle occur from pes planus to pes cavus deformity. Once the patient recovers fully and reaches disease termination, any deformity becomes a fixed deformity. A pertinent aspect of this disease is a severe equinovarus deformity, where paralysis affects the tibialis anterior, toe extensors, and the peroneus brevis and longus. The still functioning tibialis posterior, flexor hallucis longus (FHL), flexor digitorum longus (FDL), and triceps surae force the foot into equinus and cavovarus. In addition, if gastrocnemius and soleus involvement exists, then a calcaneocavus foot deformity is noted (**Fig. 1**).

Another aspect of poliomyelitis that should be considered is postpolio syndrome. This syndrome is more likely to be seen in patients whose onset was after 10 years of age. The diagnosis is based on 5 criteria, the primary one being confirmation of a history of poliomyelitis. Patients who had a "fixed" nonprogressive deformity throughout their life begin to notice progression and worsening of their existing deformity. This progression occurs owing to the remaining anterior horn cells that were initially not affected and leads to atrophy with age and increasing dysfunction.[17] Initially, the affected anterior horn cells were populated enough to allow muscle function, but as the aging process occurs, the critical population expires and leads to further weakness and the development of further muscle imbalance and deformity.[17]

Tethered Cord

Tethered cord syndrome (TCS), also known as tight filum terminale syndrome, is a condition in which the spinal cord is not able to slide normally inside the spinal canal. This condition is caused by the withdrawal of the conus medullaris and exhibits through sensory and urologic dysfunction, among others.[18] TCS can be either primary or secondary. Primary TCS is congenital and arises during the closing of the neural tube during embryonic development. Secondary TCS is caused by adhesions between the spinal cord and the surrounding tissue owing to increased tension on the postpartum spinal cord. These children typically have a normal spinal cord during

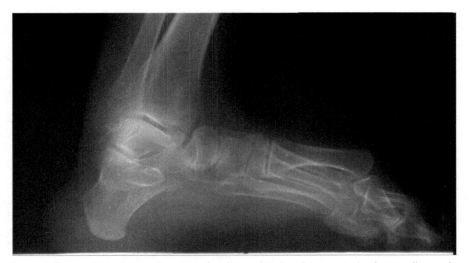

Fig. 1. Selective targeting in the case of poliomyelitis involving anterior horn cell populations in the spinal cord. Paralysis of the gastrocnemius, soleus, and peroneus longus with preservation of the deep posterior group, anterior muscle group, and peroneus brevis. Elevatus of the first ray is seen owing to unopposed tibialis anterior function secondary to loss of peroneus longus and gastrocsoleus group function. Resulting in the "pistol grip" deformity with the "bullet hole" sign of the canalis tarsi.

the initial postpartum period.[19,20] Most often, the clinical symptoms include pain, neurologic disorders, orthopedic dysfunction, and dermatologic and sphincter disorders.[21] Like the other spinal cord disorders, the diagnosis is most often made during childhood.

The clinical findings present in these patients include hairy patches or tufts in the lumbosacral region, as well as deep dimples or lipid tumors manifest at the end of the caudal spine.[21] Lower extremity symptoms are not the hallmark findings for TCS. The most common lower extremity findings include leg weakness, numbness, spasticity of lower extremities, and anisomelia. Pain, unilateral pes cavus, claw toes, and/or foot length discrepancies are further clinical manifestations. The surgical management of a tethered cord includes identifying and removing the pathology that is preventing the cephalad migration of the spinal cord through the release of compressive tissue that maintains the spinal cord in place. This process involves sectioning the filum terminale and decompressing the scar tissue.[19]

Tumors of the Spinal Cord

Spinal cord tumors may also contribute to the underlying etiology in pes cavus. Tumors of the spinal cord become a concern for pes cavus deformities in the instance of new-onset and unilateral presentation. A spinal cord tumor, also known as an intradural tumor, begins within the spinal cord. Spinal tumors make up approximately 15% of central nervous system tumors. Most commonly, spinal tumors are extradural (55%) compared with intradural tumors (40%–45%). There are 2 types of intradural tumors. The vast majority of the intradural tumors are extramedullary (40%); only 5% are intramedullary.[22,23] Intramedullary tumors begin within the cells of the spinal cord and examples of these include gliomas, astrocytomas, or ependymomas.[24] Extramedullary tumors grow in either the membrane surrounding the spinal cord or dura nerve roots. Examples include meningiomas, neurofibromas, schwannomas, and nerve sheath tumors.[24]

Spinal cord tumors can cause different signs and symptoms manifested by tumor growth. Most commonly, these patients manifest with neck or back pain, radiculopathy, paresthesia, weakness, gait abnormalities, bowl dysfunction, bladder incontinence, and in some instances Brown–Sequard syndrome.[2,24,25] Other clinical symptoms depend on the spinal level. Sciatica, loss of sensory and temperature sensation, muscle weakness, and difficulty with ambulation can occur. One must be suspicious of an adult or adolescent patient who demonstrated normal foot architecture and began to develop a progressive cavus foot. If the condition is diagnosed and treated early in its course, then the neurologic function is often preserved and the tumor is usually cured.

HEREDITARY DISORDERS

Hereditary disorders should not be overlooked in the diagnosis of the cavovarus deformity. Often, these conditions may also be associated with hereditary disorders that affect the peripheral nervous system. These patients typically present with bilateral cavus foot deformities. It is important that the foot and ankle surgeon, in conjunction with a neurologist, rule out these potential conditions in the evaluation of the undiagnosed cavovarus foot.

Friedreich's Ataxia

Friedreich's ataxia is an autosomal recessive disorder that is, caused by an abnormal gene on chromosome 9. It is the most commonly inherited ataxia in Europe.[26]

Geographically, 1 in 20,000 in Southern and Western Europe are affected, whereas 1 in 250,000 in Northern and Eastern Europe are affected.[27] The clinical phenotype is variable and expansive. Some of the most common or consistent characteristics include limb ataxia, dysarthria, loss of lower limb reflexes, and significant gait disturbances.[28] Symptoms often present between 10 and 16 years of age.[29] The most common musculoskeletal abnormalities include scoliosis, pes cavus, and ataxia.[30,31] A wide-based and uncoordinated gait is indicative of Friedreich's ataxia, often in combination with a high steppage gait secondary to weak ankle dorsiflexors.[30] Ataxia results in frequent falling and an inability to coordinate voluntary movements, which occurs secondary to spinocerebellar tract degeneration and cerebellar pathology.[30] Ataxia is often worsened in the presence of peripheral sensory neuropathy.[26]

Often children with this condition go undiagnosed until lower extremity pathology presents clinically. Cavus foot deformity often occurs in the early part of the second decade. A study conducted by Tynan and colleagues[32] compared MRI studies of normal patients with those of patients diagnosed with Friedreich's ataxia. They found that affected patients had a larger peroneal compartment in comparison with their anterior compartment. This finding suggests the dominance of the peroneus longus muscle compared with the tibialis anterior leading to a developmental cavus foot deformity.

Charcot Marie Tooth Disease

Charcot Marie Tooth (CMT) disease is a genetically heterogeneous group of diseases sharing the same clinical phenotype. CMT is the most commonly inherited neuromuscular disorder and affects 1 in 2500 individuals.[33] It presents with variable phenotypic expression and penetration. CMT is caused by gene mutations that affect proteins within different locations, compact and noncompact myelin, Schwann cells, and axons, with a wide range in function.[34] Ultimately, metabolic functions or structural defects that affect the myelin or the axon result in an axonal degenerative process.[35] From the perspective of the foot and ankle surgeon, it is the most common underlying neurologic disease causing a cavovarus deformity. Approximately two-thirds of adults with symptomatic cavovarus deformity have the underlying CMT. CMT has been broken down into several different types and classifications. CMT inheritance has significant variation, which plays directly into its classification.[35] CMT1 is an autosomal-dominant hypertrophic neuropathy with a slow progression that occurs during the first or second decade of life. CMT rarely arises in early infancy compared with some of the other hereditary disorders. However, a severe phenotype characterized by hypotonia and a delay in motor milestones can occur.[36] CMT2 presents similarly to CMT1; however, CMT2 can be autosomal dominant or recessive. CMTX or CMTX1 is X-linked, with males being more affected than females. Further, CMT3 and CMT4 present more severely than CMT1 or CMT2.[35] CMT is subclassified into demyelinating and axonal types based on the NCV.[35] The demyelinating are classified as CMT1 and CMT4 and axonal are CMT2 and CMT4 and intermediate (CMT, CTMX, and CMT2E). A more detailed description of CMT and its associated phenotypic presentation can be seen in **Table 1**. Previous literature suggested that the prevalence of cavus foot deformity in CMT, CMT1A specifically, had a near universal presentation. However, dissension within the literature demonstrated that only 11% of preadolescent children exhibited cavus foot deformity, whereas 62.5% developed during adolescent years. Moreover, the historical literature showed 33% of children younger than 5 years of age, with an increase to 55% between 5 and 10 years of age, and 87% between 10 and 20 years of age.[37] In addition to pes cavus, which is the most common skeletal deformity that presents in CMT, scoliosis is also present or noted in 10% of the affected patients.[34]

Table 1
CMT subtypes and their clinical and phenotypic characteristics

Type	Inheritance	Phenotype	Genes Affected
CMT1	Autosomal dominant	Usually typical phenotype Consistent, widespread motor and sensory NCV slowing (<38 m/s) Onion bulbs or other myelin abnormal findings on nerve biopsy	PMP22 duplication MPZ PMP22 point mutations EGR2 SIMPLE/LITAF NEFL
CMT2	Autosomal dominant or autosomal recessive	Usually typical phenotype NCV normal or near normal (>38 m/s in upper limb) with decreased amplitudes Chronic axonal neuropathy without specific diagnostic features on nerve biopsy	MFN2 MPZ NEFL HSPB1 (HSP27) HSPB8 (HSP22) RAB7 GARS GDAP1(AD/AR) LMNA (AD/AR) MED25(AR)
CMTX	X-linked	Men more affected than women Motor NCV commonly intermediate in men, in CMT2 range for women NCV nonuniform and asymmetrical Nerve biopsy shows axonal loss and demyelination	GJB1/Cx32 PRPS1
Intermediate CMT	Autosomal dominant	Mild to moderate severity NCVs between CMT1 and CMT 2 (24–45 m/s) Features both CMT1 and CMT2 phenotypic presentation	MPZ DNM2 YARS NEFL
CMT3	Autosomal dominant or autosomal recessive	Onset early in life, more severe than CMT1 Increased slowing in NCVs Dysmyelination and onion bulbs on nerve biopsy CHN	PMP22 MPZ EGR2 PRX
CMT4	Autosomal recessive	Onset earl in life, more severe than CMT1 Vocal cord weakness, partial paralysis Sensorineural deafness, facial and diaphragmatic weakness NCV slowing (<38 m/s)	GDAP1 MTMR2 SBF2/MTMR13 KIAA1985/SH3TC2 NDRG1 EGR2 PRX FGD4 FIG4

(*continued on next page*)

Table 1 (continued)			
Type	Inheritance	Phenotype	Genes Affected
CMT5	Autosomal dominant	Pyramidal involvement ranges from increased deep tendon reflexes with a positive Babinski sign to spastic paraplegia Electrophysiology - axonal loss, reduced sensory action potential amplitudes	MFN2 BSCL2 GJB1
CMT6	Autosomal dominant	Early onset Severe visual loss with optic atrophy NCVs preserved or mildly slowed	MFN2

Abbreviations: CMT, Charcot Marie Tooth disease; NCV, nerve conduction velocity.
Data from Fridman, V., Bundy, B., Reilly, M. M., Pareyson, D., Bacon, C., Burns, J., Day, J., Feely, S., Finkel, R. S., Grider, T., Kirk, C. A., Herrmann, D. N., Laurá, M., Li, J., Lloyd, T., Sumner, C. J., Muntoni, F., Piscosquito, G., Ramchandren, S., Shy, R., ... Inherited Neuropathies Consortium (2015). CMT subtypes and disease burden in patients enrolled in the Inherited Neuropathies Consortium natural history study: a cross-sectional analysis. *Journal of neurology, neurosurgery, and psychiatry*, 86(8), 873–878. https://doi.org/10.1136/jnnp-2014-308826.

The development of pes cavus associated with CMT occurs through multiple muscle-tendon units being affected by the disease. Early patterns of weakness involve the peroneus brevis, peroneus tertius, tibialis anterior and intrinsics.[38] This results in claw toes. The unopposed deep flexor group to the posterior tibialis, FDL, and FHL create the midfoot adductovarus.[39] The gastrocsoleus group is not affected, but accommodates to the varus malposition. The unopposed peroneus longus accentuates the cavus foot more and further leads a mechanical advantage to the gastroc and soleus, creating an equinus deformity.[39] The neurologic examination demonstrates characteristic signs of sensorimotor peripheral neuropathy including ataxia, hypoesthesia, and sensory loss (including loss of vibration, 2-point discrimination, and proprioception).[40] Other clinical signs owing to upper and lower limb weakness and atrophy include the main en griffe and "inverted champagne bottle" legs.[34] Additionally, a high steppage gait with foot drop is a very common motor sign and is frequently accompanied by deep tendon reflex absence or diminishment.[41] These patients may also complain of cold feet, muscle cramps, acrocyanosis, and postural tremor.

Déjèrine–Sottas Disease

Déjèrine–Sottas disease is a rare condition representing a type of CMT that is genetically heterogeneous. Compared with CMT, it has an early onset of progressive hypertrophic interstitial polyneuropathy more severe than in CMT1. It is often used to describe a severe, early childhood form of CMT. The clinical symptoms occur by the age of 2 and present with delayed motor milestones. Severe motor and sensory involvement can lead to wheelchair confinement.[35] Other features include bilateral pes cavus, scoliosis, and sensory ataxia. Respiratory insufficiency can lead to premature death.

It is important to distinguish Déjèrine–Sottas disease from other hereditary neuropathies. Tests such as a NCV test, nerve biopsies, EMG, CSF examination, brain MRI, and biochemical tests can also be helpful with differentiation. An NCV study involving patients with Déjèrine–Sottas disease can assist in the diagnosis. Patients usually present with values of significant slowing (<15 m/s). Sural nerve biopsies show marked demyelination and predominant axonal loss.[34] It is referred to as an onion bulb neuropathy owing to demyelination with reactive scarring. Clinically, the peripheral nerve can be palpable under the skin. Déjèrine–Sottas disease should be highly considered as a differential for a neurologic cause of pes cavus in the symptomatic pediatric patient.

Roussy–Levy Syndrome

Roussy–Levy syndrome is an autosomal dominantly inherited condition involving spinocerebellar degeneration.[11] It is also known as hereditary areflexic dystasia. It is a rare disorder but affects both sexes equally. Roussy–Levy syndrome is also a form of CMT disease, because it is caused by a partial duplication of the same gene that causes CMT (17p11.2). It usually becomes apparent during early childhood and has similar clinical symptoms to CMT1. Characterized by unusual weakness, atrophy, ataxia, areflexia, and pes cavus or claw foot. There is also a static tremor of the hands that differentiates the condition from CMT.[11] It is manifested as a delay in walking and bilateral pes cavus. Gait ataxia, areflexia, awkward movements, and mild cerebellar intention tremor are present without nystagmus. Also kyphoscoliosis, sensory changes, extensor plantar response, and neurologic signs of involvement are present.[11] Roussy–Levy syndrome differs in that it has an early childhood onset with slow progression and the unique characteristics of slight hand tremors in the hands. It results from a duplication of the DMD 22 gene similar to CMT 1A.

Guillain–Barre Syndrome

Guillain–Barre syndrome, also known as Landry paralysis, is an acutely progressive but self-limiting, acquired, inflammatory, demyelinating polyneuropathy resulting in rapid weakness and paralysis. The estimated incidence rate of Guillain–Barre syndrome is approximately 0.8 to 1.9 cases per 100,000 people per year, and most commonly affects those between 30 and 50 years of age.[42] In rare cases, it has occurred in children. *Campylobacter jejuni* infection is the most common cause of acute bacterial gastroenteritis. However, only 1 in 1000 patients with *C jejuni* infection develop Guillain–Barre syndrome.[43] Other bacterial and viral infections associated with Guillain–Barre syndrome include *Haemophilus influenzae*, *Mycoplasma pneumoniae*, cytomegalovirus, Epstein-Barr virus, and varicella zoster virus.[42] It was also linked to a swine flu vaccine given in 1976. At that time, approximately 45 million people were vaccinated and 450 people developed Guillain–Barre syndrome.[44] The median interval from onset of diarrhea to development of neurologic symptoms is 10 days. However, it can be as quickly as 3 days and as delayed as 6 weeks.[45]

The key findings on examination include symmetric ascending muscle weakness beginning in the distal lower extremities and progressing to the upper extremities.[46] Although sensory involvement may occur, motor weakness is always more prominent with or without decreased deep tendon reflexes.[47] Only in severe forms of Guillain–Barre syndrome is there permanent residual paralysis causing notable drop foot or cavovarus foot structure.[48] However, it is rare that a pes cavus deformity may be seen with Guillain–Barre syndrome. It should still be kept in mind, and the hallmark signs and symptoms should be correlated when making the diagnosis.

Cerebral Palsy

Cerebral palsy is a static nonprogressive neurologic condition resulting from cerebral damage occurring during the prepartum, peripartum, or postpartum periods. The prevalence of cerebral palsy is about 2 per 1000 live births in most developed countries.[16] Several types of cerebral palsy exist, but the most common is the spastic form of cerebral palsy.[49] Cerebral palsy is classified based on motor abnormalities, impairments, anatomic, and radiologic causation, as well as timing. However, the more imperative classification system is one from a musculoskeletal perspective. There are 3 principal categories: fine motor function, topographic distribution, and gross motor function.[50]

The various presentations of cerebral palsy present with multiple unique obstacles in prevalence and symptomatology. As mentioned elsewhere in this article, the most common movement disorder present in cerebral palsy is spasticity, which represents 60% to 80% of cases.[49] The other types include dyskinetic (10%–20%), mixed (10%–25%), ataxic (2%–5%), and hypotonic (2%–5%).[16] The spastic form presents with hypereflexic deep tendon reflexes and cocontraction. It is usually caused by pyramidal tract lesions and related to a loss of selective motor control and weakness.[49] The dyskinetic form is caused by extrapyramidal lesions and presents with involuntary movements of the limbs, such as dystonia, athetosis, chorea, and ballismus.[16] The next most common form is the mixed movement disorder. This is due to many children having diffuse brain involvement that involve both the pyramidal and extrapyramidal tracts. The other movement disorders including the ataxic and hypotonic types are far less common.

Limb involvement in cerebral palsy can be unilateral or bilateral. Unilateral involvement presents as monoplegia and hemiplegia. Bilateral involvement occurs as diplegia, triplegia, and quadriplegia. Most commonly hemiplegia, diplegia, and quadriplegia are the clinical presentations.[51]

The gross motor function classification system (GMFCS) is age dependent and measures the patient's level of mobility as well as groups them into 5 different levels.[52] They provide descriptors for 4 different age groups. Level I indicates the patient has minimal disability and level V indicates the patient has total dependence on caregivers as well as bracing and stability aids for posture. For example, most children between the ages of 6 and 12 demonstrating spastic hemiplegia function as GMFCS levels I and II. The patient with spastic diplegia would be considered at GMFCS levels II and III. Spastic quadriplegia usually equates to levels IV and V.[16] Understanding and classifying the patient under the GMFCS is important. The severity of foot and ankle deformities increase as the GMFCS level increases.

Three principal categories help to evaluate and manage patients with cerebral palsy. Pes cavus is often coupled with other deformity patterns, which include equinocavovarus in spastic hemiplegia, calcaneocavovalgus in hypotonia/ataxia, and calcaneocavovalgus in spasticity/dystonia.[16] Equinocavovarus deformity presents and produces abnormal tension caused by spasticity of the intrinsics. This plantarflexion of the forefoot on the hindfoot and a symmetric plantarflexion of the metatarsals presents with the first metatarsal more steeply inclined.[53] This factor leads to the cause of cavus in cerebral palsy and is the most common hemiplegic state. Associated spasticity of the tibialis posterior and Achilles produces inversion and plantarflexion of the ankle and STJ. This alters the ankle axis of rotation medially. The FHL, FDL and associated spasticity produce hallux malleus and claw toe deformities.

In summary, the abnormal tension produced by the spasticity of the flexors causes cavovarus in cerebral palsy. Spastic contracture of the tibialis posterior, FHL, FDL, and Achilles tendon lead to equinocavovarus deformity.[54] Surgical treatment includes radical plantar fascial release, lengthening of tibialis posterior, FHL, FDL, Achilles tendon, or tibialis anterior muscle transfer in a split form.[55] Understanding deforming forces is critical to successful reconstruction. Often weakness is addressed by redirection, transposition and or partial substitution (split transfer) of the agonist.[56] It is key to reestablish the equilibrium between overpowering muscle and its antagonist.

OTHER NEUROLOGIC CAUSES
Chronic Inflammatory Demyelinating Polyneuropathy

Childhood-onset chronic inflammatory demyelinating polyneuropathy (CIDP) is an immune-mediated disease of the peripheral nerves that is often misdiagnosed for more common genetic neuropathies such as CMT disease.[57] The prevalence of childhood CIDP is less than 0.5 per 100,000 compared with the CMT which is 0.82 per 100,000.[58] CIDP usually peaks during the fifth and sixth decades of life, but can be seen across all age groups.[42] Younger patients who present with this condition usually have an acute onset with a relapsing source and more prominent gait abnormalities. The common characteristics seen in patients with CIDP include symmetric motor and sensory involvement.[42] At onset, both proximal and distal limb weakness are present, with proximal involvement being slightly more pronounced.[59] Deep tendon reflexes are diffusely diminished or absent. Sensory impairment occurs in a glove–stocking pattern.[42]

Even though CMT is a more likely etiology owing to more frequent occurrence, CIDP should also be considered as a differential. Like CMT, patients with CIDP can present with bilateral pes cavus. One key laboratory marker in differentiation of CMT1 and CIDP is the presence of protein in the CSF.[60] In CIDP, the CSF protein is markedly elevated.[60] In CMT1, it is normal or only mildly elevated.[57]

Cerebrovascular Accident and Stroke

Stroke (cerebral vascular accident) has become a major cause of disability and the second most common cause of death worldwide. Studies from China have shown that approximately 70% of their 7 million stroke survivors experienced functional disabilities after 1 year.[61] Poststroke equinocavovarus foot deformity is one of the most frequent noted deformities among stroke survivors. The incidence of poststroke equinocavovarus foot deformities range from 17% to 38%.[61] About 4% to 9% of the survivors suffer disabling ambulatory function.[61] Poststroke equinocavovarus foot deformity can generally decrease one's ability to walk, sit, stand, and perform daily life activities.[62] It can also increase the risk of falls.

A stroke patient's foot deformity is present most often as hemiplegia. Post stroke cerebrovascular accident patients may present with 3 common foot deformities[1]: equinus,[2] varus,[3] and equinovarus.[63] Equinus is primarily due to spasticity of the Achilles and plantar flexors and leads to a loss of voluntary dorsiflexion.[63] The varus deformity is produced secondary to primary spasticity of the tibialis anterior. Equinovarus is the more typical hemiplegic gait pattern.[64] This pattern is caused by spasticity of the posterior tibial, FHL, and FDL. In this condition, the spasticity of the tibialis anterior has a minimal or no role in the deformity.[63] The management of these conditions may improve with the use of botulinum toxin or phenol; however, these solutions may be short lived.[65] In certain cases, surgical management is needed. This approach is considered primarily when bracing is not tolerated.

Sequelae of Compartment Syndrome

Compartment syndrome is any clinical condition in which there is increased compartment pressure of one of the fascial compartments of the leg or foot.[66] This syndrome results in decreased perfusion to the muscle and nerve owing to interstitial space and subsequent venous hypertension. Necrosis then occurs as arterial inflow is compromised, resulting in extensive fibrous and scarring.[67] This process leads to subsequent contractures, known as Volkmann's ischemic contracture. The most common cause of compartment syndrome is tibial fractures and occur most commonly in the anterior compartment of the leg.[68] Myonecrosis and irreversible ischemic nerve damage occur after ischemic insult of 8 hours or more.[69] Contracture secondary to myelofibrosis of the skeletal muscle can occur weeks or months after the initial insult.[70] Anterior compartment involvement can lead to a drop foot deformity.[71] Peroneal compartment contracture can produce an adductocavovarus deformity.[71] Superficial posterior compartment contracture of the compartment can lead to a calcaneus cavus deformity.[72] Compartment syndrome involving the foot is often secondary to high-energy injuries. Lisfranc fracture dislocations can produce an anterior cavus deformity with digital contractures. This deformity is secondary to loss of intrinsic muscle function. Calcaneal fractures can lead to hallux varus and flat foot owing to neurologic loss to the Achilles tendon and FHB.[71] This condition also leads to the loss of intrinsic foot mobility.

MUSCULAR DYSTROPHIES

Muscular dystrophy is a heterogeneous collection of diseases that have historically been grouped based on their clinical presentation. With the progression in genetic testing, these diseases have been defined more clearly based on their underlying etiology, rather than strictly their clinical manifestations. Many of the muscular dystrophies arise out of dysfunction in the production or translocation of dystrophin, a protein found within the sarcolemma that aids in strengthening the sarcolemma and plays a role in force transduction within the musculature.[73,74] This disease group affects the foot and ankle in a variety of ways, particularly in regards to contracture and the potential to develop cavus and equinus foot types.

Congenital Muscular Dystrophy

Congenital muscular dystrophy is an increasingly complex collection of conditions with onset in infancy. Infants exhibit hypotonicity as well as weakness at birth. Additionally, changes determined by muscle biopsy define congenital muscular dystrophy.[75] These individuals present with an elevated CK, which is higher in congenital muscular dystrophy in comparison with congenital myopathy.[75] Congenital muscular dystrophy and congenital myopathy are similar clinically, and are differentiated by subtle differences found in CK levels and muscle biopsy. These individuals develop contractures early. They present with ankle plantarflexion, knee flexion, hip flexion, wrist flexion, and long finger flexion.[76]

Congenital muscular dystrophy is known to have lower extremity contracture, which can include the ankle and lead to the eventual development of equinocavovarus deformity.[77] No definitive treatment exists for this patient population. Conservative management is the primary form of treatment, with physical therapy and stretching to assist in preventing contractures, as well as appropriate bracing. Release of contractures, particularly at the ankle, can be performed in rare instances to improve bracing and function.[75,77]

Duchenne Muscular Dystrophy

Duchenne muscular dystrophy (DMD) presents as a progressive weakness that affects the patient at several anatomic sites. DMD is an X-linked recessive disorder that presents with progressive weakness and wasting of skeletal muscle.[73] Onset begins at approximately 5 years of age with weakness. By ages 8 to 12, patients exhibit the inability to ambulate. DMD presents in males with 1 in 3500 newborn males affected annually worldwide.[73] Clinically, a positive Gower's sign is an early diagnostic sign when the pediatric patient is unable to rise from the floor from a sitting position. These patients often become wheelchair bound. Additionally, patients with DMD present with pseudohypertrophic calf musculature, which is secondary to fatty infiltration of the gastrocnemius and soleus muscle. Paradoxically, these patients seem to have well-developed calf musculature. Last, some patients demonstrate cognitive impairment as well as diminished activity levels.[73]

With regard to the foot and ankle surgeon, careful consideration should be given to the management of the patient with DMD. The patient with DMD not only experiences weakness and loss of muscle function, but also goes on to exhibit scoliosis, joint contractures, and pathologic fractures secondary to osteoporosis.[78] Owing to these presentations, it is important for the surgeon to understand and manage these conditions appropriately. Specifically within the lower extremity, patients develop contractures of the hip, knee, and/or ankle. The 2018 DMD Care Considerations continue to highlight the need for appropriate recognition of DMD-affected patients.[78,79] DMD can be separated into 3 phases: ambulatory stage, early nonambulatory stage, and late nonambulatory stage. In the ambulatory and early nonambulatory stages, contracture management with stretching and orthoses is critical. From a surgical standpoint, the 2018 Care Considerations consensus found that Achilles tendon lengthening in isolation may be adequate to improve gait in patients with ankle contractures, as long as they have adequate quadricep and hip extensor strength. However, surgery on the hip and knee is specifically contraindicated. In addition to Achilles tendon lengthening, the equinovarus foot deformity associated with DMD may be managed with FHL, FDL, and posterior tibial tenotomies. A posterior tibial tendon transfer to the dorsum of the foot may be beneficial in the patient with severe contractures and affect ambulation.[78,79] Outside of this parameter, the focus on late nonambulatory stages for the foot and ankle are typically limited to patient comfort, bracing, and ability to transfer.

Becker Muscular Dystrophy

Becker muscular dystrophy, also an X-linked recessive inheritance pattern, presents with a less severe presentation of dystrophinopathy. Similar in presentation to DMD, however, onset is around 12 years of age rather than the early presentation of DMD. In addition, these patients retain much more function into adulthood. However, it does exhibit a similar pattern to DMD. To contrast, there is significantly diminished cardiac involvement. From the standpoint of the foot and ankle surgeon, the similar pathology to DMD leads to a similar conservative and surgical treatment algorithm to DMD.[78,80]

Myotonic Dystrophy

Myotonic muscular dystrophy (Steinert disease or dystrophia myotonica) represents the most common type of muscular dystrophy. Patients with congenital myotonic dystrophy are affected by contractures in up to 70% of individuals. The ankle is the most commonly involved joint with contracture. Much less frequent in the hip and knee.[76] Achilles tendon lengthening with bracing can prove to be effective.

CASE REPORTS
Case 1

The patient is a 20-year-old man who presented to the outpatient clinic with progressively painful bilateral hammertoe deformities and instability during ambulation (**Fig. 2**A). Physical examination findings included fixed heel varus demonstrated by the Coleman Block test, plantarflexed first metatarsal, lower leg, and intrinsic foot atrophy; marked hammertoe deformities; and hallux malleus. Manual muscle testing

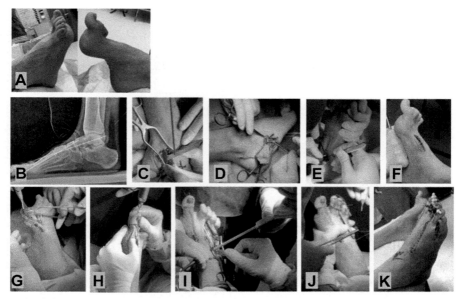

Fig. 2. (*A*) Preoperative cavus foot deformity. (*B*) Lateral view radiograph. (*C*) Dwyer calcaneal osteotomy. (*D*) Peroneal brevis to longus. (*E*) Plantar fasciotomy. (*F*) Dorsiflexory first metatarsal osteotomy. (*G*) Jones sling. (*H*) Hallux interphalangeal joint arthrodesis. (*I*) Hibbs tenosuspension. (*J*) Hammertoe corrections. (*K*) Postoperative deformity correction.

revealed intact motor function to the anterior muscle group and weakness of the peroneus brevis with lateral muscle group. The peroneus longus was intact as well as the gastrocsoleus complex. Radiographs demonstrated a Meary's angle bisecting at the first metatarsal–cuneiform indicating an anterior cavus (**Fig. 2**B), as well as plantar flexed metatarsal and contractures of the digits. Owing to the degree of deformity, a NCV test was ordered to rule out a neurologic etiology. The results from the NCV test were consistent with sensory and motor peripheral neuropathy with primarily demyelinating features.

The surgical plan included staged correction of cavus deformity by first addressing the fixed heel varus, weak peroneus brevis muscle, midfoot adductus, and plantarflexed first metatarsal. A Dwyer calcaneal osteotomy (**Fig. 2**C), transfer of the peroneus longus to brevis (**Fig. 2**D), a peroneal switch, plantar fasciotomy (**Fig. 2**E), and dorsiflexory first metatarsal osteotomy (**Fig. 2**F) were performed. The second surgery included a Hibbs tenosuspension (**Fig. 2**I) and Jones sling with a hallux interphalangeal joint arthrodesis (**Fig. 2**G, H) and correction of hammertoe deformities (**Fig. 2**J).

Case 2

A 43-year-old man presented to the author's outpatient clinic for evaluation of a painful right foot deformity (**Fig. 3**A). The patient related history of a cerebrovascular accident 2 years prior. He was previously placed in an ankle foot orthosis but, owing to the progression of the deformity, he was no longer able to tolerate ambulation in the brace. Examination revealed an equino-adductovarus deformity of the foot secondary to spasticity from an upper motor neuron lesion caused by the cerebrovascular accident. The deformity noted extensive clonus with an attempt at reduction, which gave the appearance of rigidity. There was evident spasticity of the gastrocsoleus and deep

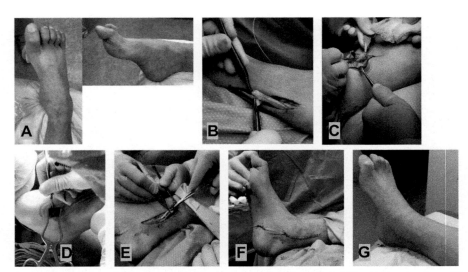

Fig. 3. (*A, B*) Preoperative equino-adductovarus deformity. (*C*) Achilles Z lengthening. (*D*) Resection of the prominent styloid process. (*E*) Deep flexor group lengthening. (*F*) Immediate postoperative correction of deformity. (*G*) Three weeks postoperative correction of the deformity.

flexor groups. The patient also had considerable discomfort with callus formation over the styloid process from chronic brace irritation. Vascular and cutaneous nerve function were normal, because a cerebrovascular accident does not lead to the loss of protective sensation. Surgical treatment was recommended to the patient with the goal of producing a pain-free, plantigrade foot that could be accommodated by bracing.

The initial approach was to lengthen the Achilles tendon via Z-plasty and perform a posterior ankle and subtalar capsulotomy (**Fig. 3**B). The patient's deformity and spasticity reduced under general anesthesia. Once this was performed, the irritated and enlarged styloid process of the fifth metatarsal base was resected (**Fig. 3**C). A plantar fasciotomy was then performed to decrease the chance of postoperative plantar fasciitis once a plantigrade foot was acquired. It also did decrease some of the arch height (**Fig. 3**D). The next approach was to lengthen the deep flexor group, which included the tibialis posterior, FDL, and FHL (**Fig. 3**E). This procedure helped to decrease the dynamic adductovarus of the foot caused by weight bearing challenge. Surgical management produced a rectus plantigrade foot that with subsequent physical therapy afforded him the ability to comfortably ambulate in an ankle foot orthosis brace (**Fig. 3**F, G).

SUMMARY

An understanding of the underlying etiology of neuromuscular conditions and disease states is imperative. Appropriate testing, referral, and early diagnosis must be performed to improve patient outcomes. Maintenance and preservation of function is a key goal in treatment of these patients. Prevention of deformity must be managed actively through conservative therapy. Surgical intervention in this patient population should be considered a final step after failure of conservative therapy. A multidisciplinary approach is critical to allow for the effective and comprehensive management of these patients.

CLINICS CARE POINTS

- A thorough evaluation must be performed in the patient with cavus foot deformity to rule out any underlying neurologic conditions.
- A multidisciplinary approach, including neurology, should be utilized to optimize timely diagnosis as well as patient outcomes.
- Progressive and spastic disorders must be thoroughly understood prior to any surgical intervention.
- Surgical intervention should be considered a final option after failure of conservative therapy.

DISCLOSURE

Drs H.J. Visser, J. Wolfe, R. Kouri, and R. Aviles have no conflicts to disclose pertaining to this article.

REFERENCES

1. Mary P, Servais L, Vialle R. Neuromuscular diseases; diagnosis and management. Orthop Traumatol Surg Res 2018;104:89–95.
2. Sabouraud P, Cuisset JM, Cances C, et al. Diagnostic approach of hyperCKemia in childhood. Arch Pediatr 2009;16(6):678–80.
3. Reilly MM. Classification of the hereditary motor and sensory neuropathies. Curr Opin Neurol 2000;13(5):561–4.
4. Bekki H, Morishita Y, Kawano O, et al. Diastematomyelia: a surgical case with long-term follow-up. Asian Spine J 2015;9:99–102.
5. Bademci G, Saygun M, Batay F, et al. Prevalence of primary tethered cord syndrome associated with occult spinal dysraphism in primary school children in Turkey. Pediatr Neurosurg 2006;42(1):4–13.
6. Alzhrani GA, Al-Jehani HM, Melançon D. Multi-level split cord malformation: do we need a new classification? J Clin Imaging Sci 2014;4:32.
7. Diastematomyelia. Can Med Assoc J 1969;100(9):439–40.
8. Gan YC, Sgouros S, Walsh AR, et al. Diastematomyelia in children: treatment outcome and natural history of associated syringomyelia. Childs Nerv Syst 2007;23:515–9.
9. Vissarionov SV, Krutelev NA, Snischuk VP, et al. Diagnosis and treatment of diastematomyelia in children: a perspective cohort study. Spinal Cord Ser Cases 2018;4(1):1–6.
10. Miller A, Guille JT, Bowen JR. Evaluation and treatment of diastematomyelia. J Bone Joint Surg Am 1993;75:1308–17.
11. Pryse-Phillips W. Companion to clinical neurology. New York: Oxford University Press; 2009.
12. Vertinsky T, Lane B. Chapter 10: radiographic evaluation of spinal canal tumors. In: Jayaraman MV, editor. Tumors of the spine. . Philadelphia: Saunders Elsevier; 2008. p. 184–282.
13. Tay VS, Cook M. Chapter 38: spine and spinal cord: developmental disorders. In: Kornberg A, editor. Neurology and clinical neuroscience. . Philadelphia: Mosby Elsevier; 2007. p. 488–506.
14. WHO. Poliomyelitis (polio). 2021. Available at: https://www.who.int/health-topics/poliomyelitis. Accessed January 15, 2021.
15. Kidd D, Williams AJ, Howard RS. Poliomyelitis. Postgrad Med J 1996;72(853): 641–7.

16. Drennan JC. Drennan's the child's foot and ankle. 2nd edition. Philadelphia: Wolters Kluwer; 2010.

17. Chu E, Lam K. Post-poliomyelitis syndrome. Int Med Case Rep J 2019;12:261–4.

18. Maurya VP, Rajappa M, Wadewkar V, et al. Tethered cord syndrome–A study of the short-term effects of surgical detethering on markers of neuronal injury and electrophysiologic parameters. World Neurosurg 2016;94:239–47.

19. Yasar S, Dogan A, Kayhan S, et al. Surgery for tethered cord syndrome: when and how? Ann Med Res 2018;25:503–10.

20. Gluncic V, Turner M, Burrowes D, et al. Concurrent Chiari decompression and spinal cord untethering in children: feasibility in a small case series. Acta Neurochir 2011;153:109–14.

21. Gharedaghi M, Samini F, Mashhadinejad H, et al. Orthopedic lesions in tethered cord syndrome: the importance of early diagnosis and treatment on patient outcome. Arch Bone Jt Surg 2014;2(2):93.

22. Arnautovic K, Arnautovic A. Extramedullary intradural spinal tumors: a review of modern diagnostic and treatment options and a report of a series. Bosn J Basic Med Sci 2009;9(Suppl 1):S40.

23. Byrne TN, Waxman SG, Benzel EC. Diseases of the spine and spinal cord, vol. 58. New York: Oxford University Press; 2000.

24. Wein S, Gaillard F. Intradural spinal tumours and their mimics: a review of radiographic features. Postgrad Med J 2013;89(1054):457–69.

25. Abul-kasim K, Thurnher MM, Mckeever P, et al. Intradural spinal tumours: current classification and MRI features. Neuroradiology 2008;50:301–14.

26. Koeppen AH. Friedreich's ataxia: pathology, pathogenesis, and molecular genetics. J Neurol Sci 2011;303(1–2):1–12.

27. Cook A, Giunti P. Friedreich's ataxia: clinical features, pathogenesis and management. Br Med Bull 2017;124(1):19–30.

28. Indelicato E, Fanciulli A, Ndayisaba JP, et al. Autonomic function testing in Friedreich's ataxia. J Neurol 2018;265(9):2015–22.

29. Parkinson MH, Boesch S, Nachbauer W, et al. Clinical features of Friedreich's ataxia: classical and atypical phenotypes. J Neurochem 2013;126:103–17.

30. Wood NW. Diagnosing Friedreich's ataxia. Arch Dis Child 1998;78(3):204–7.

31. Lee MC, Sucato DJ. Pediatric issues with cavovarus foot deformities. Foot Ankle Clin 2008;13(2):199–219.

32. Tynan MC, Klenerman L, Helliwell TR, et al. Investigations of muscle imbalance in the legin symptomatic forefoot pes cavus: a multidisciplinary study. Foot Ankle 1992;13:489–501.

33. Saporta MA. Charco-Marie-tooth disease and other inherited neuropathies. Continuum (Minneap Minn) 2014;20(5):1208–25.

34. Piazza S, Ricci G, Caldarazzo Ineco E, et al. Pes Cavus & hereditary neuropathies; when a relationship should be suspected. J Orthop Traumatol 2010;11:195–202.

35. Pareyson D. Differential diagnosis of Charcot Marie Tooth disease and related neuropathies. Neurol Sci 2004;25:72–82.

36. Chance PF, Lupski JR. Inherited neuropathies: Charcot Marie Tooth disease and related disorders. Baillieres Clin Neurol 1994;3:373–85.

37. Burns J, Redmond A, Ouvrier R, et al. Quantification of muscle strength and imbalance in neurogenic pes cavus, compared to health controls, using hand-held dynamometry. Foot Ankle Int 2005;26(7):540–4.

38. Schwend RM, Drennan JC. Cavus foot deformity in children. J Am Acad Orthop Surg 2003;11(3):201–11.

39. Ryssman DB, Myerson MS. Tendon transfers for the adult flexible cavovarus foot. Foot Ankle Clin 2011;16:435–50.
40. Szigeti k, Lupski JR. Charcot-Marie-Tooth disease. Eur J Hum Genet 2009;17: 703–10.
41. Sabir M, Lyttle D. Pathogenesis of pes cavus in Charcot-Marie-Tooth disease. Clin Orthop Relat Res 1982;(175):173–8.
42. Khadilkar SV, Yadav RS, Patel BA. Neuromuscular disorders. Singapore (Singapore): Springer; 2018.
43. Allos BM. Association between campylobacter infection and Guillain-Barré syndrome. J Infect Dis 1997;176:S125–8.
44. Hurwitz ES, Schonberger LB, Nelson DB, et al. Guillain-Barré syndrome and the 1978-1979 influenza vaccine. N Engl J Med 1981;304(26):1557–61.
45. Takahashi M, Koga M, Yokoyama K, et al. Epidemiology of Campylobacter jejuni isolated from patients with Guillain-Barré and Fisher syndromes in Japan. J Clin Microbiol 2005;43(1):335–9.
46. Ropper AH. The Guillain-Barré syndrome. N Engl J Med 1992;326:1130–6.
47. Walling AD, Dickson G. Guillain-Barré syndrome. Am Fam Physician 2013;87(3): 191–7.
48. Samelis PV, Kolovos P, Georgiou F, et al. Genu recurvatum after prolonged bracing for drop-foot in a patient with history of Guillain-Barre Syndrome. Cureus 2020;12(9):e10587.
49. Howard J, Soo B, Graham HK, et al. Cerebral palsy in Victoria: motor types, topography and gross motor function. J Paediatr Child Health 2005;41(9-10): 479–83.
50. Graham HK. Classifying cerebral palsy (On the other hand). J Pediatr Orthop 2005;25:127–8.
51. Gorter JW, Rosenbaum PL, Hanna SE, et al. Limb distribution, motor impairment, and functional classification of cerebral palsy. Dev Med Child Neurol 2004;46(7): 461–7.
52. Palisano R, Rosenbaum P, Walter S, et al. Gross motor function classification system for cerebral palsy. Dev Med Child Neurol 1997;39(4):214–23.
53. Eilert R. Cavus foot in cerebral palsy. Foot Ankle 1984;4(No.4):185–7.
54. Silver RL, Rang M, Chan J, et al. Adductor release in nonambulant children with cerebral palsy. J Pediatr Orthop 1985;5(6):672–7.
55. Karamitopoulos MS, Nirenstein L. Neuromuscular foot: spastic cerebral palsy. Foot Ankle Clin 2015;20(4):657–68.
56. Synder M, Kumar SJ, Stecyk MD. Split tibialis posterior tendon transfer and tendo-Achilles lengthening for spastic equinovarus feet. J Pediatr Orthop 1993; 13(1):20–3.
57. Tsun-Haw TOH, Kar-Foo LAU, Chee-Geap TAY, et al. Childhood-onset demyelinating polyneuropathy: challenges in differentiating acquired from genetic disease. Neurology Asia 2020;25(4):597–602.
58. McLeod JG, Pollard JD, Macaskill P, et al. Prevalence of chronic inflammatory demyelinating polyneuropathy in New South Wales, Australia. Ann Neurol 1999; 46:910–3.
59. Kuwabara S, Isose S, Mori M, et al. Different electrophysiological profiles and treatment response in 'typical' and 'atypical' chronic inflammatory demyelinating polyneuropathy. J Neurol Neurosurg Psychiatry 2015;86(10):1054–9.
60. Ryan MM, Grattan-Smith PJ, Procopisa PG, et al. Childhood chronic inflammatory demyelinating polyneuropathy: clinical course and long-term outcome. Neuromuscul Disord 2000;10:398–406.

61. Zhang Y, Liu H, Fu C, et al. The biomechanical effect of acupuncture for post-stroke cavovarus foot: study protocol for a randomized controlled pilot trial. Trials 2016;17(1):146.
62. Bensoussan L, Mesure S, Viton JM, et al. Kinematic and kinetic asymmetries in hemiplegic patients' gait initiation patterns. J Rehabil Med 2006;38:287–94.
63. Li S. Ankle and foot spasticity patterns in chronic stroke survivors with abnormal gait. Toxins (Basel) 2020;12(10):646.
64. Cioni M, Esquenazi A, Hirai B. Effects of botulinum toxin-A on gait velocity, step length, and base of support of patients with dynamic equinovarus foot. Am J Phys Med Rehabil 2006;85:600–6.
65. Esquenazi A, Moon D, Wikoff A, et al. Hemiparetic gait and changes in functional performance due to OnabotulinumtoxinA injection to lower limb muscles. Toxicon 2015;107:109–13.
66. Frink M, Klaus AK, Kuther G, et al. Long term results of compartment syndrome of the lower limb in polytraumatised patients. Injury 2007;38(5):607–13.
67. Matsen FA 3rd. Compartmental syndrome. An unified concept. Clin Orthop Relat Res 1975;(113):8–14.
68. McQueen MM, Court-Brown CM. Compartment monitoring in tibial fractures: the pressure threshold for decompression. J Bone Joint Surg Br 1996;78(1):99–104.
69. Hargens AR, Romine JS, Sipe JC, et al. Peripheral nerve-conduction block by high muscle-compartment pressure. J Bone Joint Surg Am 1979;61(2):192–200.
70. Fulkerson E, Razi A, Tejwani N. Acute compartment syndrome of the foot. Foot Ankle Int 2003;24(2):180–7.
71. Botte MJ, Santi MD, Prestianni CA, et al. Ischemic contracture of the foot and ankle: principles of management and prevention. Orthopedics 1996;19(3):235–44.
72. Thati S, Carlson C, Maskill JD, et al. Tibial compartment syndrome and the cavovarus foot. Foot Ankle Clin 2008;13(2):275–305.
73. Lovering RM, Porter NC, Bloch RJ. The muscular dystrophies: from genes to therapies. Phys Ther 2005;85(12):1372–88.
74. Petrof BJ, Shrager JB, Stedman HH, et al. Dystrophin protects the sarcolemma from stresses developed during muscle contraction. Proc Natl Acad Sci U S A 1993;90(8):3710–4.
75. Rocha CT, Hoffman EP. Limb–girdle and congenital muscular dystrophies: current diagnostics, management, and emerging technologies. Curr Neurol Neurosci Rep 2010;10(4):267–76.
76. Skalsky AJ, McDonald CM. Prevention and management of limb contractures in neuromuscular diseases. Phys Med Rehabil Clin N Am 2012;23(3):675–87.
77. Jöbsis GJ, Boers JM, Barth PG, et al. Bethlem myopathy: a slowly progressive congenital muscular dystrophy with contractures. Brain 1999;122(4):649–55.
78. Apkon SD, Alman B, Birnkrant DJ, et al. Orthopedic and surgical management of the patient with Duchenne muscular dystrophy. Pediatrics 2018;142(Supplement 2):S82–9.
79. Birnkrant DJ, Bushby K, Bann CM, et al, DMD Care Considerations Working Group. Diagnosis and management of Duchenne muscular dystrophy, part 2: respiratory, cardiac, bone health, and orthopaedic management. Lancet Neurol 2018;17(4):347–61.
80. Angelini C, Marozzo R, Pegoraro V. Current and emerging therapies in Becker muscular dystrophy (BMD). Acta Myol 2019;38(3):172.

Hallux and Lesser Digits Deformities Associated with Cavus Foot

Lawrence A. DiDomenico, DPM[a],*, Jacob Rizkalla, DPM, PGYII[b], Joelaki Cartman, DPM, PGY II[b], Sharif Abdelfattah, DPM, PGY III[b]

KEYWORDS

- Cavus foot • Digital deformity • Tendon transfer • Arthroplasty • Arthrodesis

KEY POINTS

- It is important to identify the level of the deformity or deformities.
- It is important to get the limb as close to anatomic alignment as possible.
- Many levels and multiple procedures may be involved with this reconstruction.

INTRODUCTION

Cavus foot types are due to neuromuscular causes, such as Charcot-Marie-Tooth (CMT) and post–polio syndrome, 60% to 75% of the time.[1] With neuromuscular disorders, there is an imbalance in muscle strength and spasm resulting in a cavus foot type. The anterior tibial tendon initially begins to weaken, leading to unopposed action and spasm of the peroneus longus, resulting in a plantarflexed first ray. The peroneus brevis then is weakened and overpowered by spasms of the tibialis posterior, resulting in supination of the hindfoot. At this time, there is noted paralysis of the intrinsics, leading to a biomechanical advantage for the extrinsic extensors.[2] Biomechanical imbalances are the number 1 contributing factor for digital and metatarsophalangeal joint contractures.[3] This results in an abnormal weight-bearing or muscle imbalance between the extrinsic extensor tendons and the intrinsic at the plantar foot. The recruitment of the extensor hallucis longus results in a dorsal contracture of the hallux. When there is an imbalance, with weak intrinsics as there is with CMT, the extensor digitorum longus (EDL) can act unopposed, resulting in a hyperextension at the metatarsophalangeal joint.[4] As this occurs, there is a counterbalance effect that is attempted through the flexor digitorum longus (FDL) and flexor digitorum

[a] East Liverpool City Hospital, NOMS Ankle and Foot Care Centers, St. Elizabeth Hospital, 8175 Market Street, Youngstown, OH 444512, USA; [b] East Liverpool City Hospital, 425 W 5th Street, East Liverpool, OH 43920, USA
* Corresponding author.
E-mail address: LD5353@aol.com

Clin Podiatr Med Surg 38 (2021) 343–360
https://doi.org/10.1016/j.cpm.2020.12.013
0891-8422/21/© 2020 Elsevier Inc. All rights reserved.

podiatric.theclinics.com

brevis (FDB) that results in a flexion contracture at the distal interphalangeal joints (DIPJ) and proximal phalangeal joints. The result is a claw toe and an accentuated plantarflexed forefoot on the rearfoot. In early stages of the deformity, it could be reducible; however, as the condition progresses, it can become rigid. Commonly it is referred to extensor substitution, which in the past has also been referred to as extensor recruitment[5] (**Fig. 1**).

In the cavus foot, there may be a complaint of painful distal clavus or prominences at the dorsal aspect of the proximal interphalangeal joint (PIPJ) and DIPJ rubbing on shoe gear. Another common presenting complaint is metatarsalgia/ulcers or stress reaction/fracture of the metatarsals (**Figs. 2–4**).

In addition to the digital examination, the ankle, hindfoot, and midfoot should be assessed and observed in seated, weight-bearing, and gait examination to understand the deformity in static and dynamic moments. Of note, muscle strength testing should be addressed to determine if the cause of the cavus is a neuromuscular disorder. Manual muscle testing and gait observation are commonly used to clinically evaluate muscle weakness.[6] The tibialis anterior, peroneus brevis, peroneus longus, intrinsics, triceps surae, and tibialis posterior should be assessed. Doing so can help to distinguish subtle cavus from a possible undiagnosed neuromuscular and possibly progressive disorder. If there is any question, a neurologic consult, nerve conduction studies, and electromyography study should be performed. Evidence of neurologic deficits may be evident with gait examination as well. In these cases, a high steppage gait may indicate a weakened tibialis anterior, and a wide base of gait can also be an indicator. Equinus should be assessed through the Silfverskiold examination. In the senior author's experience, there is a high degree of equinus contractures associated with a pes caves foot. Typically, this goes against initial thoughts, as many of the radiographs demonstrate a high calcaneal inclination angle, often suggesting there is not a tight posterior muscle group. Each patient should be thoroughly evaluated, as there is a high degree of association with pes caves deformities. In determination of metatarsophalangeal joint reducibility, a Kelikian push-up test should be performed. This test helps to determine if the deformity is flexible or rigid at the metatarsal phalangeal joints (MTPJ) (**Fig. 5**).

Digital deformities may present in a variety of forms, such as a mallet toe, hammertoe, claw toe, and curly toe. The deformities most commonly present in the

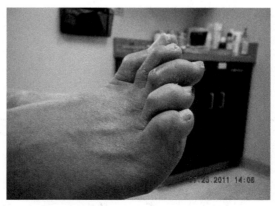

Fig. 1. A lateral clinical view demonstrating a cavus foot type with associated extensor recruitment hammertoe deformities 1 to 5.

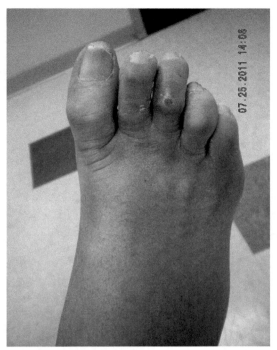

Fig. 2. A dorsal clinical view demonstrating a cavus foot type with associated extensor recruitment hammertoe deformities 1 to 5, an ulcer secondary to the pressure from at the PIPJ third toe right.

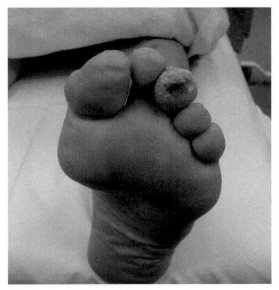

Fig. 3. A plantar clinical view with a bilateral cavus foot type with associated extensor recruitment and flexion contracture of hammertoe deformities 1 to 5 left and 2 to 5 right. An ulcer of the third toe left is secondary to the pressure from the flexion contracture.

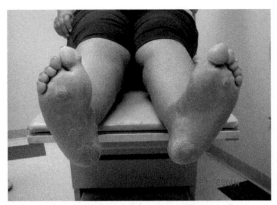

Fig. 4. A plantar clinical view with a cavus foot type with associated extensor recruitment and flexion contracture of hammertoe deformities 1 to 5 left. A preulcerative session is located to the sub third metatarsal right and a sub second metatarsal of the right foot. Note the extent of the extension and flexion contracture of the toes, resulting in an inability to see the plantar aspect of the digits because of the severe contracture of the toes.

sagittal plane; however, they also occur in the frontal and transverse plane. The literature suggests a biomechanical imbalance between the extrinsic and intrinsic musculature is the reason for the development of hammertoes. The 3 categories have been described as flexor stabilization, flexor substitution, and extensor substitution[7] (**Fig. 6**).

It is important to identify the underlying cause of the hammertoe deformity and understand the cause of the deformity. Flexor stabilization typically occurs in a pronated foot type. As the foot pronates, the FDL fires earlier in the gait cycle, gaining a mechanical advantage over the interossei muscles. An adductovarus rotation of the fourth and/or fifth digit is typically present.[8,9] Flexor substitution is often associated with a weak triceps surae. The deep posterior group musculature overpowers to accommodate for the weak triceps surae. The flexors gain an advantage over the interossei.[8]

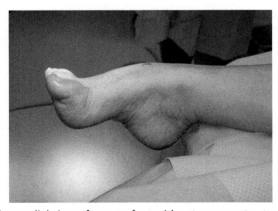

Fig. 5. Preoperative medial view of a cavus foot with extensor contracture at the MTPJ and flexion contracture at the proximal phalangeal joint resulting in increased pressure and pain at the plantar aspect of the MTPJ.

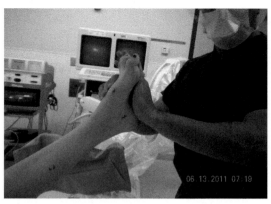

Fig. 6. A medial view of a left foot with a patient under anesthesia, demonstrating the contracture of the toes in a cavus foot deformity.

Extensor substitution occurs in the swing phase of gait with the long extensors gaining a mechanical advantage over the lumbricals.[8] Generally, there is contracture at the metatarsophalangeal joint level with bowstringing of the extensor tendons.[9] Neuromuscular disorders, such as CMT, polio, muscular dystrophies, and lumbar disc disease, may lead to contracture at the metatarsophalangeal and interphalangeal joints (IPJ) of the lesser digits,[10] manifesting most commonly as a claw toe deformity. A high-arched, cavus foot type is often exhibited with this type of deformity.[11] Hibbs[12] originally termed this foot type a "claw foot." The classic presentation consists of a high-arch foot, plantar calluses, and prominent metatarsal heads secondary to the digital deformities, resulting in retrograde increased pressure. A detailed history from the patient is necessary, as the patient may inform the surgeon of a family history of a high-arched foot type with neuropathic type symptoms. Muscle weakness with complaints of a drop foot highly associated with tripping or instability can be found.[13] Prominences at the dorsal and PIPJ can make shoe gear difficult. Callus formation secondary to prominent metatarsal heads and increased pressure leads to metatarsalgia.[14]

DIAGNOSIS/ASSESSMENT

A complete non-weight-bearing and weight-bearing examination, along with a gait analysis, should be performed. A Silfverskiold test should be performed to assess for an underlying contributory equinus contracture. The toes should be evaluated in the sagittal, transverse, and frontal plane. In most cases of hammertoe deformities associated with a pes cavus foot, the deformity is commonly in the sagittal plane. The digit can be classified whether the deformity is flexible, semirigid, or rigid. Long-standing deformities may lead to subluxation/dislocation at the level of the MTPJ.

Radiographs should consist of an anterior-posterior projection to assess the transverse and sagittal plane deformity. The "gun-barrel sign" is a hallmark of sagittal plane deformity, as one visualizes the medullary canal of the middle phalanx.[9,11] The lateral view will confirm a sagittal plane pathologic condition. An oblique view will confirm the pathologic condition and the plane or planes of deformity (**Fig. 7**).

In deformities whereby the plantar plate rupture is suspected, an MRI should be ordered. A plantar plate injury or predislocation may include MTPJ synovitis and synovitis or effusion in the flexor tendon sheath.[15]

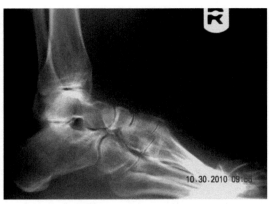

Fig. 7. A lateral radiograph demonstrating Significant contracture of the toes.

The EDL tendon acts as a dorsiflexor of the ankle through the swing phase of gait. The tendon splits once it passes the ankle into 4 separate slips, which insert on the dorsal aspect of the middle and distal phalanges of digits 2 to 5. The extensor digitorum brevis (EDB) tendon has 3 separate slips to digits 2, 3, and 4 and inserts at the extensor expansion of the corresponding EDL tendon. The extensor expansion has plantar attachments with the capsule, plantar plate, and flexor tendon sheath at the level of the MTPJ. Therefore, the pull of EDL and EDB causes significant dorsiflexor power at the level of the MTPJs and minimal power at the IPJ. The FDB originates at the medial calcaneal tuberosity. It courses distally and splits into 2 slips that attach to the plantar aspect of middle phalanx. The FDL originates in the posterior compartment of the leg and courses to the digits through the split in the FDB tendon to insert on the distal phalanx.

In a patient with neuromuscular disease, such as CMT or polio, a thorough neuromuscular examination is needed. These patients are highly associated with digital deformities, such as extensor substitution. In the CMT population, the disease process begins with atrophy of the intrinsic musculature. With loss of stability of the lumbricals at the level of the MTPJ, there is unopposed pull of the long extensor tendons and the long flexor tendons. This pull causes extension at the MTPJ and flexion of the phalanges. Subsequently, there is a generalized weakness of the tibialis anterior tendon as well as the peroneus brevis tendon. The muscle strength to the long flexors and peroneus longus is preserved. The weakness in the anterior compartment requires the EDL tendon to compensate for the lack of dorsiflexion at the level of the ankle, further creating the hyperextension, hammertoe contracture.[16]

DISCUSSION OF TRADITIONAL THOUGHTS AND PROCEDURES FOR HAMMERTOE CORRECTION

It is important to recognize the extent and severity of the cavus deformity. The surgeon must consider multiple factors: whether the deformity is flexible or rigid, muscle imbalance, and location of the deformity.[6] The foot will not be balanced with any uncorrected structure, and the deformity will recur if the foot is not balanced.[3] In order to restore MTPJ alignment, a proximal interphalangeal joint fusion, extensor hood release, EDL lengthening, FDL tendon transfer, flexor plate release, or K-wire fixation can be performed.

Soft Tissue Procedures

Digital contractures can be categorized broadly into 2 categories: flexible and rigid deformity. Procedure selection for these 2 groups can vary greatly. If a physical examination of the toes reveals it can be realigned manually, and the contracture is secondary to soft tissue imbalance, a procedure to balance the foot may be performed, which will weaken the deforming muscles and/or strengthen those which have lost their mechanical advantage.

Flexor Digitorum Longus Transfer

A procedure that can be used for a flexible contracted digit (hammertoe) is the FDL tendon transfer.[17] This procedure was first popularized by Girdlestone and Taylor in the 1940s and 1950s.[18] Now, several versions of this procedure exist, but their goal remains the same.[19] By removing the FDL distal attachment from the distal phalanx and transferring the tendon to the extensor hood at the base of the proximal phalanx, this will alleviate flexion contracture forces at the PIPJ and DIPJ that are often associated with digital contracture, while creating a plantarflexion at the MTPJ.

Jones Tenosuspension

A Jones tenosuspension is a removal of the extensor longus tendon with reattachment to the distal aspect of the first metatarsal. Its primary indication is for a flexible claw toe deformity with flexion of the great toe interphalangeal joint and extension at the first metatarsal, thus reducing the contracture at the MTPJ. The procedure can be used for abnormalities at this anatomic location in such deformities as CMT.[20]

Hibbs Tenosuspension

The EDL is recruited to help with dorsiflexion when the tibialis anterior is weak or overpowering the Achilles tendon. Often the deformity will lead to a contracture of the MTP, causing metatarsalgia and digital deformities. The Hibbs procedure is indicated for equinus with or without claw toes. Contraindication includes nonfunctioning or weakened EDL. The procedure can be performed as an isolated procedure if the digital contracture is fully reducible.[21] The procedure involves the tendon slips of the EDL being detached from their insertions combined and being reattached to either the peroneal tertius or the midfoot. The EDB tendon is then transected and reattached to the corresponding distal EDL tendon, which inserts into the toes.

Osseous Procedures

These procedures can be done isolated or in conjunction with the soft tissue procedures. Fixation may vary based on surgeon preference.

Arthroplasty

It is senior author opinion that there are better selections of surgical treatment other than arthroplasty in many cases. The downside of the procedure may make the risks larger than the benefits: most notably, a floppy toe secondary to shortening or over-resection. There is no measurable way to quantify how much bone is necessary to be resected. Resection of the head of the proximal phalanx effectively shortens the distance of the origin to insertion of the FDL and the FDB, thereby causing weakness of the flexor tendons. The extensor tendons, however, are not weakened because they functionally insert into the MTPJ via the extensor hood apparatus. Therefore, the arthroplasty is more effective at correcting flexor-induced hammertoes rather than extensor hammertoes. If an arthroplasty is used on an extensor digital deformity, then it often requires an additional extensor tendon release. This procedure has its place within the topic of digital deformity correction. Atinga and colleagues[22] found the procedure to be reliable and reproducible and to have few medium-term complications. A K-wire is commonly used for temporary fixation and is driven distally from within the joint and out through the end of the toe; then this wire is redirected back through the proximal phalanx and possibly into the head of the metatarsal based on indications.[23]

Arthrodesis

The biomechanical forces can be combated in several ways. One such method is fusion of the IPJ. Although fusion is typically reserved for a nonreducible or rigid deformity, it can be an effective procedure any time a long-lasting deformity correction is required. By fusing a joint within the toe, all of the forces are transferred to the surrounding joints, which can be used as a biomechanical advantage. In the case of a proximal interphalangeal fusion, the proximal and intermediate phalanxes are turned into a rigid lever arm, allowing the flexor tendons to act without causing a dorsiflexion deformity at the level of the metatarsophalangeal joint secondary to retrograde buckling.

There are numerous products on the market that help give compression to the fusion site. One such method is an intramedullary cannulated screw. This method was found to have long-standing deformity correction and reduction of pain by Caterini and colleagues.[24] The surgeon can also create an entirely osseous construct to provide stability via insertion of 1 phalanx into the other. One such technique is a peg-and-hole technique, as described by Alvine and Garvin.[25] The review by Lamm[26] of these procedures found no significant difference based on the osseous construct used. This procedure can be performed on the PIPJ and/or DIPJ of the lesser digits as well as the IPJ of the hallux.[27–29]

SUMMARY OF TRADITIONAL PROCEDURES

There is no concrete algorithm that can guide every digital deformity secondary to a cavus foot type with predictable desirable results. Careful physical examination is required to identify the level of the deformity, along with rigidity of the deformity. It is the authors' belief that the above procedures alone, or in conjunction with one another, can successfully be used to correct all the digital deformities that can stem from the biomechanical forces caused by a cavus foot type. Last, it is important to consider all the forces causing the deformity before committing to any distal procedures. The surgeon should work proximal to distal to help achieve optimal corrections.

THE SENIOR AUTHOR'S THEORY AND EXPERIENCE

The senior author has not performed bony surgical procedures except in very few cases, such as severe revision procedures, over the past 20 years or more. One needs to ask themselves, is there any deformity in the proximal phalanx when isolated, the middle phalanx when isolated, or the distal phalanx when isolated? The answer is overwhelmingly no. The osseous components are typically normal and not diseased, but they are contracted and sometimes are rotated and pulled by the abnormal biomechanical forces of the lower extremity, giving mechanical advantage to the soft tissue (tendons), resulting in single- or multiplane hammertoe deformities.

Before surgical intervention of a digital contracture, vascular analysis should be seriously considered. Complete vascular studies, which include digital pressures and/or toe-brachial indices, should be ordered. A neurologic workup may include an electromyographic or a nerve conduction velocity study. If the foot deformities have been progressive versus static, the foot and ankle surgeon should suggest a workup by a neurologist.[1]

The surgical patient should be educated that the digital deformity is a chronic soft tissue pathologic process that has occurred because of tendon imbalance and secondary soft tissue contracture has occurred. This contracture can occur at each segment of the involved joint/joints, consisting of either the MTPJ, PIPJ, or the DIPJ, or a combination of all. Although the digit as an entity may present as a deformity, each separate segment (proximal, middle, and distal phalanx) does not exhibit any bony pathologic condition when isolated. The goal is to balance the toe. Remove the deforming force and "weaken" the overpowering tendon and "strengthen" the weaker tendon to balance the biomechanics of the given toe. Essentially, the surgeon is taking away the deforming soft tissue attachment from the digit, putting the digit in the desired position, and then rebuilding the soft tissue attachments to the given toe via tendon transfers loaded under physiologic tension. This procedure should improve digital alignment and function, resulting in improved and more balanced biomechanics about the toe, resulting in a stable, neutrally placed toe with no loss of cubic volume of bone maintaining stability. After completing the procedure, the deforming force is gone; therefore, the patient should not get a reoccurrence.

TREATMENT/SURGICAL TECHNIQUE: MUSCLE TENDON BALANCING
The Modified Girdlestone-Taylor Procedure (Flexor Digitorum Longus Tendon Transfer)

The modified Girdlestone-Taylor procedure is used to treat flexion contractures of the DIPJ and/or PIPJ in the sagittal plane. The senior author performs the procedure through a midline incision approach on the lateral aspect of the hallux and the medial or lateral aspect of the second, third, and fourth toes and the medial aspect of the fifth toe. The senior author prefers a midline-based approach. Placing the incision in these locations provides for a good cosmetic appearance of the incision lines, as they are hidden between the toes.

The assistant surgeon should use fine double skin hooks for gentle retraction in order to avoid soft tissue compromise and irritation to the very small neurovascular structures of the toes. The incision is deepened in the same plane, with careful attention to avoid the neurovascular bundles. The dissection is carried to the fascia and to the plantar aspect of the soft tissues of the respective toe. The deep fascia tissue is incised into, and the FDL is identified. Detach the FDL tendon insertion from the distal phalanx and use an Allis clamp to pull the FDL tendon proximally toward the proximal phalanx. Attention is then directed to the FDB tendon. Detach (both the medial and lateral slips/insertions) the tendon from the base of the middle phalanx. If needed, a capsulotomy at the IPJ (for a flexion contracture of the PIPJ) and/or the DIPJ is performed, allowing the contracture to be reduced. The deforming force should now be removed, and there should no longer be a flexion contracture. Whether the deformity is classified as rigid, semirigid, or flexible, this contracture now should be completely resolved no matter the preoperative classification. A K-wire (preferably 0.062 in in size) is inserted from the distal tip of the distal phalanx through the DIPJ with the joint reduced into the middle phalanx and through the PIPJ to the base of the proximal phalanx proximal cortex if only performing an FDL transfer. If performing an FDL transfer in combination with a modified Hibbs/extensor transfer, then the K-wire will be inserted across the MTPJ into the base of the respective metatarsal. Relative to the correction of the toes, it has been the author's experience to be cautious not to overcorrect the flexion contracture in the sagittal plane by placing the DIPJ and/or the PIPJ into a neutral or extended/hyperextended position, resulting in a recurvatum at the respected joint/joints. Rather, correct the flexion contracture into a neutral to slight plantar flexion position. If an isolated FDL tendon transfer is being performed, there should not be a contracture at the metatarsophalangeal joint; therefore, there is no need to pin across the metatarsophalangeal joint with the K-wire. Next, while the toe is held in anatomic alignment and held into the desired position, the FDL tendon is tensioned and transferred and then sutured into the extensor soft tissue (extensor hood) of the proximal phalanx under physiologic tension. Although the FDL tendon is being sutured, the surgeon should be pulling dorsally on the Allis clamp that is clamped to the tip of the FDL tendon under physiologic tension. The Allis clamp will help insert the FDL tendon on under physiologic tension. The excess/remainder of the FDL is resected, and the skin is reapproximated with typical skin closure.

There are several advantages to the procedure. With the scars located on the lateral aspect of the hallux and the medial or lateral aspect of the second, third, and fourth toes and the medial aspect of the fifth toe, the procedure leaves a much more cosmetically pleasing result, essentially hiding the incisions. In addition, by performing the FDL transfer, this removes the pathologic sagittal plane force as well as any additional pathologic pull in the frontal and transverse plane from the FDL tendon, allowing the toe to be placed in a neutral position. Postoperatively, there is a much more natural clinical look in terms of the length of the toe. The digits retain stability in the transverse and frontal plane, as the medial and lateral collateral ligaments are left intact. The toe is not shortened, as there is no bone resection. In the senior author's experience, in comparison to bony procedures, there is minimal postoperative edema relative to bony procedures. The postoperative edema is relatively minimal, as the dissection consists of soft tissue only and there is no bony involvement. Any resulting bursa, hyperkeratosis, and ulceration eventually dissipate as the deforming forces are removed and the preoperative pressures to the respective joints are relieved.

Because there is no surgery on the bony structures, there is no rotation, translation, malalignment, or shortening of the digits. The tendon transfer targets and treats the underlying pathologic condition. The dynamic/static deforming force from the tendon on the toe is eliminated, and there is no need to disturb the natural ligamentous and osseous structures of the soft tissues or phalanxes of any of the toes. Postoperatively, with an isolated FDL transfer, the K-wire is removed at approximately 7 to 10 days. Because the deforming force is removed, the K-wire can be removed. If the preoperative deformity involves the extensor tendons in addition to the flexion contracture, then the K-wires are left in longer. Last, if a problem would occur postoperatively, one can always perform a bony procedure, such as an arthroplasty or arthrodesis if needed.

In terms of disadvantages, this is a more technically challenging surgical procedure in terms of dissection and suturing. The anatomic space is crowded to work in. Complications are similar to those with any other digital surgery; more unique complications to this procedure consist of overcorrection or hyperextension, leading to a sagittal plane recurvatum deformity of the corrected joints. Soft tissue maceration, and wound issues at the incision site can become an issue secondary to interdigital contact or vascular compromise as in any digital repair. In addition, loss or partial loss of a toe or foot can occur if the stretch on the vascularity of the toes goes into spasm following a significant straightening and stretch of a toe. Again, preoperative vascular studies, as discussed above, should be performed.

The Modified Hibbs Procedure (Extensor Tendon Transfers)

The modified Hibbs procedure is indicated for patients who exhibit extensor substitution/recruitment. The dorsal subluxations/dislocations often result in increased retrograde pressures/deformity at the metatarsophalangeal joints and are frequently linked with claw toes and hammertoes. These deformities typically result in the recruitment of a tight EDL (extensor substitution/recruitment) to support dorsiflexion against a tight posterior muscle group (equinus contracture).

To treat hammertoes 2 to 5 (extension pathologic condition), beginning at the second metatarsophalangeal joint, make an oblique dorsal incision proximal to the base of the fourth metatarsal. Deepen this incision in the same plane and avoid all neurovascular structures. Be sure to avoid and preserve the superficial nerves within the subcutaneous tissue, as these will be running longitudinally. Good care of the soft tissue is essential, and the senior author recommends fine double skin hooks for retraction to avoid soft tissue compromise. The assistant should only be retracting in the area of the where the surgery is being performed. Identify the extensor tendons (EDL and EDB tendons of the respected toes) and separate only these tendons from the subcutaneous tissues. There is no need to dissect any other tissues other than separating the soft tissues from the EDL and EDB tendon. The EDL and EDB tendons lie deep to the superficial nerves. The surgeon should separate and dissect the extensor tendons longitudinally. Isolate the second, third, and fourth EDL tendons, respectively, and cut these tendons as far proximal within the incision site. Clamp each one of the most distal aspects of the proximal portion of the cut EDL with a small mosquito hemostat. Clamp the most proximal aspect of the distal cut portion of the EDL tendon with an Allis clamp. The distal cut portions of the EDL tendons are then reflected from the remaining soft tissues as far distally within the incision site and retracted out of the way. The distal portion of the second EDL tendon is reflected distally and temporarily placed in the first web space of the foot. The third EDL tendon is placed similarly in the second web space, and the fourth EDL tendon is placed in third web space. The fifth EDL tendon is identified, and a Z-lengthening procedure is performed, allowing the tension and contracture to be released from the fifth EDL tendon.

Attention is directed to the second, third, and fourth metatarsophalangeal joints as far distal in the incision site. The second, third, and fourth EDB tendons are dissected as far distal within the incision site, and a tenotomy is performed as far distal as possible on the EDB. An Allis clamp is applied to the most proximal portion of the cut second, third, and fourth EDB tendons, and these tendons are retracted proximally. At this time, complete exposure of the metatarsophalangeal joint is achieved. A complete capsulotomy at the second, third, fourth, and fifth metatarsophalangeal joints is completed with a sharp no. 15 blade. This capsulotomy facilitates release of all contractures, and the use of a McGlamry elevator is used to perform a complete capsulotomy contracture release primarily in the sagittal plane but also in the transverse plane. Following this release, the surgeon should realize that all the soft tissue deforming forces have now been removed and the digits should naturally revert to a "neutral position."

In most scenarios, when a digit involves the extension contracture, there also is a flexion component in the deformity. In deformities that exhibit both flexion and extension deformities, additional soft tissue procedures need to be performed to address flexion contracture of the second, third, fourth, and fifth digits (flexor tendon transfer). The flexor tendon transfer is then performed at each toe. Once this is accomplished, insert a 0.062-in K-wire from the distal aspect of the toes through the DIPJ, the PIPJ, and the metatarsophalangeal joint to the base of the second, third, fourth, and fifth metatarsals into the respected proximal cortex. Ensure there is good anatomic alignment of the toe relative to the metatarsal. Be sure the DIPJ, the PIPJ, and the MTPJ are reduced into anatomic alignment and the toe is in the desired position.

Next, proceed back to the dorsal aspect of the foot and perform a tendon transfer via a weave graft, anastomosing the distal portion of the proximal segment of the EDB into the most proximal portion of the distal EDL stump into the digit. This procedure is done separately for digits 2, 3, and 4 under physiologic tension. This tendon transfer will essentially weaken the extensor pull of the respected toes from the larger, longer EDL muscle and tendon to the smaller EDB muscle and tendon. Suture the Z-lengthened fifth EDL with physiologic tension while maintaining good anatomic alignment. Typically, the author uses 4.0 Monocryl for the suture of choice for the tendon transfer and deep closure. Remember, the K-wire is holding all in place (similar to an internal cast); therefore, the suture is holding the tendon transfer into its new insertion site. Next, pass the most proximal portion of the distal stumps of the second and third EDL tendons deep to the soft tissue structure (to avoid pressure on the neurovascular structures) with the fourth EDL. Suture the distal stumps together (the author typically uses 0 Vicryl) of the second, third, and fourth EDL tendons and transfer them into the peroneus tertius or the periosteum of the intermediate cuneiform with the surgical assistant loading and holding the ankle at 90° relative to the leg. Again, this tendon transfer should be executed under physiologic tension. This method provides a mechanical gain in dorsiflexion. Be sure to avoid the superficial neurovascular structures when closing the tissues.

In the postoperative phase, following K-wire removal, one should emphasize physical therapy for the patient in order to help resolve any edema and soften the postoperative fibrosis and scar tissue formation. Active and passive manipulation and range-of-motion exercises of the respected joints (**Fig. 8**) are suggested.

In scenarios that involve the great toe individually or in combination, the same surgical technique and principle should be applied. The same procedures are performed, but because of a larger tendon, this makes the procedures easier (**Figs. 9–16**).

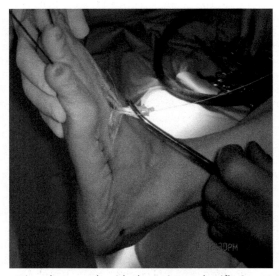

Fig. 8. An intraoperative photograph with the assistant dorsiflexing at the ankle, loading the foot, and transferring the second, third, and fourth proximal stumps of the EDL tendon into the midfoot under physiologic tension to gain balance and mechanical advantage.

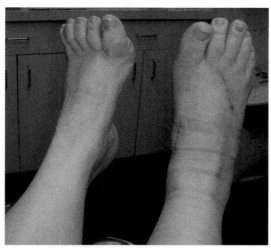

Fig. 9. A right foot postoperative dorsal clinical view versus the left preoperative view of a patient with a cavus foot deformity who underwent modified Hibbs and Girdlestone-Taylor procedures on toes 1 to 5 right.

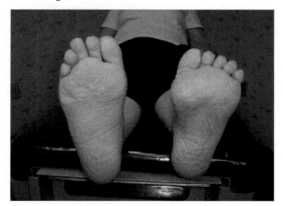

Fig. 10. A right foot postoperative plantar clinical view versus the left preoperative view of a patient with a cavus foot deformity who underwent a modified Hibbs and Girdlestone-Taylor procedures on toes 1 to 5 right.

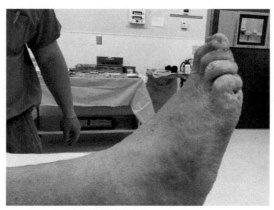

Fig. 11. A lateral and frontal preoperative view demonstrating significant contracture of toes 1 to 5 of the right foot.

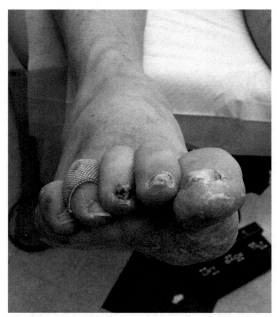

Fig. 12. A frontal plane preoperative view demonstrating a pes cavus foot with a significant contracture of the toes 1 to 5 of the right foot. Note the forefoot valgus that is often associated with a pes cavus foot type.

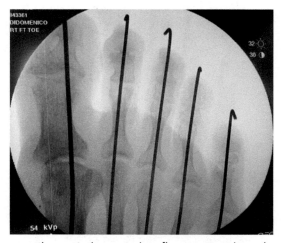

Fig. 13. An intraoperative anterior-posterior fluoroscopy view demonstrating good anatomic alignment of toes of the right foot. Note the contracted joints at the MTPJ, PIPJ, and DIPJ are all no longer contracted, and the joint spaces are visible.

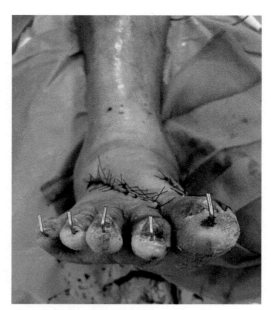

Fig. 14. A postoperative frontal view demonstrating the reduction of the digital deformities following tendon transfer and K-wire fixation following a modified Hibbs and Girdlestone-Taylor procedures to all toes of the right foot.

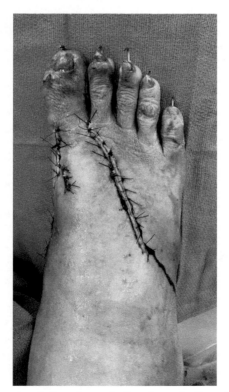

Fig. 15. A postoperative dorsal view demonstrating the reduction of the digital deformities following tendon transfer and K-wire fixation following a modified Hibbs and Girdlestone-Taylor procedures to all toes of the right foot.

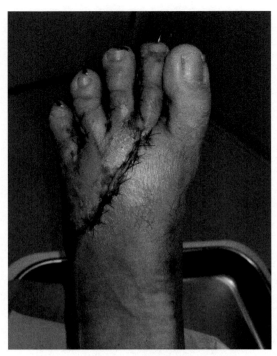

Fig. 16. A postoperative clinical view of a patient who had postoperative surgical reconstruction consisting of a Girdlestone-Taylor and modified Hibbs tendon transfer procedures.

SUMMARY

The most important component of performing tendon transfer for the correction of digital deformities is identifying which procedure to perform for the given pathologic condition. Most digit deformities are associated with an abnormal pull and biomechanics of the short and long flexor and extensor tendons that have caused the toe or multiple toes to have a pathologic tension on the toe. The objective of the surgery should be to balance the flexors and extensors in order to prevent recurrence and to treat the underlying pathologic condition. Once the surgeon removes the deforming force, a recurrence should not occur. If the surgeon evaluates and appropriately addresses the digital deformity, the appropriate procedure should be able to correct the toe in all planes.

Making a sound decision in which procedure or combination of surgical procedures (flexor tendon transfer and/or extensor tendon transfer) to perform is critical. The foot and ankle surgeon must be able to identify the appropriate pathologic process in order to perform the proper surgical procedure to address the given underlying pathologic condition. Digital deformities present in many ways. The pathologic condition can present to an isolated joint of a toe, multiple joints of a toe, a single toe, and multiple toes, unilaterally or bilaterally. These digital deformities can involve other pathologic conditions, such as an equinus contracture, pes cavus deformity associated with metatarsals deformities, systemic diseases, such as rheumatoid arthritis, diabetes mellitus, polio, and CMT disease, and other neuromuscular diseases.

When patients with a pes cavus foot deformity present with global deformities of all toes, the respected procedures can be approached for correction of each involved segment of each toe. These procedures can be performed on an isolated toe or multiple toes. Each segment of each toe needs to be appropriately assessed and addressed for predictable good long-term outcomes.

The senior author has found tendon balancing procedures to be more predictable outcomes of hammertoe surgery with successful long-term resolution, as this is treating the underlying pathologic condition. Because the underlying pathologic condition is being evaluated, identified, and directly treated, there should be little chance of reoccurrence. This approach addresses the biomechanical cause of the given deformity. Performing these forefoot joint-sparing procedures provides a long-term predictable outcome with relatively limited postoperative complications. From a cosmetic standpoint, the Girdlestone-Taylor procedure leaves scars on the medial aspect of the second to fifth digit, and on the lateral aspect of the hallux, and the Hibbs scar leaves 1 dorsal scar on the forefoot and none on the toes, resulting in a much more cosmetically pleasing result. Postoperatively, there appears to be a much more natural appearance to the digits in comparison to more traditional bony procedure with a dorsal approach. In addition, there is no shortening of the toe. The medial and lateral collateral ligaments are left intact, thus limiting frontal or transverse plane complications. The cubic volume of bone is not changed, preventing instability and shortening of the toes. Last, because dissection is limited to soft tissue, postoperative edema is minimal in relation to bony procedures.

CLINICS CARE POINTS

- Identify the underlying pathologic condition.
- Correct the underlying pathologic condition.
- Typically, this surgical reconstruction will involve multiple procedures and multiple planes of deformity correction.

DISCLOSURE

The authors have nothing to disclose.

REFERENCES

1. Piazza S, Ricci G, Caldarazzo Ienco E, et al. Pes cavus and hereditary neuropathies: when a relationship should be suspected. J Orthop Traumatol 2010;11(4):195–201.
2. Maynou C, Szymanski C, Thiounn A. The adult cavus foot. EFORT Open Rev 2017;2(5):221–9.
3. Kim BS. Reconstruction of cavus foot: a review. Open Orthop J 2017;11:651–9.
4. Joo SJ, Choi BO, Kim DY, et al. Foot deformity in charcot marie tooth disease according to disease severity. Ann Rehabil Med 2011;35(4):499–506.
5. DiDomenico L. Essential insights on tendon transfers for digital dysfunction. 2010; 23(4). Available at: https://www.podiatrytoday.com/essential-insights-on-tendon-transfers-for-digital-dysfunction. Accessed March 25, 2010.
6. Kaplan JRM, Aiyer A, Cerrato RA. Operative treatment of the cavovarus foot. Foot Ankle Int 2018;39(11):1370–82.
7. Boberg J, Eilts C. Lesser digital deformities: etiology, procedure selection, and arthroplasty. In: McGlamry's comprehensive textbook of foot and ankle surgery. Philadelphia: Lippincott; 2013. p. 117–23.

8. DiDomenico L, Rollandini J. A closer look at tendon transfers for crossover hammertoe. Podiatry Today 2014;27(6):44–51.
9. Boberg JS. Surgical decision making in hammertoe surgery. In: Vickers NS, et al, editors. Reconstructive surgery of the foot and eg: update '97. Tucker (GA): Podiatry Institute; 1997. p. 3–6.
10. Coughlin MJ. Lesser toe abnormalities. Instr Course Lect 2003;52:421–44.
11. Bouchard JL, Castellano BD. Clawtoe deformities and contractures of the forefoot. In: Camasta CA, Vickers NS, Ruch JA, editors. Reconstructive surgery of the foot and leg, update 88. Tucker (GA): Podiatry Institute Publishing; 1998. p. 14–21.
12. Hibbs RA. An operation for "clawfoot". JAMA 1919;73:1583–5.
13. Rosenbaum AJ, Lisella J, Patel N, et al. The cavus foot. Med Clin North Am 2014; 98:301–12.
14. Hansen S Jr. Transfer of the extensor digitorum communis to the midfoot. In: Functional reconstruction of the foot and ankle. Philadelphia: Lippincott; 2000. p. 451.
15. Yao L, Do H, Cracchiolo A, et al. Plantar plate of the foot: findings on conventional arthrography and MR imaging. AJR Am J Roentgenol 1994;163:641–4.
16. Schwend RM, Drennan JC. Cavus foot deformity in children. J Am Acad Orthop Surg 2003;11:201–11.
17. Filliatrault AD, Ruch JA, Weiskopf SA. Flexor digitorum longus tendon transfer. McGlamry's comprehensive textbook of foot and ankle surgery. 2012;1(4):145–53.
18. Girdlestone GR. Physiology for the foot and hand. J Bone Joint Surg 1947;29: 168–9.
19. Cove R, Cooke P, Thomason K. The Oxford procedure for the treatment of lesser toe deformities. Ann R Coll Surg Engl 2011;93(7):553–4.
20. Veljkovic A, Lansang E, Lau J. Forefoot tendon transfers. Foot Ankle Clin 2014; 19(1):123–37.
21. Grambart ST. Hibbs tenosuspension. Clin Podiatric Med Surg 2016;33(1):63–9.
22. Atinga M, Dodd L, Foote J, et al. Prospective review of medium term outcomes following interpositional arthroplasty for hammer toe deformity correction. Foot Ankle Surg 2011;17:256–8.
23. Kramer WC, Parman M, Marks RM. Hammertoe correction with K-wire fixation. Foot Ankle Int 2015;36(5):494–502.
24. Caterini R, Farsetti P, Tarantino U, et al. Arthrodesis of the toe joints with an intra-medullary cannulated screw for correction of hammertoe deformity. Foot Ankle Int 2004;25(4):256–61.
25. Alvine FG, Garvin KL. Peg and dowel fusion of the proximal interphalangeal joint. Foot Ankle 1980;1:90–4.
26. Lamm BM, Riberio CE, Vlahovic TC, et al. Lesser proximal interphalangeal joint arthrodesis: a retrospective analysis of the peg-in-hole and end-to-end procedures. J Am Podiatr Med Assoc 2001;91:331–6.
27. Moyer J, Lowery C, Knox J. Hallux IPJ fusion. Clin Podiatric Med Surg 2004;21(1): 51–64.
28. Langford JH, Fenton CF 3rd. Hallux interphalangeal arthrodesis. J Am Podiatr Med Assoc 1982;72(3):155–7.
29. Thorud JC, Jolley T, Shibuya N, et al. Comparison of hallux interphalangeal joint arthrodesis fixation techniques: a retrospective multicenter study. J Foot Ankle Surg 2016;55(1):22–7.

The Subtle Cavovarus Foot Deformity

The Nonneurologic Form of Cavus Foot Deformity

Harry John Visser, DPM, Hannan H. Zahid, DPM*,
Jared J. Visser, DPM, Brittany R. Staples, DPM,
Nicholas J. Staub, DPM

KEYWORDS

- Peek-a-boo heel sign • Nonneurologic cavus foot • Coleman block test
- Peroneal overdrive • Adjunctive operative reconstruction

KEY POINTS

- Lateral foot and ankle pathology.
- Subtle cavus foot deformity.
- Presence of equinus, heel varus, and first ray plantarflexion.

INTRODUCTION

The cavus foot has long been a complex condition known to be associated with neurologic conditions—most commonly, Charcot-Marie-Tooth disease and other hereditary motor sensory neuropathies, poliomyelitis, spina bifida, myelomeningocele, Friedreich ataxia, and spinal cord lesions or tumors.[1] Cerebral palsy and post-cerebrovascular accident (stroke) represent spastic forms of cavus conditions. Trauma may also create the cavovarus condition. It includes trauma secondary to compartment syndrome, fracture malunions of the calcaneus and talar neck, as well as common peroneal nerve injury.

Another condition in recent years found to cause loss of foot and ankle equilibrium is the subtle cavus foot (SCF). This mild variation known to possibly represent the "cavus end" of the normal distribution curve for arch height is associated with a set of symptoms and complaints.[2] Commonly associated conditions include frequent ankle sprains of which 28% had underlying rearfoot varus;[3] frequent stress fractures of the fourth and fifth metatarsals; and peroneal tendinopathy, which involved 33% of

Foot and Ankle Surgery Residency, SSM Health DePaul Hospital, 12303 DePaul Drive, Suite 701, St Louis, MO 63044, USA
* Corresponding author.
E-mail address: hannanz93@gmail.com

Clin Podiatr Med Surg 38 (2021) 361–378
https://doi.org/10.1016/j.cpm.2021.02.003
0891-8422/21/© 2021 Elsevier Inc. All rights reserved.

patients with an underlying rearfoot varus.[4] Sesamoid injury, Achilles tendon pathology, and ankle impingement syndromes are also commonly noted (**Box 1**). First described by Manoli and Graham (1993),[5] SCF has been increasingly accepted to exist without an identifiable underlying neurologic deficit.[2] Thus it has become the "idiopathic" form of the cavus condition.[2] Manoli and colleagues (1993) did cite a genetic component with a familial inheritance pattern.[6] But the genetic determinants were poorly delineated. A preliminary study in a pedorthic practice consisting of a year-long patient log noted slightly more than half of all patients were fitted with cavus-correcting foot orthotics.[2]

Awareness of these conditions increases with experience, and this was found to be the case with the "too many toes sign" description by Johnson and Strom[7] for adult-acquired flat foot (**Fig. 1**A), as there are no reliable tests or classifications that can diagnose the SCF conditions objectively. The "peek-a-boo" heel sign has become a similar clinical finding (**Fig. 1**B).

PATHOMECHANICS

The loss of foot–driven equilibrium or cotton's static triangle of support (first, fifth metatarsal, heel)[8] relates to an "underpronator" described by Manoli and colleagues.[5,6] The Varus condition of rearfoot and thus arch elevation in the SCF may be either hindfoot driven or forefoot driven.

With normal biomechanical function of the gait cycle, there is an initial flexible phase at heel strike and forefoot load (pronation of the subtalar joint [STJ], oblique midtarsal joint [OMTJ], supination of longitudinal midtarsal joint [LMTJ], and it progresses to more rigid phase at toe off [STJ, OMTJ supination, pronation of LMTJ, plantarflexed first ray [metatarsus primus pronatus]). Rear foot–driven SCF is secondary to a malposition deriving from the calcaneus and/or STJ. Theories include aberrant bone morphology with the calcaneal tuberosity excessively medial to the long axis of the calcaneal body seen on a calcaneal axial radiographic view. Also, it may present as a calcaneal varus torque of the body of the calcaneus. It may also exist with malalignment at the STJ level including postintraarticular calcaneal fracture and talar neck fracture malunions, as well as tarsal coalitions. Sequela of deep posterior compartment syndrome or poliomyelitis may also lead to cause.[5,9,10]

Biomechanically the foot fails to pronate at heel contact and remains rigid at toe off thus described as the "underpronator." The forefoot initially flexible in its

---

Box 1
Conditions commonly associated with subtle cavus foot

Metatarsalgia

Stress fractures of the lateral metatarsals 4 and 5

Sesamoiditis/fractures

Peroneus longus/brevis tendinopathy and tears

Os peroneum syndrome

Recurrent ankle sprains/instability

Achilles insertional and noninsertional tendinopathy (Haglund syndrome)

Medial tibial stress syndrome

Medial malleolus stress fracture

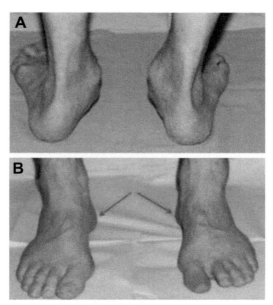

Fig. 1. (A) (*Top*) "Too many toes sign" of adult-acquired flatfoot deformity. (B) (*Bottom*) "Peek-a-boo" heel sign for subtle cavus foot deformity.

compensated pronated position becomes rigid over time.[11] The supinated STJ locks the calcaneocubid joint (OMTJ) and gives a distinct mechanical advantage to the peroneus longus to plantarflex the first ray and bring it to ground contact.

Forefoot-driven rearfoot varus in SCF relates to a flexible rearfoot compensating from a rigid plantarflexed first ray. Cause is unknown.[12] The first metatarsal contacts the ground before the rearfoot reaches full eversion. The first ray then acts as a "kickstand" and abbreviates the flexible pronatory phase of the gait cycle.[12] These factors of rearfoot or forefoot-driven rearfoot varus in SCF lead to loss of shock absorption. They increase eccentric boney loads and attenuate strain of the lateral foot and ankle soft tissue structures as well as the arthropathic lateral column.

Peroneal tendon overdrive involving the peroneus longus may also contribute to a rearfoot varus. With hyperactivity, the first ray locks the midfoot earlier in the gait cycle and swings the rearfoot into varus.[13] This condition associated with idiopathic cases demonstrated both histologic and MRI findings of peroneus longus muscle enlargement.[14] Halliwell and colleagues[14] concluded that in idiopathic forefoot pes cavus fiber hypertrophy of the peroneus longus relative to its antagonist the tibialis anterior may contribute to cavus deformity and increase the longitudinal arch height.[12]

Another pathomechanical property of the SCF is the ubiquitous presence of an isolated gastrocnemius contracture.[5] Coexistence of rearfoot varus and gastrocnemius equinus is not fully clear. However, with medial insertion of the Achilles tendon involving a rearfoot varus heel acts as a deforming inverting force that worsens the condition. The equinus condition of the ankle secondary to gastrocnemius tightness can allow a vector pull of the peroneus longus relative to the tibialis anterior, thus enhancing its mechanical advantage and allowing further flexion of the first ray **(Fig. 2)**.[5]

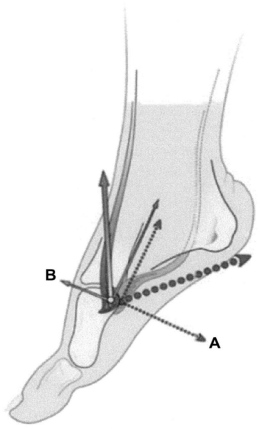

Fig. 2. Equinus causing an increase vector pull of the peroneus longus relative to tibialis anterior. (*From* Chilvers, M., & Manoli II, A., (2008). The Subtle Cavus Foot and Association with Ankle Instability and Lateral Foot Overload. *Foot and Ankle Clinics of North America*, *13*, 315–324, with permission.)

EVALUATION

Initial evaluation involves examination of the spine to rule out any evidence of a spinal dysraphism or myelodysplasia,[2] which includes presence of a nevus, hairy patch, or dimple at the lower lumbar level that would indicate posterior laminar insufficiency. Cystic structures may represent more ominous conditions such as the myelodysplasia: meningocele and myelomeningocele.

A neurologic examination is done of the lower extremity to detect any form of muscular imbalances. The medical research council muscle grading system is used. Sensory deficits and presence of spasticity, ataxia, or tremors are noted.

Next the patient's gait is examined and antalgia or aberrations are noted. The patient is then evaluated standing from the front. The presence of the peek-a-boo heel was first described as a sequela for compartment syndrome.[6,15] The medial heel when in neutral or a valgus position cannot be seen by viewing from the front. In patients who demonstrate a significant heel varus the medial heel will be clearly visible. In the SCF only the most medial edge will be visible (**Fig. 3**A). Also, a fold or bulge may be noted at the head of the first metatarsal during standing and front viewing (**Fig. 3**B).[11] When the patient is viewed from behind it is difficult to see any heel varus (**Fig. 3**C).

The Coleman block test (1977) is used to determine the flexibility of the rearfoot (**Fig. 4**).[16,17] A one-inch block is placed under the heel and lateral border of the foot. The first metatarsal is then dropped out. If the rearfoot corrects to 5° of valgus, then the rearfoot varus is forefoot driven by a rigidly plantarflexed first ray. Failure of the heel varus to reduce indicates a rearfoot-driven condition (**Fig. 5**).

The remaining examination is done in a seated position. The presence of an equinus is determined by the Silverskiöld test. Active dorsiflexion is assessed with the knee extended and flexed. Increased dorsiflexion with the knee flexed indicates a contracture of the gastrocnemius muscle. Subtalar joint range of motion and position is often done in a prone position. Failure of the STJ to evert to 6° valgus indicates restricted STJ motion and indicates a rearfoot-driven heel varus. If able to evert to 6° valgus, then the forefoot drives the heel varus.

The lateral ankle ligaments are evaluated for anterior drawer and talar tilt on ankle stress radiographs. Evaluation for peroneus longus overdrive is evaluated with the patient seated, knee extended, and the ankle maximally dorsiflexed (**Fig. 6**). One thumb is placed under the first metatarsal and the other thumb under the lesser metatarsals; the patient is then instructed to maximally plantarflex their foot against resistance. Increased and associated plantarflexion of the first ray indicates hyperactivity of the peroneus longus.[5,18]

DIAGNOSTIC IMAGING

There are no definite radiographic criteria for discriminating the SCF from other normal conditions. However, radiographic lateral views in weight-bearing stance can bear out subtle cavus parameters (**Fig. 7**).[19]

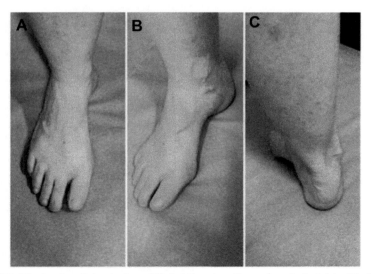

Fig. 3. (*A*) "Peek-a-boo" heel sign. (*B*) Subtle elevation of arch height. (*C*) Difficulty observing heel varus from behind.

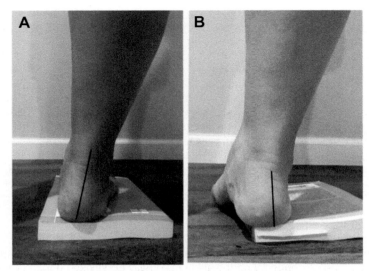

Fig. 4. (*A*) (*Left*) Heel varus position in relaxed calcaneal stance. (*B*) (*Right*) Reduction of heel varus to 6° of valgus with first metatarsal dropped off, incicating forefoot-driven hindfoot varus.

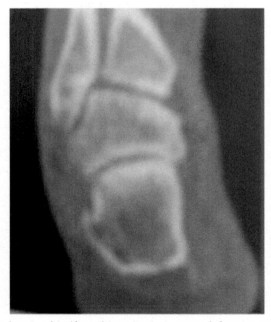

Fig. 5. Coronal CT showing hindfoot-driven intrinsic varus deformity. Note varus calcaneal position in reference to the tibia. CT, computed tomography.

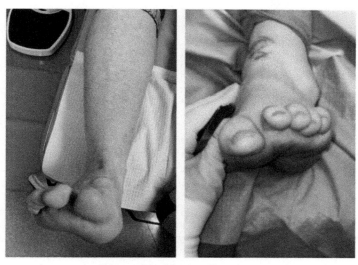

Fig. 6. Peroneus longus overdrive with ankle dorsiflexed at 90° and forefoot fully loaded noting increased plantarflexion of first metatarsal.

1. Meary's angle represents an intersection of a line through the long axis of the talus, and first metatarsal is normally 0° to 5°.[20] In the SCF Meary's angle is greater than 5° or negative.[21]
2. Arch height is another parameter noted in SCF greater than 14 mm the measurement from the medial cuneiform—first metatarsal to the fifth metatarsal.[22] Normal arch height is 10 mm. The metatarsals also appear in "stacked" conformation.[12]
3. Calcaneal inclination will just exceed 25° in normal foot and be at 30° for SCF.[23]
4. Posterior positioning of the fibula relative to the tibia (external rotation) overlaps the posterior one-third of the tibial shadow,[5,12] which was found to be 0.6 to 0.7 mm in a normal ankle and greater than 0.7 mm in an SCF. This measurement was noted by 2 parallel lines, articulation points of talus to tibia and talus to bisection of the fibula.[19]

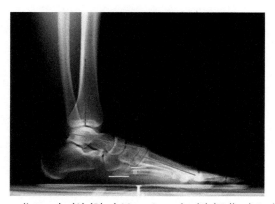

Fig. 7. Lateral view radiograph. (A) (*Blue*) Meary's angle. (B) (*Yellow*) Arch height. (C) (*Red*) Posterior positioning of fibula relative to tibia.

If there is loss of STJ motion, a computed tomography scan is advised to rule out tarsal coalition and/or intraarticular abnormality. An MRI is advised in cases of ankle instability, suspected peroneal tendon pathology, and intraarticular osteochondral lesions.

Associated Clinical Pathology

The SCF can present with a wide assortment of accompanying symptoms affecting the foot and ankle, such as stress fractures, lateral column overload, and peroneal and lateral ankle ligamentous pathology. These associated pathologies result from repetitive impact over many years.[12] This connection between arch height and overuse injuries in athletics has been established in the literature. In a 2001 study, Williams and colleagues surveyed 40 runners, 20 with high-arched feet and 20 with low-arched feet. In the study it was determined that the high-arched runners displayed a greater number of overall foot and ankle injuries. The high-arched runners also exhibited a greater incidence of lateral ankle injuries, whereas the low-arched runners had more knee injuries (Williams 2001).[24] This result was consistent with a previous study of running injuries summarized by van Mechelen.[25] A study of Army infantry recruits established a significant linear trend for an increased risk of injury with increasing arch height.[26] An association between high arches and an increased risk for incurring a stress fracture has also been established in 2 other prospective studies of military recruits.[27,28]

Patients with a cavus foot distribution walk with increased pressure to the lateral border of the foot as well as the plantarflexed first ray, which has been well established through pedobarographic studies.[29,30] There are no such similar studies available specific to the subtle pes cavus foot; however, it can be postulated that this abnormal joint pressure would continue to occur, albeit at a lesser extent.[12]

These pressure distributions will often lead to overload calluses under the first metatarsal head and the fifth metatarsal head or base (**Fig. 8**) and can further lead to hallux sesamoiditis as well as stress fractures of the fifth metatarsal.[31] Less commonly, stress fractures may be present to the other lesser metatarsals, especially at the base of the fourth metatarsal.[32] Patients may also present with a history of a Jones fracture to the fifth metatarsal, and this injury will commonly present as a chronic problem due to the uneven pressure distribution. Even after successful radiologic union of

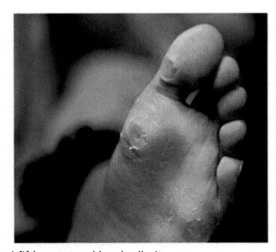

Fig. 8. Sub first and fifth metatarsal head callosity.

the fracture, those with an underlying cavus foot may continue to report pain over the fifth metatarsal if the greater deformity is not addressed.[2]

Associated peroneal tendon pathologies are common as well. These symptoms can include recurrent dislocation or subluxation, tendon splitting or inflammation, as well as an os peroneum that may also fracture resulting in increased pain.[33] In addition, an enlarged painful peroneal tubercle may be present to the lateral calcaneus.[5] A 2012 review of the surgical management of peroneal tendon pathology identified that 33% of the patients had an accompanying hindfoot varus deformity.[4,34] Because of the frequent association of SCF with a tight Achilles tendon as well as reduced shock absorption Achilles pathology as well as plantar fasciitis may develop.[25,35]

The calcaneal varus deformity may potentially lead to a prominence at the postero-lateral superior calcaneal tuberosity with retrocalcaneal bursitis or Haglund syndrome.[2] Other common presenting symptoms are ankle instability and recurrent sprains.[11] In a 2007 study of patients with chronic lateral ankle instability, undiagnosed hindfoot varus alignment abnormalities were identified in 28% of patients.[3] Chronic cases of ankle varus with resultant collateral ligament instability may also lead to ankle arthritis (**Fig. 9**).[31] More proximally, the decreased shock absorption of the pes cavus foot along with medial eccentric load can lead to a vertical stress fracture of the medial malleolus as well as tibial or fibular stress fractures.[5] In the knee, external rotation of the talus and tibia can result in pain along the lateral collateral ligament or iliotibial band.[31,36]

CONSERVATIVE CARE

Treatment of the SCF depends on the clinical findings as discussed earlier, as well as the symptomatology of the patient. As with any condition, conservative measures are the first line in treatment. Manoli discusses nonoperative treatment consisting of rigid orthoses. In cases of forefoot-driven SCF where the Coleman block test allows the calcaneus to become vertical or in valgus he describes the "cavus foot orthotic," which includes an elevated heel and cushion to accommodate a tight posterior muscle group. A cut-out under the first metatarsal head was made to accommodate the plantarflexed first ray to allow heel eversion.[5] A forefoot wedge that originates lateral to the first metatarsal recess extends to the lateral border to reenact forefoot pronation. A reduction in medial arch height is done to allow for hindfoot eversion with the case of a rearfoot-driven SCF. The medial arch height is accommodative, and there is

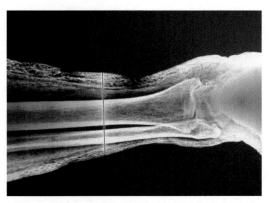

Fig. 9. Incongruous talar tilt secondary to long-standing lateral collateral ligament insufficiency.

the addition of a posterior lateral heel wedge.[5] Certainly, physical therapy involving posterior calf stretching along with the plantar fascia can be helpful; this is also done with intrinsic muscle strengthening.

SURGICAL TREATMENT

When considering surgical correction of the SCF it is advisable to work progressively from the ankle (equinus contracture), then to the rearfoot, and finally to the forefoot in the supine position. Maskill describes the technique by first addressing the equinus condition, and it is necessary to be repeated when the patient is under anesthesia. Paralyzing the patient may also prove helpful. The Silverskiöld test is performed and more reliable as the patient is relaxed. It is believed to be present when accommodated to the persistent varus position of the calcaneus. With a global contracture of gastrocnemius-soleus group, a Hoke percutaneous tendoachilles lengthening is performed (**Fig. 10**). More commonly only the gastrocnemius is contracted, and a recession is performed (**Fig. 11**).[18]

The Coleman block test, which is done preoperatively is then performed to assess the flexibility of the rearfoot. If the first metatarsal is dropped off the 1-inch block and noted correction of the heel to 5° valgus is demonstrated this represents a case of forefoot overdrive. The recommendation was a dorsiflexory wedge osteotomy of the first metatarsal (**Figs. 12** and **13**) or a first metatarsal-medial cuneiform arthrodesis.[1] In a 2010 study by Maskill and colleagues[18] who evaluated 29 feet with SCF and had persistent lateral pain after an ankle sprain found the rearfoot remained in varus with the block test. This meant that he found none of the patients went to 5° of valgus when the first metatarsal was dropped off the 1-inch block. He also found that 86% of patients after calcaneal osteotomy and equinus release required a peroneal switch procedure or first metatarsal osteotomy.

Ryssman and colleagues also thought the Coleman block test was used too frequently in planning treatment.[1] Their impression was that a first metatarsal osteotomy was rarely effective in correcting heel varus. Also, in none of those cases did the heel reduce to 5° of valgus with the block test. They performed posterior calcaneal osteotomy in all cases. Thus, if they had persistent heel varus (does not attain 5° of

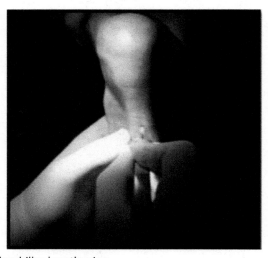

Fig. 10. Hoke tendoachilles lengthening.

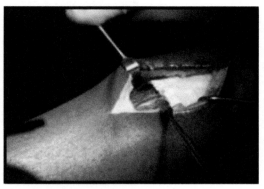

Fig. 11. Strayer gastrocnemius recession.

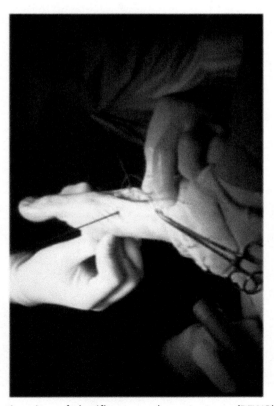

Fig. 12. Intraoperative view of dorsiflexory wedge osteotomy (DFWO). First metatarsal brought level with heel.

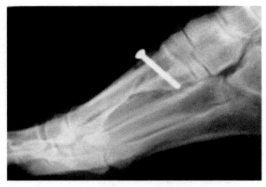

Fig. 13. Dorsiflexory wedge osteotomy (DFWO) fixated with screw.

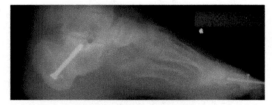

Fig. 14. Lateral displacement osteotomy of the calcaneus.

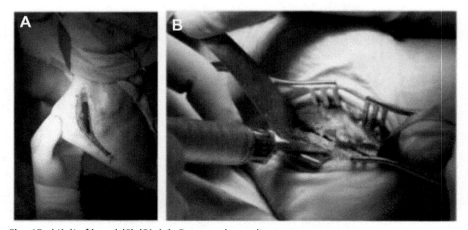

Fig. 15. (*A*) (*Left*) and (*B*) (*Right*): Dwyer calcaneal osteotomy.

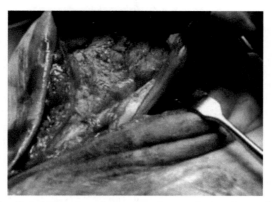

Fig. 16. "Peroneal switch." Transfer of peroneus longus to brevis proximal to the cuboid notch.

valgus with the Coleman block test) lateral displacement osteotomy of the calcaneus is performed (**Fig. 14**). The shift is normally 5 to 10 mm, with the goal to bring the heel in slight valgus.[18] Dwyer calcaneal osteotomy is also an option with a posterior calcaneal wedge resection (**Fig. 15**). This will bring the heel into slight valgus and "relax" the tarsal tunnel. It also serves to "relax" the plantar fascia. A plantar fascial release may be needed with a displacement osteotomy.

In the case of a rearfoot, heel varus most commonly is associated with a tarsal coalition. Resection of the coalition or arthrodesis of the STJ and possible double or triple

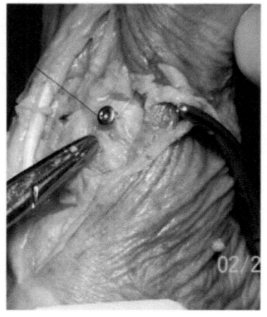

Fig. 17. Tension band screw fixation for first metatarsal elevational osteotomy.

arthrodesis may be required. Other forms of rearfoot-driven heel varus are also managed with posterior calcaneal osteotomy.

The next consideration is the forefoot, which is examined in the supine position with equinus and heel varus corrected. In approximately 14% of cases (Maskill and colleagues)[18] the first metatarsal fully reduces to a neutral position, and no surgery is required. If the first metatarsal is plantarflexed but can be reduced to neutral position at the level of metatarsals 2 to 5 then peroneal overdrive is present which indicates a flexible deformity. The flexible condition is then treated with a "peroneal switch" (**Fig. 16**) where the peroneus longus is transferred to the peroneus brevis. It is commonly done at the peroneal groove at the cuboid level. It can also be performed at the subtalar level above the peroneal/fibular groove, which serves to remove the plantarflexory force on the first metatarsal.[18]

If the first metatarsal remains plantarflexed then a rigid deformity exists. This deformity is managed by a first metatarsal dorsiflexory wedge osteotomy or first metatarsal-medial cuneiform arthrodesis, a condition where there is associated arthritis involving the joint or Meary's angle is slightly more proximal. It is normally a vertical osteotomy to allow adequate correction of the increased declination while limiting the amount of shortening. The dorsal proximal cortex is tamped down to prevent prominence and irritation. The wedge is sufficient to be brought level to the calcaneus. Fixation is a plate or a tension band screw (**Fig. 17**).

A hallux malleus may also be present secondary to weak tibialis anterior.[37] This can be managed by an interphalangeal fusion and transfer to the first metatarsal head (Jones procedure) or a flexor hallucis longus transfer to the proximal phalanx.[37] Ancillary procedures such as a Broström for lateral ankle instability, fixation of fourth or fifth metatarsal stress fractures, peroneal tendon repair, and others noted in **Box 1** may be considered.

Postoperative care based on the calcaneal and first metatarsal osteotomy is 4 weeks non–weight-bearing in a posterior splint followed by 4 weeks in a weight-bearing boot. An arthrodesis of the first metatarsal-medial cuneiform may require 6 weeks non–weight-bearing. Ancillary procedures normally fall in the similar time frame of weight-bearing and non–weight-bearing.

CASE STUDY

The association of the SCF and a secondary condition is manifested in a legal case where a 32-year-old white man gave a history of feeling a "pop" while standing on a

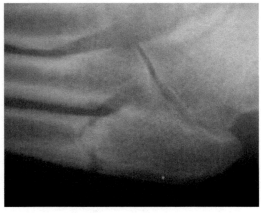

Fig. 18. Refracture of previously healed Jones fracture.

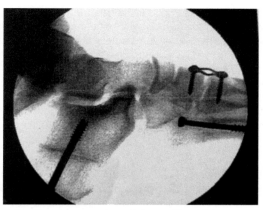

Fig. 19. Nonunion of the first metatarsal-medial cuneiform joint.

ladder doing home repair. This occurred when he went up on his toes to work on the ceiling. He had a history of a prior Jones fracture of the fifth metatarsal that had healed. The patient was 6 ft 0″ and 289 lbs. He reported to the emergency room and was diagnosed again with a Jones fracture of the fifth metatarsal.

The treating podiatric physician evaluated the radiograph and noted a refracture at the metaphyseal-diaphyseal location of the fifth metatarsal (**Fig. 18**). On examination he noted a "peek-a-boo" heel sign and a high arch indication of an SCF deformity. The surgeon then recommended a posterior calcaneal osteotomy and a first metatarsal-medial cuneiform arthrodesis along with a repair of the fifth metatarsal. The patient sought different opinions as to whether only the metatarsal fracture should be treated,

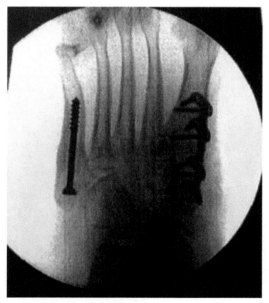

Fig. 20. Healed first metatarsal-medial cuneiform arthrodesis after third operation.

and opinions varied as to the best course of treatment. Unfortunately, he decided to proceed with the initial treating surgeon. The patient went on to a nonunion of the first metatarsal-medial cuneiform joint with complete healing of the calcaneal osteotomy and the jones fracture (**Fig. 19**). The nonunion required two further operations to attain an arthrodesis (**Fig. 20**).

As a result, the case went to litigation with the plaintiff's attorney arguing over aggressive and needless surgery. They argued only the Jones fracture should have been addressed. The defense countered with the supporting literature as well as the patient's deformity and weight. The verdict was for the defense and treating surgeon.

SUMMARY

The Subtle cavus foot deformity is an often-unrecognized condition when compared with the adult-acquired flatfoot. With the clinical finding of the "too many toes sign" it has become a commonly recognized condition. The peek-a-boo heel sign described by Manoli and Graham has become a clinical sign to present the nonneurologic SCF deformity. This deformity that causes an abnormality of foot and ankle equilibrium is associated with number of foot and ankle problems, including chronic lateral ankle instability, lateral foot column overload, peroneal tendinopathy, peroneal tendon subluxation, and chronic fifth metatarsal stress fractures to mention a few. Proper diagnosis is essential to allow better outcomes functionally while limiting associated perpetuation of the condition created by this deformity.

CLINICS CARE POINTS

- Lateral pedal pathology and ankle instability, peroneal tendinopathy, and stress fractures of metatarsal bases 4 and 5 warrant evaluations of the "peek-a-boo" heel sign (fixed calcaneal varus).
- Despite normal to mild high arch appearance of pedal structure, equinus associated with heel varus is a factor of deformity.
- Musculoskeletal unbalance without neurologic cause is central to the gastrocnemius and peroneal longus musculature.
- Heel varus generated from a plantarflexed first metatarsal nearly always requires calcaneal osteotomy.

DISCLOSURE

Dr H.H. Zahid and Dr N.J. Staub have no disclosures. Dr H.J. Visser, Dr. J.J. Visser, and Dr. B.R. Staples have no conflicts to disclose pertaining to this article.

REFERENCES

1. Ryssman DB, Myerson MS. Tendon transfers for adult flexible cavovarus foot. Foot Ankle Clin 2011;435–50.
2. Abbasian A, Pomeroy G. The idiopathic cavus foot - not so subtle after all. Foot Ankle Clin North Am 2013;18:629–42.
3. Strauss JE, Forsberg JA, Lippert FG III. Chronic lateral ankle instability and associated conditions: a rationale for treatment. Foot Ankle Int 2007;28(10):1041–4.
4. Grasset W, Mercier N, Chaussard C, et al. The surgical treatment of peroneal tendinopathy (excluding subluxations): a series of 17 patients. J Foot Ankle Surg 2012;51(1):13–9.

5. Manoli A II, Graham B. The subtle cavus foot, "the underpronator," a review. Foot Ankle Int 2005;26(3):256–63.
6. Manoli A II, Smith DG, Hansen ST Jr. Scarred muscle excision for the treatment of established ischemic contracture of the lower extremity. Clin Orthop 1993;292:309–14.
7. Johnson KA, Strom DE. Tibialis posterior tendon dysfunction. Clin Orthop Relat Res 1989;239:196–206.
8. Cotton FJ. Foot statistics and surgery. New Eng Surg Soc 1936;218(8):353–62.
9. Beals T, Bohay D, Lee C, Manoli A II: Tarsal coalitions presenting with cavovarus foot deformities. Presented at the Annual Meeting, American Orthopaedic Foot and Ankle Society, Fajardo, Puerto Rico, July 9–11, 1999. Level IV.
10. Solis G, Hennessy M, Saxby TS. Pes cavus: a review. Foot Ankle Surg 2000;6(3):145–53.
11. Chilvers M, Manoli A II. The subtle cavus foot and association with ankle instability and lateral foot overload. Foot Ankle Clin North Am 2008;13:315–24.
12. Pomeroy GC, Deben SE. Subtle cavus foot: diagnosis and management. J Am Acad Orthop Surg 2014;22:512–20.
13. Sammarco VJ. The talonavicular and calcaneocuboid joints: Anatomy, biomechanics, and clinical management of the transverse tarsal joint. Foot Ankle Clin 2004;9(1):127–45.
14. Helliwell TR, Tynan M, Hayward M, et al. The pathology of the lower leg muscles in pure forefoot pes cavus. Acta Neuropathol 1995;89(6):552–9.
15. Beals TC, Manoli A. The "peak-a-boo" heel sign in the evaluation of hindfoot varus. Foot 1996;6:205–6.
16. Coleman SS, Chesnut WJ. A simple test for hindfoot flexibility in the cavovarus foot. Clin Orthop 1977;123:60–2.
17. Kaplan J, Aiyer A, Cerrato RA, et al. Operative treatment of cavovarus foot. Foot Ankle Int 2018;39(11):1370–82.
18. Maskill MP, Maskill JD, Pomeroy GC. Surgical management and treatment Algorithm for the subtle cavovarus foot. Foot Ankle Int 2010;1057–63.
19. Lee D, Kim JH, Song SH, et al. Is Subtle cavus foot a risk factor for chronic ankle instability? Comparsion of prevalence of subtle cavus foot beteen chronic ankle instability and control group on the standing leateral radiograph. J Foot Ankle Surg 2019;26(8):907–10.
20. Steel MW III, Johnson KA, DeWitz MA, et al. Radiogrpahic measurements of the normal adult foot. Foot Ankle 1980;1(3):151–8.
21. Younger AS, Hansen ST Jr. Adult cavovarus foot. J Am Acad Orthop Surg 2005;13(5):302–15.
22. Ledoux WR, Shofer JB, Ahroni JH, et al. Biomechanical differences among pes cavus, neutrally aligned, and pes planus feet in subjects with diabetes. Foot Ankle Int 2003;24(11):845–50.
23. Eleswarapu AS, Yamini B, Bielski RJ. Evaluating the cavus foot. Pediatr Ann 2016;45(6):e218–22.
24. Williams DS III, McClay IS, Hamill J. Arch structure and injury patterns in runners. Clin Biomech (Bristol, Avon) 2001;16(4):341–7.
25. van Mechelen W. Running injuries: a review of the epidemiological literature. Sports Med 1992;12:320±35.
26. Cowan DN, Jones BH, Robinson JR. Foot morphologic characteristics and risk of exercise-related injury. Arch Fam Med 1993;2(7):773–7.
27. Simkin A, Leichter I, Giladi M, et al. Combined effect of foot arch structure and an orthotic device on stress fractures. Foot Ankle 1989;10:25–9.

28. Kaufman KR, Brodine SK, Shaffer RA, et al. The effect of foot structure and range of motion on musculoskeletal overuse injuries. Am J Sports Med 1999;27(5): 585–93.

29. Metaxiotis D, Accles W, Pappas A, et al. Dynamic pedobarography (DPB) in operative management of cavovarus foot deformity. Foot Ankle Int 2000;21(11): 935–47.

30. Nyska M, Shabat S, Simkin A, et al. Dynamic force distribution during level walking under the feet of patients with chronic ankle instability. Br J Sports Med 2003;37(6):495–7.

31. Desai SN, Grierson R, Manoli A 2nd. The cavus foot in athletes: Fundamentals of examination and treatment. Oper Tech Sports Med 2010;18(1):27–33.

32. Saxena A, Krisdakumtorn T, Erickson S. Proximal fourth metatarsal fractures in athletes: similarity to proximal fifth metatarsal injury. Foot Ankle Int 2001;22:603–8.

33. Brandes CB, Smith RW. Characterization of patients with primary peroneus longus tendinopathy: a review of twenty-two cases. Foot Ankle Int 2000;21:462–8.

34. Carlson RE, Fleming LL, Hutton WC. The biomechanical relationship between the tendoachilles, plantar fascia and metatarsophalangeal joint dorsiflexion angle. Foot Ankle Int 2000;21(1):18–25.

35. McKenzie DC, Clement DB, Taunton JE. Running shoes, orthotics, and injuries. Sports Med 1985;2:334–47.

36. Renne JW. The iliotibial band friction syndrome. J Bone Joint Surg Am 1975;57: 1110–1.

37. Ortiz C, Wagner E, Keller A. Cavovarus reconstruction. Foot Ankle Clin North Am 2009;14:471–87.

Use of Calcaneal Osteotomies in the Correction of Inframalleolar Cavovarus Deformity

Jesse R. Wolfe, DPM, AACFAS[a],*, Tyler D. McKee, DPM, AACFAS[b],
Melinda Nicholes, DPM[c,d]

KEYWORDS

- Pes cavus • Cavovarus deformity • Calcaneal osteotomy • Hind-foot alignment
- Joint-preserving surgery

KEY POINTS

- Cavovarus resulting in hind-foot deformity may be neurologic, posttraumatic, or iatrogenic in nature.
- Weight-bearing radiographs are necessary in determining procedure selection.
- Correction of inframalleolar deformity should focus on joint-preservation techniques with an emphasis on evaluation of subtalar joint and calcaneocuboid joint positioning.
- Multiple osteotomies have been described providing uniplanar, biplanar, and triplanar correction. Careful evaluation of pathologic condition is necessary in determining appropriate surgical planning and treatment course.

INTRODUCTION

Cavovarus deformity provides a challenging and complex condition for the foot and ankle surgeon, affecting 20% to 25% of the population.[1,2] In treating patients with cavovarus deformity, a thorough evaluation of the patient with a biomechanical emphasis should be performed. The cavovarus deformity is the result of a varus heel position with pronation of the first ray in stance resulting in a forefoot equinus and high longitudinal plantar arch.[3] Because of the complex nature of the forefoot and hind-foot relationship, cavovarus deformity may be the result of forefoot deformity, hind-foot deformity, or a combination of both.[3] As these deformities progress, osteoarticular malalignment secondary to intrinsic and extrinsic imbalances results in overall deformity.

[a] Northwest Iowa Bone, Joint, & Sports Surgeons, 1200 1st Avenue E, Suite C, Spencer, IA 51301, USA; [b] American Health Network Foot & Ankle Reconstructive Surgery Fellowship, 12188B North Meridian Street, Suite #330, Carmel, IN 46032, USA; [c] SSM Health DePaul Hospital Foot and Ankle Surgery Residency, St Louis, MO, USA; [d] SSM Health DePaul Hospital, 12303 DePaul Drive, Bridgeton, MO 63044, USA
* Corresponding author.
E-mail address: jwolfe@nwiabone.com

Clin Podiatr Med Surg 38 (2021) 379–389
https://doi.org/10.1016/j.cpm.2021.03.002
0891-8422/21/© 2021 Elsevier Inc. All rights reserved.
podiatric.theclinics.com

Understanding the etiologic factors of cavovarus is prudent. Neurologic, posttraumatic, or idiopathic pathologic conditions are common and should be thoroughly evaluated. Neurologic conditions tend to be the most common, and the 3 primary conditions resulting in cavovarus deformity include Charcot-Marie-Tooth (CMT) disease, cerebral palsy, and poliomyelitis.[2] In the presence of hereditary motor and sensory neurologic conditions, such as CMT disease, bilateral cavovarus deformity is often observed.[4] This imbalance affects the peroneal brevis musculature, causing a compensatory mechanism. In CMT, overdrive of the peroneal longus tendon with concomitant plantarflexion of the first ray drives a subtle varus heel position, as noted in **Fig. 1**. The forefoot driven deformity can be carefully evaluated through the previously described Coleman block test, where restoration of the hind-foot alignment is demonstrative of a reducible deformity where joint-preserving osteotomies are beneficial.

Unilateral cavovarus deformity typically occurs secondary to neurologic, posttraumatic, or idiopathic conditions. Two common neurologic conditions of consideration include cerebral palsy and poliomyelitis. In the case of cerebral palsy, deep flexor musculature spasticity secondary to upper-motor neuron deficiencies results in a severely plantar-flexed cavovarus deformity and can often be identified at an early age as a child with toe-walking. Other neurologic diseases, including poliomyelitis, spinal dysraphism, and intraspinal causes, often present unilaterally with radiographic findings of a severe calcaneal inclination angle, hyper-plantarflexion of the lesser metatarsals with posterior displacement of the fibula secondary to external rotation of the tibia.[5] This deformity results in a horizontal posterior facet with double density of the talar dome within the ankle mortise, as noted in **Fig. 2**.

Cavovarus deformity secondary to posttraumatic injuries is commonly the result of reduction malalignment, and this tends to be the case whereby comminution is present along the medial aspect of the talar neck or in intra-articular joint depression calcaneal fractures and has been well described in the literature.[6–21] Other causes of consideration include tarsal coalition, limb-length discrepancy, subtalar arthritis,

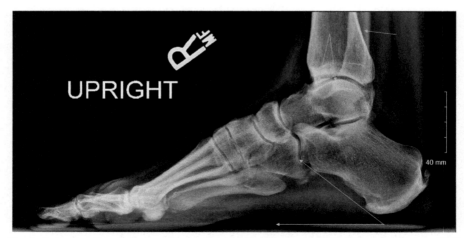

UPRIGHT

40 mm

Fig. 1. Lateral radiograph view of a patient with a cavovarus deformity secondary to CMT disease, with radiographic features, including mild posterior displacement of the fibula secondary to external rotation of the ankle mortise, double density of the talar dome with significant calcaneal inclination angle.

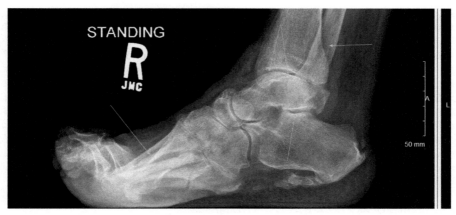

Fig. 2. Lateral radiographic view of a patient with a history of poliomyelitis presenting with a hind-foot cavovarus deformity as demonstrated with external rotation of the ankle noted by posterior displacement of the fibula, hyperflexion of the lesser metatarsals, and horizontal presentation of the posterior facet with double density of the talar dome.

or spasticity. In some cases, no underlying cause can be identified, resulting in an idiopathic cavovarus deformity.

The purpose of this article is to address inframalleolar cavovarus deformity with an emphasis on radiographic evaluation for joint-preserving calcaneal osteotomy techniques.

PREOPERATIVE EVALUATION

On evaluation of a patient with a suspected cavovarus deformity, a thorough history and physical examination are imperative in determining the cause of the deformity. Discussion with the patient on the deformity characteristics is essential. In the case of a progressively worsening deformity, timing of when the deformity initially occurred is prudent in ascertaining the specific pathologic condition involved. In the case of Hereditary Motor Sensory Neuropathy (HMSN), variable penetrance of disease progression and variable age of disease onset occur. Discussion with the patient on likelihood for worsening of the condition should be performed as well as the possibility of future surgery, which may be required.

IMAGING

Standard bilateral 3-view weight-bearing radiographs and long tibia calcaneal axial views are essential in the evaluation of the inframalleolar cavovarus deformity. Identifying the center of rotation of angulation (CORA) is necessary when determining the level of involvement of the cavovarus deformity. This level of deformity often occurs at the Chopart joint and is best visualized on the lateral radiograph. If a more proximal deformity is present, further evaluation of supramalleolar cavovarus deformity should be performed. In the case of inframalleolar deformity, standard radiographic assessments are helpful in identifying the level of deformity as well as uniplanar, biplanar, or triplanar involvement. Key identifying features include a Meary angle of 18°, a Hibbs angle of 90°, and a calcaneal pitch of greater than 30°.[5,22]

Two additional radiographic tools can be beneficial when evaluating the severity of a cavus deformity: evaluation of the length of the lateral column on the lateral radiographic view and evaluation of the posterior facet on weight-bearing computed tomography (CT).[3] The calcaneocuboid joint acts as the CORA in evaluation of surgical correction for the hind-foot deformity through either joint-preserving calcaneal osteotomies or shortening calcaneocuboid arthrodesis.[2] Following correction of the deformity, a reduction of the calcaneocuboid joint can be noted with a decreased calcaneal inclination angle. Because of recent advances with weight-bearing CT, a screw-shaped morphology has been described of the subtalar joint with the posterior facet presenting neutral, with a progressive worsening varus position of the middle and anterior facet on serial images.[3] Although the relationship is not fully understood, screw-shaped morphology secondary to subtalar joint compensation is thought to correlate with supramalleolar deformity, and further evaluation should be performed to determine the appropriate level of correction.[3,23–27]

INFRAMALLEOLAR CALCANEAL OSTEOTOMIES

Several inframalleolar calcaneal osteotomies have been described resulting in uniplanar, biplanar, or triplanar correction.

Uniplanar Osteotomies

Posterior displacement osteotomy

Historically used in cases of anterior poliomyelitis deformity, the posterior displacement osteotomy is used to increase the lever arm of the Achilles tendon.[28] Since the near eradication of poliomyelitis, the posterior displacement osteotomy has rarely been documented.

The osteotomy is performed through a lateral approach, whereby a plantar release of the soft tissues to the calcaneal tubercles should be performed. Next, an oblique transverse osteotomy of the calcaneus is made, allowing for displacement of the posterior fragment superiorly and posteriorly restoring the lateral column length in the sagittal plane.[28]

Dwyer osteotomy

When the heel is in a varus position with frontal plane involvement, the Achilles tendon becomes an inverter, resulting in contracture of the plantar fascia and adduction of the forefoot.[29] The Dwyer osteotomy is a useful correction technique in restoring the Achilles tendon from an inverter to a neutral position as well as overall hind-foot position under the tibia.

When performing a Dwyer osteotomy, a curved incision is made over the lateral calcaneal tuberosity with dissection carried to the periosteum. In the original description, Dwyer[29] recommended a subcutaneous division of the plantar fascia in order to reduce contraction of the forefoot. Following a plantar fascia release, the tendon of the peroneus longus is exposed and used as a guide to create an 8- to 12-mm closing wedge osteotomy proximal and parallel to the tendon. The osteotomy is tapered and passed through the medial cortex to ensure adequate closure of the osteotomy. Once the wedge is removed, the forefoot is pressed into dorsiflexion to allow for reduction of the osteotomy.[29] One additional benefit of the Dwyer osteotomy is the large contact surface available for fixation and stabilization of the osteotomy site.[30]

On an important note, overshortening the Dwyer osteotomy can result in an antalgic gait. If the calcaneus is significantly shortened, the lever arm of the Achilles tendon is decreased, resulting in weak plantarflexion. Appropriate shortening of the calcaneus may be advantageous to the patient, as this results in lateral column shortening, a decrease in arch height, and a natural lengthening of the Achilles tendon.[31,32] When performing the Dwyer osteotomy, a surgeon pearl includes performing the osteotomy anteriorly, allowing a large degree of correction because of the osteotomy being closer to the apex of the deformity.[33]

Lateralizing Osteotomies

A lateralizing osteotomy also allows for further correction of hind-foot varus deformity in the transverse plane by increasing ground reactive forces to the lateral aspect of the heel. Although it is a simple oblique osteotomy that helps to maintain calcaneal length,[30] there is a limited amount of translation able to be achieved by the calcaneus because of soft tissue restrictions. In addition, as the posterior aspect of the calcaneus is translated laterally, the inverter force becomes restored in a more neutral alignment. An important surgeon recommendation when performing a lateralizing calcaneal osteotomy is if significant translation is being required, careful evaluation of the neurovascular soft tissues should be performed.[34–36]

Biplanar Osteotomies

When the Dwyer and lateralizing osteotomy is used in combination, the osteotomy provides a biplanar correction in the frontal and transverse plane. The biplane correction osteotomy is useful in the HMSN cavovarus deformity where forefoot overdrive is the underlying result of the hind-foot varus deformity.[30]

Triplanar Osteotomy

Z-osteotomy

Although the Z-osteotomy is a more technically demanding technique, it allows for powerful triplane correction while maintaining a large contact surface across the osteotomy site to increase stability.[2,30,37] The osteotomy is performed with a horizontal orientation to the lateral aspect of the calcaneus, parallel to the weight-bearing surface. Vertical osteotomies are placed on either side of the horizontal osteotomy. Here, the anterior osteotomy purchases the plantar cortex directly in front of the tubercle. Next, the posterior osteotomy purchases the dorsal cortex in the concavity of the tuberosity. An osseous wedge is then removed, allowing for triplanar correction, which is achieved through translation of the calcaneal tuber in the transverse plane, rotational correction in the frontal plane, and shortening for correction in the sagittal plane.[31] Cavovarus deformity has been recognized as a triplanar deformity, and in the case of non-HMSN, severe calcaneal inclination is often present and the Z-osteotomy provides powerful correction.

Percutaneous Osteotomies

For patients at risk of wound dehiscence or with poor vasculature blood flow, percutaneous osteotomies may be a viable option. The osteotomy can be created through multiple perforations of the cortex or through the use of a Gigli as has been previously described.[38] The use of a burr allows for a controlled corticotomy that helps to minimize the amount of soft tissue contact, potential tissue damage, and periosteal stripping.[38] Use of an external fixator device may be applied following a percutaneous osteotomy in order to allow for triplanar correction without overall shortening of the foot.[39–42]

When evaluating minimally invasive calcaneal osteotomy versus open calcaneal osteotomy techniques, studies have demonstrated minimally invasive osteotomies have a mean displacement of 9.4 mm, whereas open techniques provide 10.2 mm of correction.[38,43] An additive benefit of the minimally invasive osteotomy technique includes a decreased complication rate in both patient hospitalization and decreased postoperative infections.[38,43] In addition, multiple studies have shown open procedures to have a higher risk for damage to the sural nerve.[43–47]

SURGEON PEARLS

Calcaneal osteotomies in the correction of cavovarus deformity have been demonstrated as a useful technique. Considerations should be made in regards to the adjacent neurovascular structures. In the authors' experience, consideration of the following surgical pearls may be beneficial in order to achieve satisfactory outcomes.

Neurovascular Compromise

Cavovarus deformity of the hind foot often presents as a long-standing deformity. Because of this, the amount of lateral translation required to correct the deformity may be significant. In cases of severe cavovarus deformity, lateralizing calcaneal osteotomies pose a risk to injuring the medial neurovascular bundle. A prophylactic tarsal tunnel release may be required as an adjunctive procedure to mitigate an iatrogenic neurovascular complication. When performing the calcaneal osteotomy, the authors recommend using a saw and osteotome technique. This technique is performed using subperiosteal dissection whereby the sagittal saw is used for the initial two-thirds of the osteotomy. The osteotomy should then be completed using an osteotome and mallet with care taken to not injure the medial neurovascular bundle.

Evaluating Equinus Deformity for Concomitant Achilles Lengthening

Following completion of the osteotomy, proximal retraction of the calcaneal tuber is likely to occur secondary to the shortened Achilles tendon. The equinus deforming force should be evaluated preoperatively, and in cases whereby the ankle dorsiflexion is unable to achieve a neutral position, an Achilles tendon-lengthening procedure should be performed. Another surgical pearl includes using a sterile triangle intraoperatively to provide flexion on the knee when completing the osteotomy and during lateral translation of the calcaneal tuber to prevent proximal displacement of the calcaneus.

When fixating the calcaneal osteotomy, a rigid stable construct should be used. Because of the inverter deforming force of the Achilles tendon in cavovarus deformity, 2 points of fixation should be performed to prevent an inadvertent frontal plane malalignment of the calcaneal osteotomy. The rotational force of the Achilles tendon is particularly worrisome in the isolated lateralizing calcaneal osteotomy.

Surgical Templating for Lateralizing Calcaneal Osteotomies

When assessing calcaneal osteotomy correction, evaluation of the plane involvement of the cavovarus deformity should be performed. A wide variety of heel osteotomies exist for the correction of the varus hind foot. The primary goal is to appropriately place the heel underneath the weight-bearing surface along the middiaphyseal line of the tibia.[29,33,48–53]

A common concern among new surgeons is determining the appropriate size wedge resection for the lateralizing calcaneal osteotomy. If undercorrection occurs, residual cavovarus deformity persists, whereas if overcorrected, excessive shortening of the calcaneus and valgus deformity may occur. Templating for calcaneal osteotomies has been previously described as a helpful technique in order to estimate level of deformity correction required; however, it has been

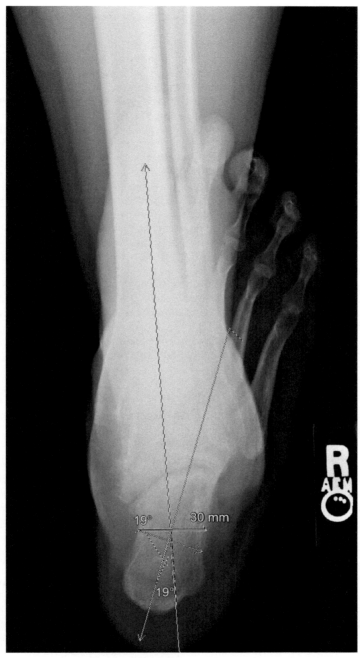

Fig. 3. Evaluation of cortical resection when performing Dwyer calcaneal osteotomy. The CORA of the calcaneus is identified through bisection of the tibia and bisection of the calcaneal tuber providing the angle of deformity correction required ($\alpha°$). A perpendicular line to the bisection of the tibia is made at the CORA level. The width of the calcaneus is measured (y) and through establishing a right triangle, an equation using the law of tangents $x = y(\tan(\alpha°))$ allows for an estimation of the amount of cortical resection to achieve adequate

described as less useful because of the difficulty in reproducing intraoperative results.[33,54,55]

Following evaluation of the patient for a calcaneal osteotomy, the corresponding author (J.W.) recommends a 2-pin technique in order to determine the appropriate placement of the osteotomy as well as the level of osseous wedge resection.[33] The corresponding author (J.W.) presents a modification of the 2-pin technique in order to assist newer surgeons in appropriate osseous wedge resection in a lateralizing calcaneal osteotomy through prudent evaluation of the calcaneal CORA.

First, a long leg calcaneal axial view should be obtained whereby a parallel line through the bisection of the tibia extending through the calcaneus is made using standard radiographic software. Next, a bisection line should be created through the calcaneal tuber extending into the posterior facet. The angular relationship between the bisection of the tibia and the bisection of the calcaneus is used to determine the degree of deformity correction required and represents the CORA of the calcaneal varus deformity ($\alpha°$). This angle relationship can also be measured through standard radiographic software. Second, a perpendicular line to the bisection of the tibia is made between the medial and lateral wall of the calcaneus at the calcaneal CORA; this allows for measuring the width of the calcaneus (y).

When performing the osteotomy intraoperatively, the placement of the second pin will establish a right triangle with 3 known values: the width of the calcaneus in millimeters (y), the angle necessary for correction of the calcaneal varus deformity ($\alpha°$), and the formation of a 90° triangle (**Fig. 3**).

The width of cortical resection necessary for adequate correction can be closely estimated through the trigonometry law of tangents, whereas

$$Tan\ (\alpha) = \frac{x}{y}$$

Therefore, the amount of cortical wedge resection can be estimated through the following equation:

$$x = y(Tan\ (\alpha))$$

By using the above equation, the surgeon can appropriately determine the amount of cortical resection and placement of the second pin for appropriate correction of the deformity. Intraoperatively, the 2 pins act as a cut guide when performing the Dwyer osteotomy. Further studies should be performed in order to assist in determining the reproducibility of deformity correction using the above equation, and to the corresponding author's (J.W.) knowledge, no other studies have used the described equation when performing a Dwyer lateralizing calcaneal osteotomy.

In summary, cavovarus deformity presents a challenge to the physician in cause as well as in biomechanical correction. In young and active patients, joint preservation surgery is recommended in the case of nonrigid deformity and often involves both soft tissue and osseous procedures.[2] In the case of neurologic conditions, progression of deformity is likely to occur because of continued progression of the disease process, and patient education is paramount on the

---

correction of the deformity. In the example, a 19° varus deformity is observed. At the level of the CORA, the calcaneus measures 30 mm. Therefore, the estimated amount of cortical resection would be 30(tan (19°)), or 10.32 mm.

necessity for future surgical procedures. Inframalleolar osteotomies in the cavovarus deformity prove to be a useful joint-sparing technique and following clinical and radiographic evaluation prove helpful in restoration of hind-foot alignment, reducing pain and instability.

CLINICS CARE POINTS

1. Equinus deformity correction should be addressed before a performing a calcaneal osteotomy to reduce proximal migration of the calcaneal osteotomy.
2. Two-screw fixation across the calcaneal osteotomy should be used to prevent frontal plane rotation of the calcaneal osteotomy.
3. Evaluation of forefoot-driven pathologic condition using the Coleman block test is pertinent to appropriately addressing hind-foot cavovarus deformity in determining procedure selection.

DISCLOSURE

The authors have no disclosures.

REFERENCES

1. Aminian A, Sangeorzan BJ. The anatomy of cavus foot deformity. Foot Ankle Clin 2008;13(2):191–8.
2. Usuelli FG, Manzi L. Inframalleolar varus deformity: role of calcaneal osteotomies. Foot Ankle Clin 2019;24(2):219–37.
3. Krähenbühl N, Weinberg MW. Anatomy and biomechanics of cavovarus deformity. Foot Ankle Clin 2019;24(2):173–81.
4. Nagai MK, Chan G, Guille JT, et al. Prevalence of Charcot-Marie-Tooth disease in patients who have bilateral cavovarus feet. J Pediatr Orthop 2006;26(4):438–43.
5. Akoh CC, Phisitkul P. Clinical examination and radiographic assessment of the cavus foot. Foot Ankle Clin 2019;24(2):183–93.
6. Calvert E, Younger A, Penner M. Post talus neck fracture reconstruction. Foot Ankle Clin 2007;12(1):137–51.
7. Rammelt S, Zwipp H. Talar neck and body fractures. Injury 2009;40(2):120–35.
8. Suter T, Barg A, Knupp M, et al. Talar neck osteotomy to lengthen the medial column after a malunited talar neck fracture. Clin Orthop Relat Res 2013;471:1356–64.
9. Hawkins LG. Fractures of the neck of the talus. J Bone Joint Surg Am 1970;52(5):991–1002.
10. Canale ST, Kelly FB Jr. Fractures of the neck of the talus. Long-term evaluation of seventy-one cases. J Bone Joint Surg Am 1978;60(2):143–56.
11. Rammelt S, Winkler J, Heineck J, et al. Anatomical reconstruction of malunited talus fractures: a prospective study of 10 patients followed for 4 years. Acta Orthop 2005;76(4):588–96.
12. Rammelt S, Winkler J, Grass R, et al. Reconstruction after talar fractures. Foot Ankle Clin 2006;11(1):612–84.
13. Huang PJ, Cheng YM. Delayed surgical treatment of neglected or mal-reduced talar fractures. Int Orthop 2005;29(5):326–9.
14. Fortin PT, Balazsy JE. Talus fractures: evaluation and treatment. J Am Acad Orthop Surg 2001;9(2):114–27.
15. Monrole MT, Manoli A. Osteotomy for malunion of a talar neck fracture: a case report. Foot Ankle Int 1999;20(3):192–5.

16. Sproule J, Glazebrook M, Younger A. Varus hindfoot deformity after talar fracture. Foot Ankle Clin N Am 2012;17(1):117–25.

17. Sangeorzan BJ, Wagner UA, Harrington RM, et al. Contact characteristics of the subtalar joint: the effect of talar neck misalignment. J Orthop Res 1992;10(4): 544–51.

18. Daniels T, Smith J, Ross T. Varus malalignment of the talar neck. J Bone Joint Surg 1996;78A(10):1559–67.

19. Barg A, Suter T, Nickisch F, et al. Osteotomies of the talar neck for posttraumatic malalignment. Foot Ankle Clin N Am 2016;21(1):77–93.

20. Matsumara T, Sekiya H, Hoshino Y. Correction osteotomy for malunion of the talar head: a case report. J Orthop Surg 2008;16(1):96–8.

21. Younger AS, Hansen ST Jr. Adult cavovarus foot. J Am Acad Orthop Surg 2005; 13(5):302–15.

22. Neumann JA, Nickisch F. Neurologic disorders and cavovarus deformity. Foot Ankle Clin 2019;24(2):195–203.

23. Krähenbühl N, Tschuck M, Bolliger L, et al. Orientation of the subtalar joint: measurement and reliability using weightbearing CT scans. Foot Ankle Int 2016;37(1): 109–14.

24. Krähenbühl N, Horn-Lang T, Hintermann B, et al. The subtalar joint: a complex mechanism. EFORT open Rev 2017;2(7):309–16.

25. Krähenbühl N, Siegler L, Deforth M, et al. Subtalar joint alignment in ankle osteoarthritis. Foot Ankle Surg 2019;25(2):143–9.

26. Wang B, Saltzman CL, Chalayon O, et al. Does the subtalar joint compensate for ankle malalignment in end-stage ankle arthritis? Clin Orthop Relat Res 2015; 473(1):318–25.

27. Burssens A, Peeters J, Buedts K, et al. Measuring hindfoot alignment in weight bearing CT: a novel clinical relevant measurement method. Foot Ankle Surg 2016;22(4):233–8.

28. Mitchell GP. Posterior displacement osteotomy of the calcaneus. J Bone Joint Surg Br 1977;59(2):233–5.

29. Dwyer FC. Osteotomy of the calcaneum for pes cavus. J Bone Joint Surg Br 1959;41(1):80–6.

30. Cody EA, Kraszewski AP, Conti MS, et al. Lateralizing calcaneal osteotomies and their effect on calcaneal alignment: a three-dimensional digital model analysis. Foot Ankle Int 2018;39(8):970–7.

31. Bariteau JT, Blankenhorn BD, Tofte JN, et al. What is the role and limit of calcaneal osteotomy in the cavovarus foot? Foot Ankle Clin 2013;18(4):697–714.

32. Kraus JC, Fischer MT, McCormick JJ, et al. Geometry of the lateral sliding, closing wedge calcaneal osteotomy: review of the two methods and technical tip to minimize shortening. Foot Ankle Int 2014;35(3):238–42.

33. Lamm BM, Gesheff MG, Salton HL, et al. Preoperative planning and intraoperative technique for accurate realignment of the Dwyer calcaneal osteotomy. J Foot Ankle Surg 2012;51(6):743–8.

34. Bruce BG, Bariteau JT, Evangelista PE, et al. The effect of medial and lateral calcaneal osteotomies on the tarsal tunnel. Foot Ankle Int 2014;35(4):383–8.

35. VanValkenburg S, Hsu RY, Palmer DS, et al. Neurologic deficit associated with lateralizing calcaneal osteotomy for cavovarus foot correction. Foot Ankle Int 2016; 37(10):1106–12.

36. Stødle AH, Molund M, Nilsen F, et al. Tibial nerve palsy after lateralizing calcaneal osteotomy. Foot Ankle Spec 2019;12(5):426–31.

37. Knupp M, Horisberger M, Hintermann B. A new z-shaped calcaneal osteotomy for 3-plane correction of severe varus deformity of the hindfoot. Tech Foot Ankle Surg 2008;7(2):90–5.

38. Kendal AR, Khalid A, Ball T, et al. Complications of minimally invasive calcaneal osteotomy versus open osteotomy. Foot Ankle Int 2015;36(6):685–90.

39. Hani EM. Assessment of percutaneous V osteotomy of the calcaneus with Ilizarov application for correction of complex foot deformities. Acta Orthop Belg 2004;70: 586–90.

40. Kocaoğlu M, Eralp L, Atalar AC, et al. Correction of complex foot deformities using the Ilizarov external fixator. J Foot Ankle Surg 2002;41(1):30–9.

41. Paley D. Principles of foot deformity corrections. In: Gould JS, editor. Operative foot surgery. Philadelphia: Saunders; 1994. p. 476–514.

42. Suresh S, Ahmed A, Sharma VK. Role of Joshi's external stabilisation system fixator in the management of idiopathic clubfoot. J Orthop Surg 2003;11(2): 194–201.

43. Gutteck N, Zeh A, Wohlrab D, et al. Comparative results of percutaneous calcaneal osteotomy in correction of hindfoot deformities. Foot Ankle Int 2019;40(3): 276–81.

44. Myerson MS, Badekas A, Schon LC. Treatment of stage II posterior tibial tendon deficiency with flexor digitorum longus tendon transfer and calcaneal osteotomy. Foot Ankle Int 2004;25(7):445–50.

45. Catanzariti AR, Lee MS, Mendicino RW. Posterior calcaneal displacement osteotomy for adult acquired flatfoot. J Foot Ankle Surg 2000;39(1):2–14.

46. Eastwood DM, Atkins RM. Lateral approaches to the heel A comparison of two incisions for the fixation of calcaneal fractures. Foot 1992;2(3):143–7.

47. Wacker JT, Hennessy MS, Saxby TS. Calcaneal osteotomy and transfer of the tendon of flexor digitorum longus for stage-II dysfunction of tibialis posterior: three-to five-year results. J Bone Joint Surg Br 2002;84(1):54–8.

48. Ayres MJ, Bakst RH, Baskwill DF, et al. Dwyer osteotomy: a retrospective study. J Foot Surg 1987;26(4):322–8.

49. Gleich A. Beitrag zur operation plattfuss behandlung. Arch Klin Chir 1893;46:358.

50. Schouwenaars B, Fabry G. Dwyer-osteotomy of the calcaneus: indications, literature review and follow-up study. Acta Orthop Belg 1979;45(4):446–58.

51. Weseley MS, Barenfeld PA. Mechanism of the Dwyer calcaneal osteotomy. Clin Orthop Relat Res 1970;70:137–40.

52. Bremer SW. The unstable ankle mortise–functional ankle varus. J Foot Surg 1985; 24(5):313–7.

53. Kleiger B, Mankin HJ. A roentgenographic study of the development of the calcaneus by means of the posterior tangential view. JBJS 1961;43(7):961–9.

54. Krackow KA, Hales D, Jones L. Preoperative planning and surgical technique for performing a Dwyer calcaneal osteotomy. J Pediatr orthopedics 1985;5(2):214–8.

55. Boffeli TJ, Collier RC. Surgical technique for combined Dwyer calcaneal osteotomy and peroneal tendon repair for correction of peroneal tendon pathology associated with cavus foot deformity. J Foot Ankle Surg 2012;51(1):135–40.

Management of Midfoot Cavus

John F. Grady, DPM, FACFAOM, FRCPS(G)[a,b,c,d,]*, Jaclyn Schumann, DPM[e],
Clare Cormier, DPM[f], Kathryn LaViolette, DPM[g], Austin Chinn, DPM[f]

KEYWORDS

- Midfoot cavus • Pes cavus • Conservative treatment • Surgical treatment • Cole
- Japas

KEY POINTS

- Conservative therapy is recommended for asymptomatic midfoot pes cavus and the initial treatment of symptomatic idiopathic midfoot pes cavus.
- When surgically addressing midfoot pes cavus, flexible deformities can be corrected with tendon transfers, but rigid deformities should be treated with osseous procedures.
- The Japas and the Cole are two classic osseous procedures that have been popularized for the surgical treatment of rigid midfoot cavus.
- Treating a concomitant equinus is patient-dependent in non-neurologic idiopathic cases.
- Additional deforming forces and patient symptoms presenting with midfoot pes cavus may require subsequent surgical osseous procedures to be performed.

INTRODUCTION

Pes cavus is a multiplanar deformity with the primary abnormality occurring in the sagittal plane. Defining a pes cavus deformity is multifactorial and current literature does not agree on a universal definition. However, defining pes cavus usually begins with determining the location of the anterior, midfoot, or hindfoot cavus. Midfoot cavus is characterized as a cavus deformity with an apex at the tarsal level between the Lisfranc joint and Chopart joint.[1] Furthermore, a pes cavus deformity also is classified as either flexible or rigid. The flexibility or rigidness of the deformity refers to the

[a] Podiatric Residencies, Advocate Christ Medical Center and Advocate Children's Hospital, 4650 Southwest Highway, Oak Lawn, IL 60453, USA; [b] Rosalind Franklin University (Adjunct Track), North Chicago, IL, USA; [c] Foot and Ankle Institute of Illinois, 4650 Southwest Highway, Oak Lawn, IL 60453, USA; [d] Foot and Ankle Institute for Research (FAIR), 4650 Southwest Highway, Oak Lawn, IL 60453, USA; [e] Podiatric Medicine and Surgery Residency Program PGY3, Advocate Christ Medical Center, 4440 West 95th Street, Oak Lawn, IL 60453, USA; [f] Podiatric Medicine and Surgery Residency Program PGY2, Advocate Christ Medical Center, 4440 West 95th Street, Oak Lawn, IL 60453, USA; [g] Podiatric Medicine and Surgery Residency Program Graduate, Advocate Christ Medical Center, 4440 West 95th Street, Oak Lawn, IL 60453, USA
* Corresponding authors. Advocate Christ Medical Center and Advocate Children's Hospital, 4650 Southwest Highway, Oak Lawn, IL 60453.
E-mail address: john.grady@footandankleinstitute.com

Clin Podiatr Med Surg 38 (2021) 391–410
https://doi.org/10.1016/j.cpm.2021.02.004
0891-8422/21/© 2021 Elsevier Inc. All rights reserved.

reducibility of the deformity. The most important aspect of defining pes cavus, however, is to determine if the deformity is progressive or static in nature.[2-4]

Universally, literature has demonstrated that the treatment of pes cavus foot is multifactorial and dependent on location, flexibility, and developmental nature of the deformity.[2,3,5] The goal of treatment is to alleviate symptoms, lessen deforming forces, and provide a stable plantigrade foot. When determining the appropriate course of treatment of a patient, the entire clinical picture needs to be reviewed thoroughly. To date, there is no established gold standard for the treatment of the cavus foot. Additionally, there is little research support for a standardized method of measuring pes cavus (**Table 1**). The goal of this article is to perform a literature review of the management of the cavus foot and provide a treatment algorithm for midfoot cavus deformity.

PATIENT WORK-UP

The initial work-up of pes cavus should include a thorough clinical examination comprised of a physical examination, gait observation, and radiographic assessment. It is important to determine the etiology of the cavus deformity, and a thorough medical history helps determine whether the deformity is progressive or static.[2-4]

Table 1 Literature definitions of pes cavus	
Burns et al,[16] 2006	Foot posture index (score of −2 or less)
Chatterjee and Sahu,[26] 2009	Paralytic pes cavus deformity (no measurable criteria stated)
de Palma et al,[45] 1997	Definition not provided
Dreher et al,[7] 2014	Cavovarus foot structure secondary to CMT with component of foot drop (no measurable criteria stated)
Haritidis et al,[44] 1994	Definition not provided
Jahss et al,[27] 1980	Equinus deformity, clinically evident idiopathic pes cavus from mild to moderate deformity, residual clubfoot deformity, compartment, neurologically related (no measurable criteria stated)
Johnson et al,[22] 2009	Cavovarus foot structure secondary to CMT (no measurable criteria stated)
Leeuwesteijn et al,[29] 2010	Cavovarus foot structure secondary to CMT (no measurable criteria stated)
Maskill et al,[34] 2010	Subtle cavovarus foot of non-neurologic origin (no measurable criteria)
Pechecva et al,[46] 2018	Definition not provided
Sammarco and Taylor,[30] 2001	Cavovarus foot deformity secondary to neurologic disease (no measurable criteria stated)
Tullis et al,[8] 2004	Definition not provided
Vienne et al,[35] 2007	Pes cavovarus deformity with associated clinical symptoms
Wetmore and Drennan,[42] 1989	Cavovarus foot structure secondary to CMT (no measurable criteria stated)
Wülker and Hurschler,[1] 2002	Cavus deformity with associated clinical symptoms
Zhou et al,[19] 2014	Abnormally high arch medially in the sagittal plane of the foot

Visual inspection of the patient may demonstrate findings, such as a high arched foot, a tripod foot structure (with associated hyperkeratoses), an adducted forefoot, hammer toes or claw toes, an inverted calcaneus, lateral ankle joint instability, and calf atrophy.[6]

Muscle strength testing can identify if a muscle imbalance is contributing to the deformity. Joint range of motion of the foot should be performed to determine the degree of flexibility/rigidity of the deformity. In the setting of calcaneal varus, a Coleman block test should be performed to determine the influence of the first ray on the hindfoot varus and the flexibility of the rearfoot deformity.[4,6,7] A comprehensive neurologic work-up also may be necessary to identify any concurrent neuromuscular components of pes cavus.

Although no standardization exists for radiographic findings of pes cavus, lateral, anteroposterior (AP), and standing hindfoot radiographs generally have been accepted. Lateral radiographs usually show an increased first metatarsal calcaneal angle (Hibbs angle), an increased Meary angle, a bullet-hole sinus tarsi, an increased calcaneal inclination angle (calcaneal pitch angle), a decreased talar declination angle, and a decreased talocalcaneal angle[7] (**Fig. 1**). The location of the intersection between the longitudinal axis of the first metatarsal and the talus determines the apex of the cavus deformity. In the setting of a midfoot cavus, this apex is located at the navicular-cuneiform joint.[2,5,8] AP radiograph characteristic findings include an apparent shortened first metatarsal, overlapping or stacking of the lateral metatarsal bones, and global metatarsus adductus.[3,7,8] With a standing hindfoot view, the relationship between the calcaneus and tibia can be measured to determine the severity of calcaneal varus.[9,10]

TREATMENT

The authors' treatment algorithm begins with differentiation of asymptomatic and symptomatic patients.

Asymptomatic Patients

Asymptomatic patients may present to a podiatric physician's office for concerns unrelated to cavus foot structure, such as in cases of trauma, soft tissue pathology, nail

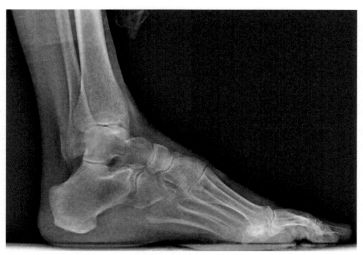

Fig. 1. Cavus foot radiograph. (*From* Ethics Committee of Foot & Ankle Associates, LTD., with permission.)

pathology, and so forth. Although literature has shown proactive surgical intervention to be beneficial for progressive neurologic asymptomatic pes cavus, such as Charcot-Marie-Tooth (CMT),[11] there is no literature that demonstrates early preventative surgery is advantageous in the treatment of non-neurologic asymptomatic pes cavus. In cases of a non-neurologic cavus deformity, education is of utmost importance. Patients should be educated on the inherent foot structure and commonly associated pathology.

Symptomatic Patients

More commonly, the podiatric physician encounters a patient who presents with symptoms from an underlying midfoot cavus foot structure. Patients may complain of difficulty fitting into shoe gear, chronic ankle sprains, heel pain, arch pain, and forefoot pain and hyperkeratoses. Physical examination may reveal muscle weakness, lateral ankle instability, pain along peroneal tendons, fifth metatarsal fractures, sesamoiditis, dorsally contracted digits, hyperkeratoses, and ulcerations.

Conservative Treatment

The goal of conservative care in symptomatic patients is to alleviate pain, correct pedal biomechanics, and provide a plantigrade foot.[8,12,13] Initial conservative treatment of an idiopathic symptomatic midfoot cavus should consist of custom molded orthotics with the appropriate modifications.[7,13–15] When treating a pes cavus foot with custom molded orthotics, the shell should be flexible enough to alleviate pain.[16] Specific modifications can be made to orthotics depending on the specific patient complaint, summarized in **Table 2**.[14,16]

Burns and colleagues,[16] in a single-blind randomized controlled study, demonstrated statistically significant improvement in foot pain and function in those patients who received custom molded orthotics over those who received placebo over a 3-month time frame. This study demonstrates that mildly symptomatic patients with bilateral cavus of any etiology can experience decreased pain with the use of custom molded orthotics.

Furthermore, custom ankle-foot orthoses and bracing can be beneficial for the pes cavus foot with concurrent lateral ankle instability, chronic ankle inversion sprains, drop foot, or muscle weakness.

Table 2	
Conservative care pes cavus orthotic modifications	
Deformity	**Orthotic Correction**
Equinus	Heel lift
Lateral ankle instability calcaneal varus	Flat rear foot posting Lateral heel post flare Lateral clip
Lateral column pain	Lateral forefoot ramp
Metatarsalgia	Metatarsal bar/pad
Plantarflexed first ray	First ray cutout Sub-second through fifth metatarsal bar post
Sesamoiditis	First ray cutout dancer pad

Surgical Intervention

The symptomatic midfoot pes cavus is a complex and challenging foot structure to treat. After conservative options have been exhausted and failed to provide pain relief, numerous surgical options are available to treat flexible versus rigid and forefoot versus rearfoot pathologies. Soft tissue procedures have their place in pes cavus reconstruction and can be performed in the presence of flexible deformities or as an adjunct to osseous procedures in rigid pes cavus deformities.[6,17] Tendon transfers generally are accepted as the first-line surgical treatment option for flexible cavus deformities and may be performed for two reasons: to reestablish lost function and to weaken deforming forces.[18] In the context of the inevitable rigid, arthritic deformity, however, soft tissue procedures are insufficient in correcting the underlying deformity. At this time, osseous procedures are favored and should be carried out. An important note to be made when performing midfoot osteotomies, the location of the osteotomy should be made through osseous structures, with great care taken to preserve surrounding joints. In the primary author's opinion (JG), by salvaging the midfoot joints, motion still can take place, allowing for more functionality of the foot.

OSSEOUS PROCEDURES
Midfoot Osseous Procedures

Once a deformity is determined to be rigid or correction is unattainable by soft tissue intervention alone, osseous surgical procedures must be performed, at times in conjunction with soft tissue procedures, in order to correct the deformity. Research has highlighted primarily two midfoot osteotomies for the correction of midfoot cavus: the Cole and the Japas.

Cole

The Cole osteotomy is the most commonly reported midfoot osteotomy for management of patients with a symptomatic rigid midfoot cavus deformity. The procedure is performed with a continuous transverse wedge osteotomy through the first cuneiform navicular joint medially to the midcuboid laterally (**Fig. 2**).[19] The wedge then is removed and the distal foot is elevated to close down the osteotomy site. Variations of this osteotomy cut can be effective for deformities that require multiplanar correction. Saunders[20] suggests a wider resection laterally to correct a cavo-adductus deformity, whereas Alvik and colleagues[21] recommended a larger medial cuneiform wedge to correct an excessive plantarflexion deformity of the first ray.

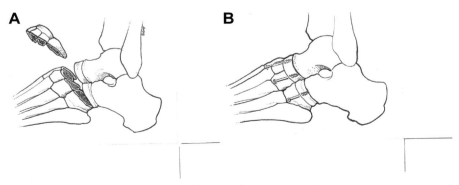

Fig. 2. (A) Dorsal wedge osteotomy. (B) Screw fixation across the osteotomy.

Literature supports the Cole osteotomy as an acceptable treatment of midfoot cavus despite continued pain as a common postoperative complication. Wülker and Hurschler[1] identified the Cole osteotomy as satisfactory for realignment of the foot with improvement in symptoms. One-quarter of patients, however, were dissatisfied and complained of mild to moderate pain that limited their daily activities at 46 months' follow-up.[1] Tullis and colleagues[8] found statistically significant decrease in the lateral talo–first metatarsal angle (Hibbs angle), calcaneal inclination angle, metatarsus adductus angle, and talo–first metatarsal angle. Additionally, 87.5% of the patients experienced occasional to no pain with activities of daily living (ADLs) or high-impact activities.[8] Zhou and colleagues[19] performed a prospective study of the midfoot osteotomy and found all patients had improved foot appearance and gait after the procedure. Furthermore, a statistically significant increase in American Orthopaedic Foot and Ankle Society (AOFAS) scores was demonstrated as was statistically significant decrease in Meary angle, calcaneal pitch angle, tibiotalar angle, and Hibbs angle postoperatively.[19] Most literature finds the Cole osteotomy to correct radiographic angles, but pain at the osteotomy postoperatively is not a rare occurrence.

This dorsal closing wedge osteotomy often is combined with supplemental procedures to address concomitant deformities, long-standing contractures, and muscular imbalance. Gastrocnemius recessions or Achilles tendon lengthening procedures frequently are necessary to correct the accompanying equinus deformity.[2,4] Other common soft tissue procedures to consider are plantar fascial release, Steindler stripping, and tendon balancing procedures. It is believed that a plantar soft tissue release can reduce the deformity and lessen the size of bone resection required in the osteotomy.[22] Johnson and colleagues[22] performed the Cole osteotomy in conjunction with Steindler stripping and a posterior tibial tendon transfer. This prospective study found patients had improved pain and increased function with a plantigrade foot postoperatively. Furthermore, this study demonstrated that transferring the posterior tibial tendon out of phase decreased the tendon's deforming advantage over the weakened peroneus brevis while augmenting the weak tibialis anterior.[22]

Although the Cole osteotomy has been widely accepted as effective and relatively safe for treatment of midfoot cavus, it is important to note its contraindications, complications, and risks. Contraindications for the Cole osteotomy include pes cavus where the apex is not localized to the midfoot, progressive neuromuscular disease, gross motor weakness, vascular compromise, and a skeletally immature foot.[20,23,24] Although the most common associated complications are minor, such as superficial skin infection, wound dehiscence, fixation failure, and pain, patients also may experience marked foot shortening, joint destruction and stiffness of adjacent joints, and decreased ankle joint range of motion postoperatively.[19,23]

Japas

Following popularization of the Cole osteotomy, Japas developed the midfoot V-osteotomy in an attempt to evade the complications observed with the Cole osteotomy. This V-shaped osteotomy is performed at the midtarsal-to-tarsometatarsal joints with the apex oriented proximally at the highest point of the cavus. The osteotomy is completed with the cuts angled distal-medial and distal-lateral, staying proximal to the first and fifth tarso-metatarsal joints. The distal part of the foot then is elevated and the osteotomy site is compressed without a wedge resection and without risk of extensive extremity shortening.[25]

Similar to the Cole osteotomy, the Japas often is performed in conjunction with a plantar fasciotomy and/or Steindler stripping. The primary author recommends the Japas also can be performed in conjunction with a tendo-Achilles lengthening or gastrocnemius recession to address any symptomatic equinus deformity. This procedure has indications and contraindications similar to those of the Cole osteotomy. Chatterjee and colleagues[26] evaluated the outcomes of a Japas osteotomy in conjunction with a Steindler stripping on postpolio patients who often are predisposed to a residual global cavus deformity. Patients were followed for a mean of 5.4 years with outcomes of very good, 33%; good, 44%; and poor in 22%. These findings are some of the first to suggest that satisfactory results can be obtained with the use of Japas when managing with a global cavus foot, although limited research is available in regard to utilization of this procedure in the long term.[26]

Additional Osseous Procedures

Many times, additional osseous procedures must be performed in order to decrease deforming forces and to alleviate focal symptoms secondary to pes cavus deformity.

Lesser metatarsalgia

As a cavus foot progresses from flexible to rigid, the lesser metatarsal heads are plantarflexed by intrinsic and plantar soft tissue contractures, similar to the first ray. Extension deformity and shortening of the metatarsophalangeal joint capsules additionally displace the plantar fat pad anteriorly, thus predisposing the patient to metatarsalgia.[4,27] Jahss and colleagues[27] described a truncated wedge arthrodesis of the tarsometatarsal joints to correct for painful metatarsalgia across the first through fifth metatarsal heads. This surgical approach removes dorsal wedges from the first, second, and third metatarsal cuneiform joints as well as the fourth and fifth metatarsocuboid joints. No fixation was utilized in the original description of this technique because the investigators felt the tarsometatarsal joint provided superior stability as the apex of the cavus deformity with a wider contact area for osseous union. It should be stressed that consideration of this procedure requires extremely close attention to detail intraoperatively and postoperatively in casting technique to maintain adequate compression at the arthrodesis site and to keep the metatarsal heads entirely level. Although this study found excellent results in relief of metatarsal pain, the investigators observed complications of rotary valgus deformity, transfer calluses and pain to localized metatarsal heads, incomplete correction of deformity, rocker bottom deformity and pain to the plantar fifth metatarsocuboid, and nonunion.[27]

Despite the fact that this procedure has been shown to reduce painful symptoms, few patients experience pain equivalently distributed across all metatarsal heads. In the primary author's experience, many patients experience pain localized to one or multiple metatarsal heads. Therefore, the authors recommend consideration of dorsiflexory osteotomies limited to the symptomatic metatarsals as the preferred method for treatment of lesser metatarsalgia.

Plantarflexed first ray

In pes cavus deformity, a plantarflexed first ray commonly occurs as a result of muscle imbalance as the peroneus longus tendon overpowers a weakened tibialis anterior tendon.[1,2,4,5] Two procedures have been discussed and decrease the plantarflexory nature of the first ray: a dorsiflexory wedge osteotomy at base of the first metatarsal and a fusion of the first metatarsal and tarsal joint.[2,4,5,28] Care should be taken to preserve the length of the first metatarsal. Therefore, the dorsiflexory wedge osteotomy of the first metatarsal is the primary author's (JG) preference to avoid excessive shortening with arthrodesis and additionally preserve the mobility across the first metatarsal-cuneiform joint. Although this procedure can correct the first ray adequately, these procedures do not address a true midfoot cavus deformity as a standalone procedure. When indicated, first metatarsal osteotomies and fusion of the first metatarsal-cuneiform joint should be performed concomitantly with midfoot specific osteotomies and adjunctive soft tissue procedures.[17]

A retrospective review by Leeuwesteijn and colleagues[29] investigated short-term and midterm results of a dorsiflexory wedge osteotomy of the first ray in combination with appropriate soft tissue procedures. This research demonstrated an 81% decrease in pressure calluses and an increase in foot function by 84% postoperatively. Additionally, the study's results found 90% of patients were satisfied with correction of the deformity.[29] Furthermore, Sammarco and Taylor[30] evaluated patients with symptomatic metatarsalgia secondary to pes cavovarus deformity who underwent a lateral calcaneal slide elevating osteotomy, Steindler stripping, and first metatarsal dorsolateral closing wedge osteotomy. Select cases had osteotomies of the second through fifth metatarsals performed. The investigators found this combination of procedures to provide patients with a decreased cavus, symptom-free, and plantigrade foot with adequate ankle joint range of motion.[30]

Hindfoot correction

Many midfoot cavus deformities have a concurrent hindfoot varus. As literature suggests, this deformity is prone to lateral column overloading with resultant pain, increased risk of ankle inversion injuries, and chronic lateral ankle instability.[31] By redistributing ground reactive forces through the hindfoot laterally, calcaneal osteotomies can normalize biomechanics during gait and reduce symptoms. To improve the lever arm of the Achilles tendon and to create a plantigrade heel during stance, the calcaneal osteotomy is translated laterally. Lateralizing the insertion of the Achilles tendon is especially beneficial in patients with a weak triceps surae.[32,33] Additionally, in the absence of arthritic changes to the hindfoot joints, osteotomies have the significant advantage of being joint-sparing and lessen subsequent damage to adjacent joints.

Calcaneal slide osteotomy

A calcaneal slide osteotomy frequently is indicated when there is a true rigid hindfoot deformity.[14] Research suggests a lateral translation of 5 mm to 10 mm is necessary for adequate correction of the hindfoot varus deformity.[14,34] Maskill and colleagues[34] evaluated patients who underswent a calcaneal slide osteotomy with adjunctive peroneus longus transfer, dorsiflexory first metatarsal osteotomy, and gastrocsoleal lengthening when indicated. Preoperatively, all patients complained of lateral column pain, inversion ankle injuries, or ankle instability. The average calcaneal translation seen in this study was 7.5 mm. After 4.4 years, AOFAS ankle hindfoot scores and radiographic parameters were improved significantly, and 87% of patients were extremely satisfied with their surgery.[34]

Vienne and colleagues[35] observed similar outcomes in patients treated with a lateralizing calcaneal osteotomy and peroneus longus-to-brevis tendon transfer for recurrent and chronic lateral ankle instability. Some additionally underwent an adjunctive Broström ligament reconstruction. In this study, AOFAS ankle hindfoot score demonstrated a statistically significant improvement from 57 points preoperatively to 87 points postoperatively, and all patients reported satisfaction with the surgery at 43 months following.[35] This osteotomy generally is recognized in literature as safe and effective with few complications, although patients may experience pain secondary to plantar hardware with weight bearing.[14,34,35]

The calcaneal slide procedure is additionally highly versatile for pes cavus and can provide biplanar correction. Elongating the calcaneus is done by moving the capital fragment superiorly and posteriorly, which decreases the calcaneal inclination angle[4,6,32] (Fig. 3).

Dwyer osteotomy

The Dwyer osteotomy (DWO), or lateral calcaneal closing wedge osteotomy, is used to treat a calcaneal varus deformity. Literature suggests that a true DWO be reserved for mild hindfoot deformities because it has limited lateral translation due to the intact medial cortex.[36,37] This osteotomy provides predominantly transverse plane correction; however, it can provide triplanar correction if the medial cortex is breached and the capital fragment is shifted superiorly.[6,7,38] Multiple calcaneal osteotomies were directly compared in studies by An and colleagues[39] and Cody and colleagues,[39] who concluded that the use of a DWO with lateralization of the capital fragment achieved greatest correction of a hindfoot varus.[39,40]

Calcaneal Z osteotomy

A calcaneal Z osteotomy provides stable triplanar correction for severe hindfoot varus deformities[6,11,33] (**Fig. 4**).[33] The osteotomy is performed more proximally than a DWO, providing two major advantages. First, this osteotomy does not shorten the calcaneus and second, it offers greater correction of the calcaneal tuberosity.[6,11] This correction moves the lever arm of the Achilles tendon laterally and increases its mechanical advantage. This osteotomy is inherently stable and provides both translational and rotational correction for severe hindfoot varus deformities, making it an attractive option in pes cavus reconstruction.

Lateral column shortening procedures

In the primary author's opinion, when complete correction of forefoot varus and adduction is unable to be achieved, lateral column shortening can be performed. This wedge-shaped osteotomy has been described through the cuboid, calcaneus, or the calcaneal-cuboid joint itself.[4,36]

Arthrodesis

The triple arthrodesis generally is considered a salvage procedure for patients with severe rigid hindfoot deformity or degenerative changes in rearfoot.[41,42] Historically, this procedure was thought to have satisfactory short to midterm postoperative results; however, the long-term functional outcomes on the cavus foot generally are poor, with a high incidence of residual deformity, pseudarthrosis, and degenerative changes to adjacent joints. Wetmore and Drennen[42] followed patients with CMT for 21 years

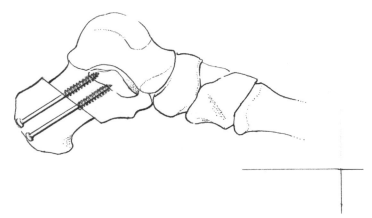

Fig. 3. Biplanar correction.

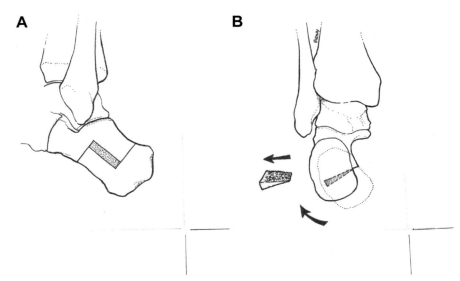

Fig. 4. (*A*) Osteotomy with lateral closing wedge. (*B*) Closing wedge removed. Rotational and translational correction of varus deformity is achieved.

after a triple arthrodesis, with only 24% with satisfactory outcomes. Long-term complications of this study were residual deformity and advanced ankle arthritis.[42] Mann and Hsu[43] evaluated the outcomes of this procedure on pediatric CMT patients and found a residual deformity rate of 33% and 25% incidence of pseudarthrosis at 7 years' follow-up. In another long-term study, Saltzman and El-Khoury[10] evaluated 57 patients with mixed underlying etiologies for an average follow-up of 25 years. The findings in regard to incidence of residual deformity and of pseudarthrosis were 78% and 19%, respectively, whereas 100% of patients were noted to have some degree of degenerative changes of the ankle joint.[10]

Some studies suggest better outcomes of the triple arthrodesis, however, in patients with static neuromuscular diseases.[42,43] In support of this, Haritidis and colleagues[44] investigated 42 patients with poliomyelitis who underwent triple arthrodesis for pes cavus treatment. After 25 years, the patient satisfaction was high, there were no reports of pseudarthrosis, and severe degenerative changes were seen in only 1 patient. Despite these positive findings, Haritidis and colleagues reported only 31% of patients with good outcomes. Therefore, although there was low incidence of pseudoarthrosis and severe degenerative joint disease, the results of this study were suboptimal to conclude that improved outcomes with the triple arthrodesis can be seen in poliomyelitis patients.[44]

Because much research reveals poor long-term outcomes, the authors recommend that arthrodesis should remain a salvage procedure for those with severe rigid deformity and those who have failed alternative conservative and surgical options. Additionally, if there are severe degenerative changes noted to one or several of the hindfoot joints, it may serve to eliminate pain associated with motion of these joints. If considering this procedure, careful and meticulous planning is emphasized to achieve accurate correction of the deformity. With a high rate of residual deformity, it also is recommended that arthrodesis be performed in conjunction with muscle and tendon balancing procedures.[41–44]

Table 3
Surgical intervention of cavus deformity with osteotomies of the forefoot and midfoot

Article	Level of Evidence/ Type of Study	No. Of Participants/ Limbs	Osteotomy Performed	Adjunct Procedures	Treatment Outcomes	Radiographic Postpperative Findings	Patient Satisfaction	Follow-up Time
Chatterjee and Sahu,[26] 2009	Prospective	18 patients; 18 feet—17 with polio and 1 with meningocele	Japas osteotomy with Steindler Stripping	No additional procedures performed	14 feet very good or good results according to Japas criteria; 4 feet had poor correction/complications according to Japas criteria and these patients went on to have triple arthrodesis or calcaneal DWO.	Unspecified	Unspecified	64.8 (range: 36–156) mo
Jahss et al,[27] 1980	Prospective	25 patients; 34 feet	DWO at Lisfranc joint	No additional procedures performed	33 feet had excellent/satisfactory results; 1 foot had fair results.	Unspecified	Unspecified	75.5 (range: 12–168) mo

(continued on next page)

Table 3
(continued)

Article	Level of Evidence/ Type of Study	No. Of Participants/ Limbs	Osteotomy Performed	Adjunct Procedures	Treatment Outcomes	Radiographic Postoperative Findings	Patient Satisfaction	Follow-up Time
Johnson et al,[22] 2009	Prospective	3 patients	Cole osteotomy with external fixation	If needed, performed Steindler stripping, posterior tibial tendon transfer, calcaneal DWO, subtalar joint arthrodesis	No statistical significance found in postoperative questionnaire, but all patients experienced improved biomechanical function and decreased pain postoperatively.	No statistically significant improvement; however, qualitative improvement noted in relaxed calcaneal stance position, talocalcaneal angle, talo-first metatarsal angel, calcaneal inclination angle, talar declination angle, and malleolar valgus index.	Unspecified	At least 12 mo
Leeuwesteijn et al,[29] 2010	Retrospective review	33 patients; 52 feet—all with CMT	DWO at base of first metatarsal	If needed, performed percutaneous Achilles tendon lengthening, dorsal release of metatarsophalangeal joints, hallux interphalangeal joint fusion,	Dutch Foot Function Index: improvement in pain and disability were statistically significant. QUOTE Questionnaire: 77% expressed a decrease in pain and foot	Unspecified	90% satisfied	56.9 (range: 13–153) mo

				extensor hallucis longus transfer, flexor to extensor tendon transfer of lesser digits, extensor digitorum longus tendon transfer, tibialis posterior tendon transfer, and tibialis anterior tendon transfer, Steindler stripping, and lateral calcaneal osteotomy	function better after surgery in 84%.			
Tullis et al,[8] 2004	Retrospective review	8 patients; 11 feet	Cole osteotomy	If needed, performed releases of abductor hallucis, flexor digitorum brevis, abductor digiti minimi, long plantar ligaments, and soft tissue stripping	4 feet no pain with ADLs, no problems completing ADLs, no difficulty with uneven terrain; 2 feet with occasional pain with high impact activity; 1 foot with moderate pain with high impact activity	Statistically significant decrease in lateral talo–first metatarsal angle and calcaneal inclination angle (sagittal plane), metatarsus-adductus angle and AP talo–first metatarsal angle (transverse); 100% radiographic fusion rate	75% satisfied, 25% indifferent	23 (range: 11–29.5) mo

(continued on next page)

Table 3
(continued)

Article	Level of Evidence/Type of Study	No. Of Participants/Limbs	Osteotomy Performed	Adjunct Procedures	Treatment Outcomes	Radiographic Postoperative Findings	Patient Satisfaction	Follow-up Time
Wülker and Hurschler,[1] 2002	Prospective	12 patients; 13 feet	Cole osteotomy	If needed, patients with severe extensor digiti contracture underwent closed manipulation prior to osteotomy.	3 feet pain-free at follow-up, 6 feet complained of mild occasional pain; 3 patients with moderate pain, no patient with permanent severe pain; 3 patients with normal alignment with well-aligned midfoot/plantigrade position clinically, no progression of deformity postoperatively	Meary angle at follow-up average 14° (range: −5 to 26°).	75% satisfied, 25% unsatisfied	46 (range: 24–80) mo
Zhou et al,[19] 2014	Prospective	17 patients; 17 feet	Cole osteotomy	No additional procedures performed	Statistically significant improvement of AOFAS score at final follow up with mean 75.8 (range 63–90); Japas criteria outcomes were very good or good in 88.2% of feet.	Statistically significant improvement in mean Meary angle, calcaneal pitch, tibiotalar angle, Hibbs angle	94.1% very satisfied/satisfied	25.3 (range 10–50) mo

Abbreviation: QUOTE, Quality of Care Through the Patients' Eyes.

Table 4
Studies evaluating the outcomes of lateral displacement osteotomies in the setting of pes cavus

Article	Level of Evidence/ Type of Study	No. Of Participants/ Limbs	Osteotomy Performed	Adjunct Procedures	Treatment Outcomes	Radiographic Postoperative Findings	Patient Satisfaction	Follow-up Time
Maskill et al,[34] 2010	Case Control Study	23 patients; 29 feet	Lateral displacement calcaneal osteotomy	If needed, performed Achilles tendon lengthening, peroneus longus to brevis transfer, and dorsiflexory first metatarsal osteotomy	Statistically significant improvement in AOFAS ankle hindfoot score	Statistically significant improvement: talo–first metatarsal angle, calcaneal inclination angle, and the medial cuneiform height	20 patients were extremely satisfied and returned to ADLs; Three patients had pain postoperatively and were unsatisfied with surgical results, although all three patients' preoperative pain had improved	52.8 (range: 12–121.2) mo

(continued on next page)

Table 4
(continued)

Article	Level of Evidence/ Type of Study	No. Of Participants/ Limbs	Osteotomy Performed	Adjunct Procedures	Treatment Outcomes	Radiographic Postoperative Findings	Patient Satisfaction	Follow-up Time
Sammarco and Taylor,[30] 2001	Prospective	13 patients; 19 feet—pes cavus deformity is secondary to underlying neurologic disease	Lateral displacement calcaneal osteotomy	If needed, performed soft tissue stripping, DWO of first metatarsal, DWO of metatarsals 2–5, Jones tendon transfer, osteotomy of fourth metatarsal head, and hammertoe correction	Statistically significant improvement in Maryland foot and ankle scores and AOFAS ankle/hindfoot and midfoot scores	Statistically significant improvement: talo–first metatarsalangle, talocalcaneal angle, calcaneal first metatarsalangle, calcaneal pitch, arch height, talosecond metatarsal angles, and calcaneus second metatarsal angle	All patients were satisfied with procedures performed.	49.8 (range: 8–101) mo
Vienne et al,[35] 2007	Prospective	8 patients; 9 feet	Lateral displacement calcaneal osteotomy with peroneus longus to brevis transfer	If needed, performed a Broström ligament reconstruction	Statistically significant improvement in AOFAS ankle hindfoot scores; statistically significant improvement in pain relief from preoperative to postoperative	Radiographic preoperative hindfoot alignment of 15° to 5° valgus postoperatively	All patients were satisfied with procedures performed.	43 (range: 30–53) mo

Abbreviation: OUOTE, Quality of Care Through the Patients' Eyes.

SUMMARY

The authors of this article conducted an extensive literature review centered on surgical correction of midfoot cavus. Studies of prospective, retrospective, and case series were included. Opinion articles and review articles were excluded from this review. The authors found that there is a deficiency in research as well as a lack of higher-level studies on this topic. This can be attributed to the varying etiology and disease progression and complexity of midfoot cavus. Clearly, there is no standard definition for the diagnosis of this deformity. The absence of firm diagnostic criteria for midfoot pes cavus has led to discrepancy in treatment protocols. In the primary author's opinion, it is important to establish a firm definition of pes cavus for research and treatment moving forward. The authors suggest examining Meary angle radiographically and implementing the Coleman block test clinically to evaluate this complex deformity. It can be concluded from literature that surgical decision making generally is determined by the apex of the cavus deformity and the extent of rearfoot varus. The research demonstrates that a majority of patients are satisfied with the Cole osteotomy and the dorsiflexory first metatarsal osteotomy for treatment of midfoot cavus (**Table 3**). In the setting of pes cavus with a concomitant rearfoot varus, studies have focused primarily on lateralizing calcaneal osteotomies. Data suggests high patient satisfaction in the short-term to midterm follow-up when treating these patients (**Table 4**).

The lack of supportive data, concurrent deformity, and variability of causes of midfoot cavus make establishing a treatment algorithm challenging. The authors suggest that when considering asymptomatic and minimally symptomatic idiopathic pes cavus, conservative treatment options should be the first line of care. Surgical intervention may be considered if conservative treatments fail to relieve symptoms. The aim of surgery is to improve cavus-related foot pain and achieve a mobile, plantigrade foot. As outlined throughout this article, there are many different procedures as well as procedure combinations that are utilized in practice to treat cavus deformities. It is the primary author's opinion that isolated fusions and osteotomies often are sufficient to resolve mild to moderate symptoms with low risk of vascular damage and complications. Although performed infrequently, the literature continues to support high patient satisfaction for the Cole osteotomy and first metatarsal dorsiflexion osteotomy in cases of the apex of the deformity at the midfoot. When rearfoot deformity is rigid, a lateralizing calcaneal osteotomy should be considered with adjunctive soft tissue and osseous procedures. The triple arthrodesis has provided poor long-term functional outcomes and should remain reserved for only end-stage arthritis or as consideration for revisional intervention. The authors believe this treatment course can provide assistance in the surgical decision-making process when faced with a symptomatic cavus patient; although further research is necessary.

CLINICS CARE POINTS

- There is insufficient evidence in literature to establish a treatment algorithm for symptomatic midfoot pes cavus.
- Asymptomatic midfoot pes cavus should be treated conservatively.
- Research has demonstrated poor long-term outcomes with prophylactic surgical intervention. The authors of the article recommend symptom-focused management.
- When surgically treating midfoot pes cavus, flexible deformities can be corrected with tendon transfers, but rigid deformities should be treated with osseous procedures.

> • With a wide variety of deforming forces and presenting symptoms, the treatment course for management of midfoot cavus should be individualized.

ACKNOWLEDGMENTS

The authors want to thank Maria Bidny, DPM, for her dedication and contribution to the illustrations within this publication.

DISCLOSURE

No authors have any commercial or financial conflicts of interest or funding of any kind.

REFERENCES

1. Wülker N, Hurschler C. Cavus foot correction in adults by dorsal closing wedge osteotomy. Foot Ankle Int 2002;23(4):344–7.
2. Groner TW, DiDomenico LA. Midfoot osteotomies for the cavus foot. Clin Podiatr Med Surg 2005;22(2):247.
3. Akoh CC, Phisitkul P. Clinical examination and radiographic assessment of the cavus foot. Foot Ankle Clin 2019;24(2):183–93.
4. Younger ASE, Hansen ST Jr. Adult cavovarus foot. J Am Acad Orthop Surg 2005; 13(5):302–15.
5. Maynou C, Szymanski C, Thiounn A. The adult cavus foot. EFORT Open Rev 2017;2(5):221–9.
6. Ortiz C, Wagner E, Keller A. Cavovarus foot reconstruction. Foot Ankle Clin 2009; 14(3):471–87.
7. Dreher T, Wolf SI, Heitzmann D, et al. Tibialis posterior tendon transfer corrects the foot drop component of cavovarus foot deformity in Charcot-Marie-Tooth disease. J Bone Joint Surg Am 2014;96(6):456–62.
8. Tullis BL, Mendicino RW, Catanzariti AR, et al. The cole midfoot osteotomy: a retrospective review of 11 procedures in 8 patients. J Foot Ankle Surg 2004; 43(3):160–5.
9. Cobey JC. Posterior roentgenogram of the foot. Clin Orthop Relat Res 1976;(118): 202–7.
10. Saltzman CL, El-Khoury GY. The hindfoot alignment view. Foot Ankle Int 1995; 16(9):572–6.
11. Barton T, Winson I. Joint sparing correction of cavovarus feet in charcot-marie-tooth disease: what are the limits? Foot Ankle Clin 2013;18(4):673–88.
12. Deben SE, Pomeroy GC. Subtle cavus foot: diagnosis and management. J Am Acad Orthop Surg 2014;22(8):512.
13. Kaplan JRM, Aiyer A, Cerrato RA, et al. Operative treatment of the cavovarus foot. Foot Ankle Int 2018;39(11):1370.
14. Manoli A II, Graham B. The subtle cavus foot, "the underpronator," a review. Foot Ankle Int 2005;26(3):256–63.
15. LoPiccolo M, Chilvers M, Graham B, et al. Effectiveness of the cavus foot orthosis. J Surg Orthop Adv 2010;19(3):166–9.
16. Burns J, Crosbie J, Ouvrier R, et al. Effective orthotic therapy for the painful cavus foot. Australas J Podiatric Med 2006;40(3):61.
17. Weiner DS, Jones K, Jonah D, et al. Management of the rigid cavus foot in children and adolescents. Foot Ankle Clin 2013;18(4):727–41.

18. Ryssman DB, Myerson MS. Tendon transfers for the adult flexible cavovarus foot. Foot Ankle Clin 2011;16(3):435–50.
19. Zhou Y, Zhou B, Liu J, et al. A prospective study of midfoot osteotomy combined with adjacent joint sparing internal fixation in treatment of rigid pes cavus deformity. J Orthop Surg Res 2014;9(1):122–35.
20. Saunders JT. Etiology and treatment of clawfoot. Arch Surg 1935;30:179–98.
21. Alvik I. Operative treatment of pes cavus. Acta Orthop Scand 1953;23(2):137.
22. Johnson BM, Child B, Hix J, et al. Cavus foot reconstruction in 3 patients with charcot-marie-tooth disease. J Foot Ankle Surg 2009;48(2):116–24.
23. Cole WH. The treatment of clawfoot. J Bone Joint Surg Am 1940;22:895–908.
24. Ergun S, Yildirim Y. The Cole midfoot osteotomy: clinical and radiographic retrospective review of five patients (Six feet) with different etiologies. J Am Podiatr Med Assoc 2019;109(3):180.
25. Japas LM. Surgical treatment of pes cavus by tarsal V-osteotomy. J Bone Joint Surg Am 1968;50(5):927–44.
26. Chatterjee P, Sahu M. A prospective study of Japas' osteotomy in paralytic pes cavus deformity in adolescent feet. Indian J Orthop 2009;43(3):281–5.
27. Jahss MH. Tarsometatarsal truncated-wedge arthrodesis for pes cavus and equinovarus deformity of the fore part of the foot. J Bone Joint Surg Am 1980;62(5):713–22.
28. Camasta CA, Cass AD. Pes cavus surgery. In: McGlamry's comprehensive textbook of foot and ankle surgery, vol. 1, 4th edition. Philadelphia, PA: Lippincott Williams & Wilkins; 2001. p. 525–40.
29. Leeuwesteijn AE, de Visser E, Louwerens JWK. Flexible cavovarus feet in Charcot-Marie-Tooth disease treated with first ray proximal dorsiflexion osteotomy combined with soft tissue surgery: a short-term to mid-term outcome study. Foot Ankle Surg 2010;16(3):142–7.
30. Sammarco GJ, Taylor R. Cavovarus foot treated with combined calcaneus and metatarsal osteotomies. Foot Ankle Int 2001;22(1):19–30.
31. Larsen E, Angermann P. Association of ankle instability and foot deformity. Acta Orthop Scand 1990;61(2):136–9.
32. Mitchell GP. Posterior displacement osteotomy of the calcaneus. J Bone Joint Surg Br 1977;59(2):233–5.
33. Coughlin MJ, Saltzman CL, Anderson RB, et al. Pes cavus. In: Mann's surgery of the foot and ankle, 1, 9th Edition. Philadelphia, PA: Saunders/Elsevier; 2014. p. 1361–82.
34. Maskill MP, Maskill JD, Pomeroy GC. Surgical management and treatment algorithm for the subtle cavovarus foot. Foot Ankle Int 2010;31(12):1057.
35. Vienne P, Schöniger R, Helmy N, et al. Hindfoot instability in cavovarus deformity: static and dynamic balancing. Foot Ankle Int 2007;28(1):96–102.
36. Krause FG, Iselin LD. Hindfoot varus and neurologic disorders. Foot Ankle Clin 2012;17(1):39–56.
37. Dwyer FC. The present status of the problem of pes cavus. Clin Orthop Relat Res 1975;(106):254–75.
38. DeVries JG, McAlister JE. Corrective osteotomies used in cavus reconstruction. Clin Podiatr Med Surg 2015;32(3):375–87.
39. An TW, Michalski M, Jansson K, et al. Comparison of lateralizing calcaneal osteotomies for varus hindfoot correction. Foot Ankle Int 2018;39(10):1229.
40. Cody EA, Kraszewski AP, Conti MS, et al. Lateralizing calcaneal osteotomies and their effect on calcaneal alignment: a three-dimensional digital model analysis. Public Finance Rev 2018;46(5):970–7.

41. Lee MC, Sucato DJ. Pediatric issues with cavovarus foot deformities. Foot Ankle Clin 2008;13(2):199–219.

42. Wetmore RS, Drennan JC. Long-term results of triple arthrodesis in Charcot-Marie-Tooth disease. J Bone Joint Surg Am 1989;71(3):417–22.

43. Mann DC, Hsu JD. Triple arthrodesis in the treatment of fixed cavovarus deformity in adolescent patients with Charcot-Marie-Tooth disease. Foot Ankle 1992;13(1):1–6.

44. Haritidis JH, Kirkos JM, Provellegios SM, et al. Long-term results of triple arthrodesis: 42 cases followed for 25 years. Foot Ankle Int 1994;15(10):548–51.

45. de Palma L, Colonna E, Travasi M. The modified Jones procedure for pes cavovarus with claw hallux. J Foot Ankle Surg 1997;36(4):279–333.

46. Pecheva M, Devany A, Nourallah B, et al. Long-term follow-up of patients undergoing tibialis posterior transfer: is acquired pes planus a complication? Foot 2018;34:83–9.

Principles of Triple Arthrodesis and Limited Arthrodesis in the Cavus Foot

Kalli E. Mortenson, DPM, Lawrence M. Fallat, DPM*

KEYWORDS

- Arthrodesis • Cavus • Cavovarus • Deformity • Hindfoot • Reconstruction
- Triple arthrodesis • Limited arthrodesis

KEY POINTS

- Proper preoperative assessment of clinical and radiographic findings is critical to determine the correct surgical procedure for adequate reduction of a cavus foot deformity.
- Triple arthrodesis is reserved for end-stage deformity with evidence of osteoarthritic changes of the rearfoot with a goal of a stable, plantigrade foot.
- Meticulous anatomic dissection and joint preparation with stable internal fixation is vital to achieve superior postoperative outcomes.
- In severe, global cavus deformity a triple arthrodesis may not be sufficient to adequately reduce the deformity, thus requiring additional procedures, such as calcaneal and midfoot osteotomies.

INTRODUCTION

Cavus foot deformity is characterized by a high arch seen on clinical and radiographic examination. Clinically, patients often present with varus of the hindfoot and clawing of the toes, in addition to an elevated arch.[1] The cause of cavus foot may be considered neurologic or idiopathic, with Charcot-Marie-Tooth disease (CMT) being the most common neurologic cause of these presenting symptoms.[1,2] Although CMT has been reported to be the most common cause of neurologic-associated cavus foot, one must always assess the patient for additional neurologic etiologies.[3] Important diagnostic work-up is necessary in surgical decision making to obtain the best outcomes. Often times the cause of cavus foot may be progressive, seen in cases of CMT, in which the deformity progresses in severity over time creating suboptimal surgical outcomes with joint-sparing techniques alone. Joint-sparing techniques are

Beaumont Health Wayne Podiatric Foot and Ankle Surgical Residency, Beaumont Hospital Wayne, 31555 Annapolis Street, Wayne, MI 48184, USA
* Corresponding author. 20555 Ecorse Road, Taylor, MI 48180.
E-mail address: lfallatdpm@aol.com

Clin Podiatr Med Surg 38 (2021) 411–425
https://doi.org/10.1016/j.cpm.2020.12.014
0891-8422/21/© 2020 Elsevier Inc. All rights reserved.

podiatric.theclinics.com

often favored in surgical treatment of cavus foot deformity, but one must consider the pertinent muscular imbalances, the flexibility of the deformity, and the apex of the deformity to correctly determine the surgical technique.

CLINICAL EXAMINATION

Cavus foot deformity is often progressive in nature, which may present with subtle or drastic clinical findings depending on the extent of the deformity. Patients often present with pain to the lateral aspect of the foot and may report recurrent ankle sprains or injuries. Lateral column overload is common in cavus foot deformity caused by the inherent muscle imbalances. Weakened intrinsic muscles of the foot are overpowered by the extrinsic muscles leading to clawing of the digits (**Fig. 1**). The first ray also presents in a plantarflexed position with varus of the hindfoot caused by the peroneus longus tendon overpowering the tibialis anterior.[3] Additionally, hindfoot varus is exaggerated because of the further adduction deformity caused by the tibialis posterior tendon overpowering the peroneus brevis.[3]

Because of the characteristic muscle imbalances seen in a cavus foot deformity patients may report difficulty fitting in shoe gear secondary to contracted digits, pain along the peroneal tendons, ankle instability, gait disturbances, fifth metatarsal fractures, or arthritic-type hindfoot pain in the more severe type cases.[2,3] Other common presentations include hyperkeratoses on the plantar aspect of the first metatarsal head, lesser metatarsal heads, and/or the fifth metatarsal base because of the plantarflexed and supinated forefoot (**Fig. 2**). These findings may also be present in the patient's family members because of the hereditary nature of CMT and other neurologic causes of cavus. When a hereditary neurologic disease is suspected, genetic counseling for your patient and their family may be considered and warranted.

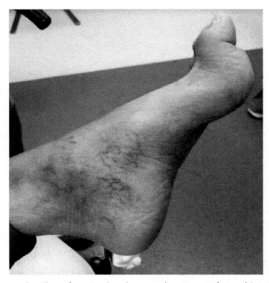

Fig. 1. On clinical examination claw-toeing is seen due to weakened intrinsic muscles of the foot. An equinus deformity of the forefoot on the rearfoot may also be noted and visualized by a plantarflexed first ray as seen in this photograph.

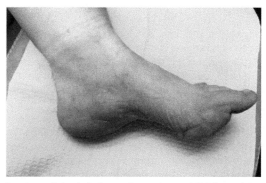

Fig. 2. Clinical examination of the left foot of a patient with idiopathic cavus foot deformity reveals a significantly increased plantar arch with a plantarflexed first ray, with hyperkeratosis plantar to the first metatarsal head.

In addition to the elevated arch and hindfoot varus that may be noted on clinical examination, there are several other reported findings that may help to determine the severity and flexibility of the cavus deformity. The "peek-a-boo heel" sign was first described in 1993, where the examiner can easily see the patients heel pad medially when observing from the front while the patient is standing in their normal angle and base of gate.[4] The average population has slight valgus of the heel in which the heel pad aligns with the rearfoot, which cannot be seen when examining the feet in front of the patient. It has been found that extremely small degrees of hindfoot varus are observed with the "peek-a-boo heel" sign in comparison with examining the heel from posterior only.[4]

Another commonly known test to be performed during the physical examination is the Coleman Block test, used to assess the rigidity of the hindfoot, an extremely important examination finding when determining the surgical procedure. Coleman first reported this clinical finding in 1977 in which he described a test to determine if the hindfoot was flexible during stance phase. It has been thought that a plantarflexed first metatarsal has been the driving force in cavus deformity, causing a pronated forefoot and subsequent supinated hindfoot.[5] If the hindfoot is found to be flexible, then corrective measures at the driving force of the plantarflexed first metatarsal result in correction of the secondary varus deformity of the hindfoot. If the hindfoot deformity is noted to be rigid, forefoot correction alone is not sufficient to correct the hindfoot deformity.[5] The test is performed by having a patient stand on a 1-inch-thick wooden block while dropping their hallux and first metatarsal over the medial side of the block.[4,5] The examiner then evaluates the heel to determine if the rearfoot has reduced to neutral or slight valgus. If the rearfoot has been found to reduce then the examiner can draw two conclusions: the deformity is considered flexible, meaning that the subtalar joint (STJ) is likely free of end-stage arthritic changes; and that the plantarflexed first ray is the driving force of the hindfoot deformity.[4]

Muscle strength should routinely be performed to assess the strength of the extrinsic muscles of the leg. It has been shown that a tendon should have strength of 4/5 on the Medical Research Council Manual Muscle Testing Scale when determining if it is a viable option for tendon transfer. Again, a thorough history and physical examination with emphasis on the neurologic examination and evaluation of muscle strength is warranted to determine the proper soft tissue balancing required during reconstruction.[6]

RADIOGRAPHIC EXAMINATION

Weight-bearing radiographs should routinely be obtained on patients presenting with foot pain and suspected underlying deformity. Standard weight-bearing anteroposterior, lateral, and oblique images are obtained for further assessment after clinical examination. On the weight-bearing lateral view Meary angle may be assessed to determine the plantarflexion deformity of the first metatarsal. Meary angle is formed by the bisection of the longitudinal axis of the talus and the longitudinal axis of the first metatarsal. In a neutral foot, Meary angle is seen as 0°, representing a talus and first metatarsal that are in line. An angle of greater than 5°, or bisections that are convex upward, typically indicate a cavus-type deformity.[7] Calcaneal inclination or calcaneal pitch can also be assessed on the lateral weight-bearing image (**Fig. 3**). Calcaneal inclination angle is formed from the bisection of the weight-bearing surface and a line drawn from the inferior most aspect of the calcaneal tuberosity and inferior distal point of the calcaneus. The average calcaneal inclination angle has been reported at 22°. An angle of greater than 30° indicates a cavus deformity of the hindfoot.[7] Furthermore, Hibb angle may also be assessed on the lateral image. Hibb angle is formed from the longitudinal bisection of the calcaneus and longitudinal bisection of the first metatarsal. A normal Hibb angle is typically less than 45°, with greater than 90° indicating a cavus deformity. Additional findings on the lateral weight-bearing images may be a decreased talocalcaneal angle, decreased talar declination angle, and posterior fibular translation because of external rotation.[8] Lastly, one may identify the apex of the deformity on lateral images, whether it be anterior involving primarily the forefoot; posterior involving the rearfoot via increased calcaneal inclination; or global, meaning a combination of deformity seen anteriorly and posteriorly (**Fig. 4**). Identifying the apex of the deformity is helpful to determine the location of surgical intervention required to reduce the present deformity.

Assessment of the anteroposterior weight-bearing images may show a decreased talocalcaneal angle, or kite angle, because of hindfoot varus and forefoot adduction.[3,7] Increased overlap of the metatarsal bases may also be seen indicating forefoot protonation.[7] Weight-bearing ankle radiographs should also be routinely evaluated, specifically the anteroposterior view, to assess for possible varus tilt of the ankle joint and end-stage arthritic changes.

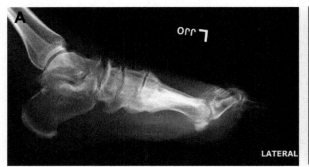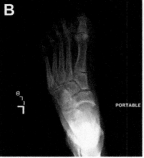

Fig. 3. (*A*) Lateral and (*B*) anteroposterior non–weight bearing radiographs of the left foot with cavus deformity secondary to cerebral palsy. Evidence of an increased calcaneal inclination angle and adaptive osteoarthritic changes of the subtalar joint, talonavicular joint, calcaneocuboid joint, and tarsometatarsal joints are noted. Characteristic clawing of the digits is also evident.

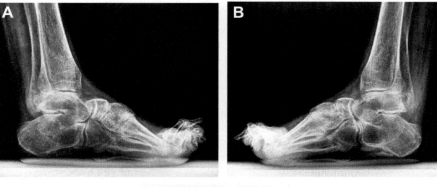

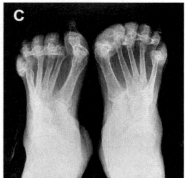

Fig. 4. Weight-bearing lateral radiographs of the right foot (*A*) and left foot (*B*) reveal a significant anterior apex of deformity located at the tarsometatarsal joints bilaterally. (*C*) Weight-bearing anteroposterior radiograph of the right and left foot.

Advanced imaging is not routinely ordered for the evaluation of cavus foot deformity; however, computed tomography scans may aid in determining the extent of hindfoot arthritic changes, and rule out rare tarsal coalitions that may be contributing to the deformity (**Fig. 5**). MRI may also be ordered to evaluate for soft tissue

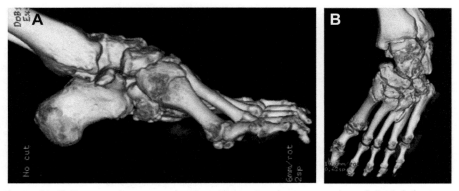

Fig. 5. (*A, B*) Computed tomography three-dimensional reconstruction of the left foot performed to assist in preoperative planning. Significant cavus deformity present at the midfoot with first ray plantarflexion and severe adductovarus.

pathologies, such as peroneal tendon tears, lateral ankle ligament injury, and articular degeneration.[3,9]

CONSERVATIVE TREATMENT

In the early stages of cavus the deformity is often flexible and therefore responsive to conservative measures. Patients with milder symptoms and mild deformity should be evaluated for conservative treatment. The goal of conservative treatment is to reduce pain by realigning the foot into a more neutral plantigrade position, thus reducing force and overload on the lateral column.[9] Additional conservative treatment options include anti-inflammatory medication, activity modification, and shoe modifications in addition to bracing and orthotics.[3] Common shoe modifications include extradepth shoes to accommodate for a high arch, tall toe box to accommodate for claw toe deformity, and lateral flare.[10] Custom orthotics with a deep heel cup, lateral rearfoot posting, and first ray cutout have proven to be successful in patients with flexible deformity.[3] Bracing and ankle-foot-orthoses are reserved for more advanced cases in which severe deformity is noted at the level of the ankle joint, or in patients with excessive neurologic weakness.[3]

SURGICAL TREATMENT

Soft tissue and joint-sparing techniques are most commonly reserved for patients in which a flexible cavus deformity has been identified clinically with lack of advanced-stage arthritic changes radiographically. Common procedures for flexible deformity include tendon transfers, first ray osteotomies, and calcaneal osteotomies. A surgeon must consider the progressive nature of the deformity and incidence of recurrence when evaluating for these joint-sparing procedures. When patients present with a rigid deformity and/or hindfoot arthritic changes present at the STJ, one must consider reliable surgical treatment options to obtain a stable, plantigrade foot. As with all osseous procedures of the foot and ankle, it is important for the surgeon to fully work-up the patient preoperatively including evaluation for age, comorbidities, osteoporosis, smoking status, history of steroid use, and many others that may hinder the probability of achieving soft tissue healing and osseous union. Surgical procedures should be chosen based on patient-centered goals, underlying cause, and the extent of deformity, thus making each cavus foot treatment unique and exclusive.

SURGICAL TECHNIQUE FOR TRIPLE ARTHRODESIS

The triple arthrodesis procedure was first described by Ryerson[11] in 1923 in which the procedure was designed to correct a variety of deformities of the foot including pes planus and pes cavus deformities. Today, triple arthrodesis remains a routinely used surgical procedure for treatment of a wide range of podiatric deformities including the cavus foot. The aim of the triple arthrodesis is to provide the patient with a plantigrade foot that improves function, stability, pain, and deformity. Cavus deformity is often times a complicated and progressive disease leaving recurrence of symptoms, or lack of adequate correction a common concern for podiatric surgeons. Triple arthrodesis, when performed with meticulous and precise dissection and preparation of the joint surfaces, can yield predictable and superior outcomes.

The beak triple arthrodesis was described by Siffert and colleagues in 1966 as a procedure specific for correction of cavus foot deformity.[3,6,12] Goals of the beak triple arthrodesis were to provide stabilization while preserving the structure of the anterior ankle joint and maintaining the length of the foot. Technique includes a partial osteotomy performed through the midtarsal joint, extending into the talar head. A dorsal ledge is intentionally left within the talar head creating a "beak." The dorsal cortex of the navicular is excised and the STJ is prepared in typical fashion. The forefoot is then displaced plantarly, so that the navicular rests just below the talar beak. This positioning locks the forefoot under the talus allowing for correction of the deformity and depression of the plantar arch.[12]

Classically, the Ollier lateral incisional approach has been described in which a single incision is performed from the tip of the lateral malleolus extending transversely and medially to the talonavicular (TN) joint allowing full access to the STJ, calcaneocuboid (CC) joint, and TN joint.[13] Over the years this incisional technique has fallen out of favor because of the significant amount of vital structures that one must avoid at the anterior midfoot, including the extensor tendons and superficial and deep neurovascular structures.[13] Incision planning is ultimately up to surgeon preference; however, a medial and lateral incisional approach is most commonly favored to allow for adequate exposure of the rearfoot while adhering to an atraumatic surgical dissection.

Our method includes a lateral curvilinear incision extending from the distal tip of the fibula to the base of the fourth metatarsal. This incision allows for visual access to the STJ and the CC joint. Dissection should be performed in layers with care taken to identify and retract the sural nerve and peroneal tendons plantarly. To gain access to the sinus tarsi often times the muscle belly of the extensor digitorum brevis requires retraction dorsally. A lamina spreader or Hintermann retractor can then be used to distract the STJ to allow for cartilage denudation (**Fig. 6**). To obtain full visualization of the posterior and medial STJ facets, the interosseous ligament is sharply transected with a scalpel, rongeur, or key elevator. Many different techniques are used to denude the cartilage down to the level of the subchondral plate. These include curettage, power burr or rasp, and osteotome/mallet. Our preference for cartilage denudation of the STJ includes a combination of hand curettage and using either a straight or curved osteotome. After the cartilage has been removed it is important to penetrate through the subchondral plate to enhance osseous union. This is achieved by fish-scaling with an osteotome and mallet and/or fenestrating the prepared joint surfaces with a smaller pitched drill or Kirschner wire (**Fig. 7**). Next, the CC joint may be prepared in similar fashion, through the same lateral incision. A lamina spreader or retractor may be used once again to distract and visualize the articular surfaces to allow for exposure to adequately denude the cartilage and prepare the joint surfaces.

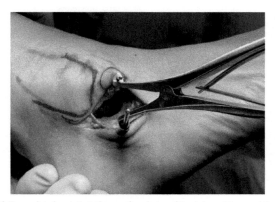

Fig. 6. Exposure of the subtalar joint through a lateral incision. Here a Hintermann retractor is used to gain visual access to the posterior and medial facets of the subtalar joint.

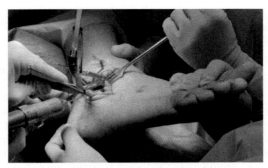

Fig. 7. Subchondral drilling is performed to the subtalar joint with a 3.0-mm drill bit. The subchondral plate is additionally fish-scaled with an osteotome and mallet to promote osseous union.

A medial incision is then performed from the medial gutter of the anterior ankle extending to the medial and inferior aspect of the naviculocuneiform joint. This linear incision provides full access and exposure of the TN joint. During dissection care must be taken to identify and retract the saphenous vein from the surgical field. The tibialis anterior tendon may also be retracted laterally to safely incise the joint capsule of the TN joint. Preparation of the TN joint is the most technically challenging because of the convex shape of the talar head. One must avoid excessive bone resection at the TN joint because the medial column is often short in a cavus foot deformity. Curettage and a curved osteotome with mallet are beneficial techniques to denude the cartilage from the joint surfaces while maintaining the convex contour of the talar head. Again, fish-scaling with an osteotome is vital to penetrate the subchondral plate, an important step during joint preparation.

After precise joint preparation of the STJ, CC, and TN joints, reduction is performed with temporary pin fixation. To properly reduce the varus deformity of the hindfoot, the surgeon may apply an abductory and dorsiflexory force at the level of the TN joint. The heel should be examined with a goal of a slight valgus position, often aiming for 5° of STJ valgus. Correction is then temporarily fixated with K-wires. To achieve adequate correction and reduction of the deformity we routinely perform a Steindler stripping procedure where the plantar fascia, abductor hallucis, flexor digitorum brevis, and abductor digiti minimi are released from their proximal origin on the calcaneal tuberosity. Releasing the contracted plantar fascia and associated structures allows for an increased dorsiflexory force at the midfoot, thus reducing the varus and cavus deformity of the foot. Often times additional wedge resection is required at the STJ to achieve adequate correction. A sagittal saw may be used for wedge resection from either the inferior lateral talus or the superior lateral calcaneus to reduce a significant varus deformity. Lateral-based wedge resection may also be necessary at the CC joint to reduce the midfoot. The surgeon must additionally be mindful that a Dwyer calcaneal osteotomy may be required if a varus position of the heel persists after reduction from joint preparation alone. From our experience, a weight-bearing heel varus deformity of 10° to 15° typically requires wedging of the STJ and an additional Dwyer calcaneal osteotomy to achieve a neutral hindfoot. A Dwyer lateral closing wedge osteotomy typically consists of an oblique wedge osteotomy within the posterior calcaneus just proximal and parallel to the peroneal tendons with removal of an 8- to 12-mm wedge to correct for heel varus (**Fig. 8**).[14,15] If correction cannot be fully achieved after preparation and reduction of the hindfoot,

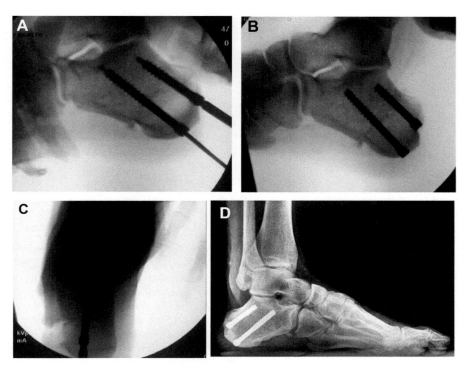

Fig. 8. (*A–C*) Intraoperative fluoroscopy of a Dwyer calcaneal wedge osteotomy with internal fixation via two partially threaded cannulated cancellous screws. (*D*) Postoperative weight-bearing lateral radiograph of the left foot after a Dwyer calcaneal osteotomy was performed for correction of a varus hindfoot.

a midfoot osteotomy may also be considered as an additional correctional procedure.

Fixation of the STJ is performed first with two 6.5 partially threaded cannulated cancellous screws. Guidewires are inserted from the posterior and plantar calcaneus into the body of the talus. Small stab incisions are made posterior to the weight-bearing surface of the heel to allow for screw placement. Intraoperative fluoroscopy with lateral and axial projections is used to confirm placements of the parallel guidewires. Standard Arbeitsgemeinschaft fur Osteosynthesefragen technique is then performed for insertion of the two partially threaded screws (**Fig. 9**).

Many different techniques of fixation have been used to fixate the TN joint including single compression screws, crossing compression screws, and staples. Our technique includes use of two crossing 4.0-mm or 4.5-mm partially threaded cannulated cancellous screws. One guidewire is directed from the distal, inferior, and medial aspect of the navicular through the talar neck and body and into the lateral aspect of the talar dome. Using an additional point of fixation decreases rotational forces and is achieved with a second compression screw. In a crossing pattern a guidewire is inserted from the distal lateral navicular body and driven into the talar neck and body. Intraoperative fluoroscopy is again used to ensure proper positioning of the guidewires. Following Arbeitsgemeinschaft fur Osteosynthesefragen guidelines, two 4.5-mm partially threaded cannulated screws are inserted overlying the guidewire to achieve stable fixation across the STJ (**Fig. 10**).

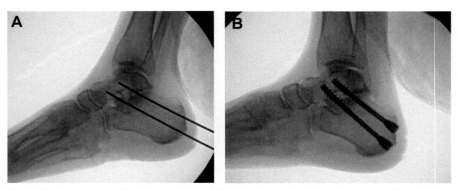

Fig. 9. (*A, B*) Intraoperative fluoroscopy of the right foot showing placement of two 6.5-mm partially threaded screws across the subtalar joint after guidewire placement.

Fixation of the CC joint is not necessary during triple arthrodesis after stable fixation of the STJ and TN joint. However, if subluxation of the CC joint is noted intraoperatively fixation should be considered to reduce the subluxation to avoid increased pain plantar to the cuboid postoperatively. If deformity correction is carried out through the CC then fixation is recommended. Fixation of the CC joint is ultimately up to surgeon preference. If fixation is desired one may use compression screws or staples. In our experience a two- or four-pronged nitinol staple applies stability and compression across the CC joint while remaining a low profile to avoid any irritation to the lateral peroneal tendons (**Fig. 11**).

Wound closure is a vital aspect of the surgical technique during a triple arthrodesis procedure. Wound dehiscence, notably higher with the lateral incision, is a complication one must attempt to avoid with wound closure that focuses on each individual anatomic layer. Deep closure of capsule and retinaculum is generally achieved with larger absorbable suture, such as 3–0 Vicryl, to avoid any dead space or hematoma formation. Subcutaneous skin closure is then completed with 4–0 Vicryl and skin

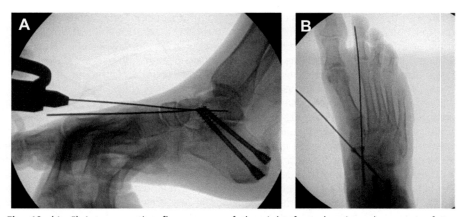

Fig. 10. (*A, B*) Intraoperative fluoroscopy of the right foot showing placement of two crossing 4.0-mm partially threaded screws from the navicular body into the talus. Correct guidewire placement is confirmed before insertion of the screws via standard Arbeitsgemeinschaft fur Osteosynthesefragen technique.

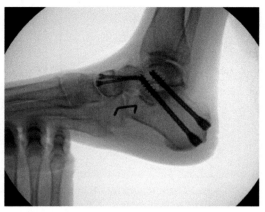

Fig. 11. Intraoperative fluoroscopy of the right foot showing placement of a two-pronged staple across the calcaneocuboid joint.

closure may be completed with nylon or absorbable suture depending on surgeon preference. A silastic drain has been proven to be useful when inserted into the lateral surgical incision to allow for adequate drainage and reduce risk of maceration and wound dehiscence.

Limited Arthrodesis in the Cavus Foot

Midfoot arthrodesis is often considered for patients in which an anterior cavus deformity is noted with goals of achieving a more dorsiflexed forefoot. If an anterior cavus deformity is noted with an equinus position of the forefoot at the level of the midfoot, then a triple arthrodesis would not sufficiently correct the more anterior apex of deformity. The traditional and historically known midfoot osteotomies were described by Cole and Japas, in which an osteotomy is performed at the level of the naviculocuneiform joints and cuboid.[6,16,17] In 1940 Cole[16] described an osteotomy performed from the central aspect of the navicular through the cuboid in a linear fashion. A second osteotomy is made just anterior and creates a dorsal wedge of bone that connects with the first osteotomy plantarly. The wedge of bone is removed and the forefoot is dorsiflexed out of an equinus position, closing the gap from the wedge removal.[16] Japas[17] described an additional midfoot osteotomy in 1968 in which a V-osteotomy is created at the level of the midfoot with a medial and lateral arm extending distally while sparing the tarsometatarsal joints. The apex of the V-shaped osteotomy is often performed at the midline of the foot within the navicular. The medial arm is then extended through the medial cuneiform, and the lateral arm through the cuboid. The distal foot is then displaced dorsally in relation to the posterior foot, allowing for correction of the cavus deformity without shortening the foot.[17] In patients in which a global cavus deformity is noted, a triple arthrodesis and midfoot osteotomy may be performed in conjunction to achieve adequate reduction (**Fig. 12**). Midfoot osteotomies may also be combined with a Dwyer calcaneal osteotomy and soft tissue procedures in patients that present with a flexible cavus deformity without evidence of adaptive arthritic changes (**Fig. 13**).

One may also choose to perform a medial double arthrodesis in comparison with triple arthrodesis for correction of hindfoot deformity. A medial double arthrodesis, where the STJ and TN joint are prepared and fixated through a singular medial

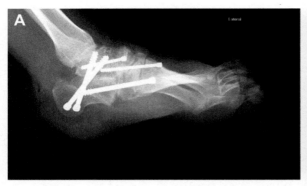
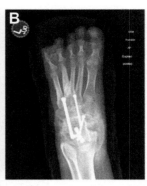

Fig. 12. Postoperative non–weight bearing lateral (A) and anteroposterior (B) radiographic view of the left foot after a calcaneal osteotomy, triple arthrodesis, and midfoot arthrodesis for treatment of severe cavus deformity secondary to poliomyelitis.

incision, is as effective in reducing hindfoot deformity.[18] Astion and colleagues[19] had previously described reserved motion of the hindfoot after specific fusion. Arthrodesis of the TN joint has been found to reduce hindfoot motion significantly, reducing the motion of the CC joint to 2° postoperatively.[19] The minimal motion reserved at the CC joint brings into question the need for fusion. In our experience, if reduction cannot be achieved alone through the STJ and TN joint, preparation and fusion of the CC joint may allow for better correction. If evidence of osteoarthritic changes is noted to the CC joint, or if a plantarflexed cuboid is seen clinically or radiographically, arthrodesis is preferred to reduce postoperative pain.

Postoperative Management

Following meticulous wound closure patients are placed in a sterile surgical dressing and a well-padded, bivalved, below knee fiberglass cast to allow for postoperative swelling. Initially patients are to remain non–weight bearing to the surgical limb with use of crutches, knee scooter, or walker for assistance. Patients are encouraged to

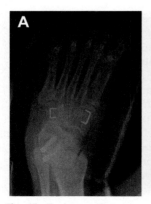
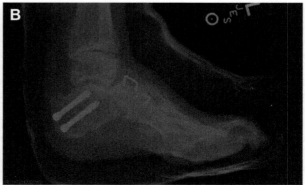

Fig. 13. Postoperative non–weight bearing anteroposterior (A) and lateral (B) views of the left foot. A tendo Achilles lengthening, Steindler stripping, Dwyer calcaneal osteotomy and a Cole midfoot osteotomy was performed because of painful cavus foot deformity. Two 6.5-mm cannulated screws and two staples were used for the calcaneal and midfoot fixation.

perform knee flexion and extension exercises postoperatively for deep vein thrombosis prophylaxis, supplemented with oral anticoagulation for the length of their non–weight bearing status. Deep vein thrombosis prophylaxis is up to physicians discretion as well as postoperative pain management. Patients are followed closely during the postoperative period with routine plain film radiographs taken to monitor osseous union across the hindfoot. Adequate consolidation is often seen by 6 to 8 weeks, but may vary because of patient comorbidities, medications, bone quality, and compliance. Once partial consolidation has been noted with stable hardware fixation, patients may be transitioned into partial weight bearing in a controlled ankle motion walker with use of crutches or a walker. This typically occurs after 4 weeks postoperatively, but may vary depending on the patient bone quality and body mass index. Once osseous consolidation has been achieved to all fusion sites the patient may begin to transition out of the controlled ankle motion boot into supportive shoe gear as tolerated. Patients are often prescribed a course of physical therapy with goals to reduce pain and inflammation, and increase strength to the surgical limb.

Complications

As with all foot and ankle surgeries one must perform careful anatomic dissection with thorough wound closure in layers to avoid wound complications. Wound dehiscence and postoperative infection are complications surgeons face during their career that require close patient monitoring. Delayed union and nonunion are two additional complications associated with arthrodesis procedures. The use of a medial and lateral incisional approach for triple arthrodesis allows for better visual access to the joints of the hindfoot and ultimately more precise joint preparation to reduce the incident of nonunion. Orthobiologics should be considered for patients where a gap or void is present post–joint preparation to facilitate osseous union. Autogenous grafting is superior but exposes the patient to additional surgical exposure and possible donor site morbidity. Numerous allograft orthobiologics have been deemed successful to promote osteoconduction and osteoinduction at surgical sites. Recurrence of deformity or residual postoperative pain can often be avoided by proper surgical planning with the correct procedure of choice to accommodate the deformity. Triple arthrodesis has been proven to be a superior surgical option for significant hindfoot deformities by allowing correction and pain reduction while providing the ability to achieve a stable plantigrade foot.

SUMMARY

Surgical treatments should vary from patient to patient depending on the apex of deformity, reducibility, progression of underlying neuromuscular disease, and evidence of osteoarthritic changes. No cavovarus foot deformity is the same, which requires well thought out surgical planning to achieve the desired postoperative outcome. A detailed conversation should be had with patients preoperatively with emphasis on goals of treatment, anticipated surgical outcomes, and postoperative protocols. Mild to moderate cavus foot deformity may be adequately treated surgically with soft tissue procedures, such as tendon balancing, in addition to joint-sparing osteotomies. Triple arthrodesis has proven to be an effective surgical option for patients experiencing rigid cavus foot deformity with a posterior apex and/or hindfoot joint adaptations from long-standing deformity. Arthrodesis of the STJ, TN, and CC joint allows for satisfactory reduction while providing the patient with a stable, plantigrade foot. Intraoperatively one must assess the extent of deformity, because a triple arthrodesis may not be sufficient in itself for correction of more severe deformities. A

Dwyer calcaneal osteotomy, and/or a midfoot arthrodesis may additionally be considered to provide a more neutral midfoot and hindfoot. Patients requiring significant hindfoot reconstruction, such as a triple arthrodesis, necessitate close monitoring in the postoperative period to ensure proper soft tissue and osseous union.

CLINICS CARE POINTS

- Goals of surgical treatment of a cavus foot include reduction of deformity to establish a pain free, plantigrade foot.
- Surgeons should be aware of the difficulty to obtain full correction in patients with significant deformity and must be conscious of surgical techniques including soft tissue procedures, joint-sparing procedures, and arthrodesing procedures.
- It is important to recognize when one may not be able to obtain full correction with a triple arthrodesis and may require additional correction through a Dwyer calcaneal osteotomy and/or midfoot osteotomy.
- To avoid maceration and wound dehiscence of the lateral surgical incision for a triple arthrodesis a silastic drain inserted within the incision is recommended to avoid postoperative incision healing complications.

DISCLOSURE

The authors have nothing to disclose.

REFERENCES

1. Bernasconi A, Cooper L, Lyle S, et al. Pes cavovarus in Charcot-Marie-Tooth compared to idiopathic cavovarus foot: a preliminary weightbearing CT analysis. Foot Ankle Surg 2020. https://doi.org/10.1016/j.fas.2020.04.004.
2. Sraj SA, Abdulmassih S, Abdelnoor J. Medium to long-term follow-up following correction of pes cavus deformity. J Foot Ankle Surg 2008;47(6):527–32.
3. Kaplan JRM, Aiyer A, Cerrato RA, et al. Operative treatment of the cavovarus foot. Foot Ankle Int 2018;39(11):1370–82.
4. Manoli A, Graham B. The subtle cavus foot, "the underpronator," a review. Foot Ankle Int 2005;26(3):256–63.
5. Coleman SS, Chestnut WJ. A simple test for hindfoot flexibility in the cavovarus foot. Clin Orthopaedics Relat Res 1977;123:60–2.
6. Zide JR, Myserson MS. Arthrodesis for the cavus foot: when, where, and how? Foot Ankle Clin N Am 2013;18:755–67.
7. Akoh CC, Phisitkul P. Clinical examination and radiographic assessment of the cavus foot. Foot Ankle Clin N Am 2019;24:183–93.
8. Kim BS. Reconstruction of cavus foot: a review. Open Orthop J 2017;11(1):651–9.
9. Maynou C, Szymanski C, Thiounn A. The adult cavus foot. EFFORT Open Rev 2017;2:221–9.
10. Rosenbaum AJ, Lisella J, Patel N, et al. The cavus foot. Med Clin North Am 2014;98:301–12.
11. Ryerson EW. Arthrodesing operations on the feet. J Bone Joint Surg Am 1923;5:453–71.
12. Siffert RS, Forster RI, Nachamie B. "Beak" triple arthrodesis for correction of severe cavus deformity. Clin Orthopaedics Relat Res 1966;45(1):101–6.

13. McGlamry ED, Ruch JA, Mahan K, et al. Triple arthrodesis. The Podiatry Institute: seminars, surgery courses, board review materials. Available at: https://www.podiatryinstitute.com/pdfs/Update_1987/1987_30.pdf. Accessed May 2020.

14. Dwyer FC. A new approach to the treatment of pes cavus. Societe International De Chirurgie Orthopedique et de Traumatologie, Imprimerie Lielens, Bruxelles; 1955. p. 551–8.

15. Lamm BM, Gesheff MG, Salton HL, et al. Preoperative planning and intraoperative technique for accurate realignment of the Dwyer calcaneal osteotomy. J Foot Ankle Surg 2012;51(6):743–8.

16. Cole WH. The treatment of claw-foot. J Bone Joint Surg 1940;22(4):895–908.

17. Japas LM. Surgical treatment of pes cavus by tarsal V-osteotomy. J Bone Joint Surg 1968;50(5):927–44.

18. DeVries JG, Scharer B. Hindfoot deformity corrected with double versus triple arthrodesis: radiographic comparison. J Foot Ankle Surg 2015;54(3):424–7.

19. Astion DJ, Deland JT, Otis JC, et al. Motion of the hindfoot after simulated arthrodesis. J Bone Joint Surg Am 1997;79:241–6.

Tendon Transfers and Their Role in Cavus Foot Deformity

Thorsten Q. Randt, MD, MBA[a], Joshua Wolfe, DPM, MHA[b],*,
Emily Keeter, DPM[c], Harry John Visser, DPM[b]

KEYWORDS

- Tendon transfer • Pes cavus • Cavus foot deformity • Spasticity • Dropfoot

KEY POINTS

- Management of the cavus foot deformity requires a comprehensive approach to patient evaluation, conservative therapy, and surgical intervention.
- History and physical examination of the patient with a cavus foot deformity should focus on their current disease state as well as evaluate underlying neurologic, congenital, and traumatic diagnoses and related events.
- Evaluation of foot deformity for rigidity and spasticity is imperative before any surgical intervention.
- Patient education on potential complications and postoperative expectations is imperative to optimize surgical outcomes.

INTRODUCTION

The simplest definition of pes cavus is a high arched foot, which occurs only in the sagittal plane. Cavus foot type may be a congenital variant, an acquired progressive neurologic or non-neurological condition, or a component of a triplane disorder as in pes cavovarus.[1] Pes cavus is also further broken down into the 3 most commonly accepted subgroups of pes cavus: anterior cavus, posterior cavus, and mixed/combined cavus. Before surgical consideration, appropriate evaluation and conservative measures should be attempted and a proper clinical evaluation and radiographic evaluation should be performed. In addition, the plane of deformity should be identified and the deformity should be examined for flexibility. Tendon transfer as a means of

[a] Department of Foot Surgery, Clinics of Traumatology and Orthopedics, St. George Hospital, Lohmühlenstrasse 5, Hamburg D-20099, Germany; [b] SSM Health DePaul Hospital, Foot and Ankle Surgery Residency, 12303 DePaul Drive, Suite 701, St Louis, MO 63044, USA; [c] American Foundation of Lower Extremity Surgery and Research, 2301 Indian Wells, Suite A, Alamogordo, NM 88310, USA
* Corresponding author.
E-mail address: joshua.wolfe.dpm@gmail.com

Clin Podiatr Med Surg 38 (2021) 427–443
https://doi.org/10.1016/j.cpm.2021.02.005
0891-8422/21/© 2021 Elsevier Inc. All rights reserved.

treatment for cavus foot deformity has been a longstanding and accepted practice for flexible cavus variants. Understanding the planes of deformity and the respective deforming forces is essential to allow for appropriate selection of tendon transfers to counteract these forces. Furthermore, it is crucial to determine whether the patient's pes cavus is of progressive or nonprogressive etiology. Tendon transfers are only indicated in flexible, nonprogressive pes cavus.[2–6]

CLINICAL EVALUATION FOR TENDON TRANSFERS
History

As with any surgical evaluation, the history and physical are the starting points for tendon transfer consideration for a cavus foot. The history is especially important in this case because of the onset of the deformity and any inciting events. Consideration should be given to the precipitating factors leading to the cavus deformity, such as neurologic conditions, motor or sensory neuropathies, traumatic events, or idiopathic causes.[7] More than 50% of symptomatic pes cavus feet are the result of a neurologic disorder stemming from the brain, spinal cord, or peripheral nerves.[8]

The level of the neurologic disorder is important for the type of muscle imbalance. A lower motor neuron (LMN) lesion can produce a flaccid paralysis, whereas an upper motor neuron lesion (UMN) can result in spasticity. **Fig. 1** presents a patient with peroneal nerve palsy. The analysis of a flaccid paralysis is less difficult and the effect of transfers more predictable. When spasticity is present, the lack of selective voluntary control makes diagnosis more difficult and the procedure susceptible for new deformities. In such cases, it is even more essential to have a thorough clinical and neurophysiological evaluation of the patient.[9–12]

Physical Examination

During the physical examination, the practitioner must check range of motion of all joints to help determine flexibility versus rigidity. Examination of the patient's foot, with and without weight bearing, is necessary to assess changes in the medial longitudinal arch, as well as to elucidate the presence of contracture to the lesser digits. From a weight-bearing stance, clinicians should pay attention to a possible "peek-a-boo" heel sign, indicative of heel varus and any callosity patterns present.[6,8,9] Examination the lower extremity should include calf wasting, atrophy, and any muscle hypertrophy.[2] Tendon transfers are applicable in only a flexible, nonprogressive pes

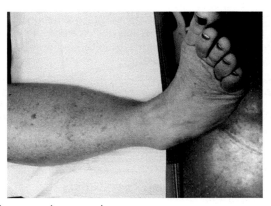

Fig. 1. Patient with peroneal nerve palsy.

cavus foot type. Failure to determine this early on, will likely lead to failure and complications in the future. As with any pes cavus, the Coleman Block test should be performed to determine the rigidity of the rearfoot to the forefoot.[13,14] If the rearfoot corrects with plantarflexion of the first ray, this is indicative of a flexible cavus foot type. Flexible cavus typically results from muscular imbalances among the antagonist muscles in the lower extremity, and preferred treatment is tendon transfers, soft tissue releases, and osteotomies.[2,15]

Manual muscle testing is an essential step in the physical examination. Muscle imbalance occurs when the antagonist or agonist muscles over power one another. Manual muscle testing should be assessed and graded according to the Medical Research Council scale, as it is not recommended to transfer less than grade 4, as seen in **Table 1**.[16] While transferring muscles in the same phase, 1 grade is lost. If transferring out-of-phase muscles, 2 grades of strength are lost.[17]

TYPES OF CAVUS

Once the surgeon has determined progressive versus nonprogressive deformity, radiographic evaluation should be performed for further evaluation. The thorough radiographic evaluation of the cavus foot is outside of the scope of this article. On lateral weight-bearing foot films, Hibbs angle (N < 45), Meary angle (N = 0), Calcaneal Pitch angle (N = 15–20), Talar declination angle (N < 21), and tibiotalar angle (N = 110) should all be evaluated to help determine the type of cavus foot present, as well as the level of deformity. Use of calcaneal axial radiographs is critical to elucidate the degree of hindfoot varus present. With anterior cavus, the forefoot is lower or more plantar than the rearfoot. On a lateral view, the apex of the deformity is distal to the talonavicular joint. With posterior cavus, the apex of the deformity on a lateral view is proximal to the talonavicular joint with a high calcaneal pitch angle and the deformity isolated to the rearfoot. Combined or global cavus, has elements from both anterior and posterior cavus.[18–21] It is important to always evaluate the patient's foot both in weight bearing and non–weight bearing to determine the type of cavus present. Some patients will present with what is referred to as "collapsible cavus" in non–weight bearing, but on weight-bearing examination, a rectus foot is formed.[22,23]

UNDERSTANDING DEFORMING FORCES

Examination of the cavus foot should include evaluation of the deforming forces causing the deformity. In the flexible cavus foot, this is important to understand to prevent

Table 1 Manual muscle testing scale	
Grade	**Muscle Activity**
0	No contraction
1	Visible or palpable contraction, but no movement
2	Movement with gravity eliminated
3	Movement against gravity
4	Movement against gravity with some resistance
5	Movement against gravity with full resistance

Data From: Bohannon, R. W. (2019). Considerations and practical options for measuring muscle strength: a narrative review. *BioMed research international, 2019.*

recurrence and to properly address the etiology of the deformity. These conditions can provide valuable information to interpret where deficits may occur and to predict whether the patient may experience a progressive or spastic deformity. This is primarily done through tendon augmentation to alleviate the deforming force. As with bony procedures, the main goal in tendon transfers is to reestablish a balanced muscle function around the foot and ankle to create a plantigrade foot. Tendon transfers should help to reorient the foot axis in gait after successful bony reconstruction to a correct lever arm. A tendon transfer will never achieve a correct alignment if there are underlying structural (bony) deformities hindering the contracture of across these joints.[24–31]

The subtalar joint axis and the ankle joint axis define 4 quadrants within the foot's geometry. According to the anatomic position of the tendon, the surgeon can deduce the function of this tendon or conversely the "loss" of function of this tendon. Tendons lying posteriorly to the ankle joint serve as plantar flexors of the ankle joint, whereas those anteriorly are dorsiflexors. The subtalar axis defines the forces for eversion and inversion. Tendons lying lateral to this joint work as evertors and medially work as inverters. All of the extrinsic muscles of the foot cross both the ankle joint and subtalar joint and therefore will have an effect in both axes. For example, the peroneus longus works both as a strong plantar flexor (with emphasis on the first metatarsal) as well as an evertor of the rearfoot.

According to Silver and colleagues,[32] equilibrium of power is even more complex with stronger plantar flexors and invertors compared with dorsiflexors and evertors. Based on their strength percentage system, which was based on fiber length of muscles and their respective mass, it was shown that the relative strength percentage of dorsiflexors is 9.4% in comparison with 54.5% of plantarflexors. With eversion and inversion, the strength percentages were 8.1% to 12%, respectively. Only the bony architecture (eg, positioning of the bones in relation to each other in the 3 dimensions) and the modulating effect of the central nervous system (via physiologic innervations) will keep the shape and function of the foot as seen in a rectus foot. This helps to explain the development of pes cavus in UMN diseases like cerebral palsy or polio.[32]

It is well established that the peroneus longus (PL) tendon has a key role in cavus foot deformity. Overactivity of the PL in combination with weakness of the tibialis anterior, its antagonist, is cited as the primary driver of plantar flexion of the first ray, resulting in forefoot-driven cavus, and can be demonstrated with the Coleman block test.[6,13,33,34]

A secondary deforming force can be found through the posterior tibial (PT) tendon. When the PT tendon overpowers its antagonist, the peroneus brevis (PB) tendon, it also can contribute to the cavus foot deformity. This becomes particularly important in a combined etiology of flexible cavus, which can be seen with overpowering by both PL and PT, which results in a more severe deformity. Depending on the etiology of the patient's cavus, this is seen in patients with drop foot deformities often seen in Charcot-Marie-Tooth (CMT) disease.[35–37]

The third deforming force to consider is equinus. Equinus is a rare contributor to the cavus foot deformity, but should be evaluated to obtain proper musculotendon balancing of the cavus foot.[1,38]

ADDRESSING CAVUS THROUGH TRANSFERS

Determining tendon transfers to address cavus foot is a complicated process. As previously mentioned, the deforming force related to the cavus deformity is a primary consideration when planning a tendon transfer. In addition, it is advisable to also identify and keep in mind the type of cavus that is being addressed. Cavus can primarily be considered in 3 phases related to tendon transfers: anterior cavus, posterior cavus, and mixed/combined cavus. Although these have been discussed previously, it is important to understand the effects of the deforming force, its relationship to the type of cavus being addressed, and the agonist-antagonist relationships of the musculotendinous units before transfer. Much of the work of Hansen, Manoli, and Myerson, among others have been critical in the development of treatment algorithms when considering tendon transfers.[1,6,15,35,39–41]

BASICS OF TENDON TRANSFERS

Understanding the principles of tendon transfers and their application to the foot and ankle is important to promote patient outcomes. Tendon transfers should accomplish 3 goals:

- improve motor function for restoration of balance and prevention of contractures
- eliminate deforming forces
- stabilize the alignment of the foot

Tendon selection should take into account if the harvested muscle is strong enough to perform its new function. In addition, the loss of its normal physiologic effect on foot alignment should not lead to undesired new deformities or imbalance.

As previously stated, tendons lose one grade of strength with in-phase transfers, and 2 grades with out-of-phase transfers. Therefore, a transfer of a muscle/tendon with a strength less than grade 4 or 5 is rarely useful if you want to achieve motor function. Transferring a tendon with a grade 3 or less will be helpful only in the case of a tenodesis. Even so, it is still questioned whether a stance phase muscle can truly convert to a swing phase muscle.

Close and Todd[42] showed in 1959 that muscles of the same phase would most of the time rapidly regain their activity in 7 to 8 weeks, whereas muscles from out-of-phase were generally unable to do so. However, clinical experience has shown that a patient can obtain a kind of functional conversion (eg, posterior tibialis tendon transfer for dorsiflexion) instead of a phase conversion. Especially patients with an LMN can bring about active dorsiflexion on a voluntary basis. This provides one more reason as to why an active and refined rehabilitation protocol for the patient with a tendon transfer must be followed for success.[42]

Timing is another important issue for transfer procedures. First, the underlying disease may set the point of surgery when it is a dynamic condition like in CMT with progressive loss of motor function or after brain damage where one has to wait for decreasing spasticity. Second, age is important for all osseous procedures. In the pediatric patient, early tendon transfer can prevent the further development of deformities. It is important to ensure that the patient has as much mature bone stock as possible, correlating this with the disease process and weighing this against the risks and benefits of the procedure. In addition, it is advantageous if the patient is old enough to understand the rehabilitation protocol.[43,44]

The principle of atraumatic technique should always be used to preserve viability (eg, blood supply), gliding mechanism, and sound soft tissue coverage of the tendon. Careful planning starting with precise skin incision and respecting the eventuality of scar tissue formation is therefore essential. The exposure time to air during surgery should be kept as short as possible. Absolute hemostasis will prevent adhesions as well as constant irrigation of the wound, preferably with Ringer solution.

The fixation of the tendon should maintain the physiologic length of the corresponding muscle, which means care should be taken to prevent over tensioning the tendon.

Too little tension on the other hand will lead to loss of power because of shortening of the muscle. Whenever a split tendon technique is used, one should be cautious to ensure that the tension is shared equally between the 2 branches, unequal forces will result in asymmetry and ineffective force on the less tensioned side.

There are principally 3 ways to fix tendons in transfer procedures:

- tendon to tendon
- tendon to periosteum
- tendon to bone

The technically easiest methods are tendon to tendon with a side-to-side anastomosis or Pulvertaft technique. However, there is a high risk of slippage, which is similarly seen when suturing a tendon to the periosteum. In most procedures, it is advisable and possible to use either suture anchor systems to decrease the pull-out force on the new insertional point of the tendon or to use an interference screw to create a reliable tendon bone interface.

TENDON TRANSFERS AMENABLE IN PES CAVUS SURGERY

Tendon transfers in the flexible pes cavus foot can be simplified into compartments and their respective pathology. Using a simplified approach with an understanding of the deforming forces previously mentioned will aid the surgeon to avoid pitfalls and allow for reproducible results.

FOREFOOT/ANTERIOR COMPARTMENT TENDON TRANSFERS

The forefoot or anterior cavus can be addressed through a variety of transfers and releases. In the consideration of tendon transfers, there are multiple avenues that can be pursued to address this deformity depending on whether the cavus is isolated to the first ray or is present through the lesser metatarsals as well.

JONES TENDON TRANSFER

When the anterior tibialis tendon is weakened, the other anterior compartment muscles overcompensate to help dorsiflex the ankle, creating overpowering of the extensor tendons leading to contracted lesser digits and a cocked-up hallux. The dorsal contracture of the digits creates greater plantarflexion of the metatarsal heads, enhancing the cavus deformity. The Jones tendon transfer releases the extensor hallucis longus (EHL) tendon from the distal phalanx and reinserts into the neck of the first metatarsal, lifting it from a plantarflexed position.[15,36,45]

The sub capital insertion in the first metatarsal can be realized either by a sling technique (drilling a horizontal hole in the metatarsal, passing the EHL tendon sling through it and suturing it back to itself) or with the easier interference screw technique. The distal stump is sutured to the extensor hallucis brevis to correct or prevent a cocked-up toe position of the hallux and in most instances an interphalangeal arthrodesis is advisable.

HIBBS TENDON TRANSFER

The Hibbs tendon transfer is primarily useful in the reducible claw toe deformity. The Hibbs tendon transfer specifically is a transfer of the extensor digitorum longus (EDL) to the lateral cuneiform. **Fig. 2** demonstrates clinical examples of the Hibbs tendon transfer. This is performed to correct claw toe deformities secondary to the overpull of the EDL (extensor substitution). In addition, the transfer of the EDL to the lateral

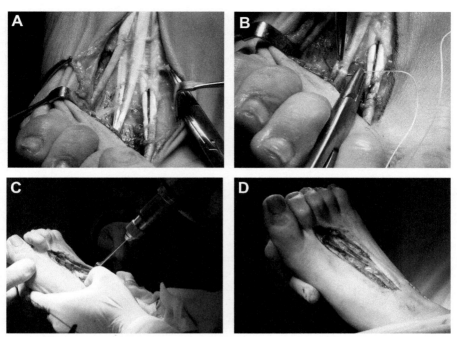

Fig. 2. (*A*) Initial exposure of extensor tendons for Hibbs tendon transfer. (*B*) Anastomosis of distal EDL to EDB before transection of EDL. (*C*) Transfer of EDL to lateral cuneiform. (*D*) Completion of Hibbs tendon transfer.

cuneiform allows for the EDL to continue to aid in dorsiflexion of the foot. It is important to use the Kelekian push-up test after transfer, as it aids in evaluating if additional metatarsophalangeal joint release and proximal interphalangeal joint fusion of the lesser toes is necessary.[46]

The approach is a curvilinear incision starting from 2 cm proximal to the head of the third metatarsal ending near to the calcaneocuboid joint. The distal stumps of the EDL are attached to the corresponding extensor digitorum brevis (EDB) tendons. The proximal stump is sutured together and fixed preferably with an interference screw in the lateral cuneiform or the cuboid.

TIBIALIS ANTERIOR TENDON TRANSFER/SPLIT TIBIALIS ANTERIOR TENDON TRANSFER

With transfer of the tibialis anterior tendon, the supinatory forces in the foot are reduced. In the case of a split tibialis anterior tendon transfer (STATT) the tendon transfer works like a check rein, balancing the supinatory and pronatory effects. With a total tibialis anterior tendon transfer, depending on its lateral point of reinsertion (eg, intermediate or lateral cuneiform or even cuboid), it is possible to not only contribute dorsiflexion but eversion is possible as well.[47–50]

A STATT needs 3 incisions. It starts with an incision over the insertion at the medial cuneiform and base of the first metatarsal. The second incision is at the anterior surface of the ankle joint just above the extensor retinaculum. The tendon is then split in half and the lateral half of the tendon is subcutaneously routed laterally underneath the retinaculum. The third incision is made over the peroneus tertius approximately 2 cm proximal to its insertion. Fixation is accomplished in a side-to-side technique or in the case of absence of the peroneus tertius with a tenodesis screw in the cuboid.[47] The foot is held in slight eversion and neutral to 5-degree dorsiflexion during fixation for adequate tensioning. By splitting the tibialis anterior tendon in half, you are weakening the strength of the tendon, therefore decreasing the varus pull of the tendon.

LATERAL COMPARTMENT TENDON TRANSFERS

Transfers of the lateral compartment are perhaps the most common, and one of the most important tendon transfers in the flexible cavus foot. This is significant, as the posterior compartment antagonists on the medial aspect of the foot often overpower the lateral compartment agonists. This is commonly due to the shared innervation of the lateral compartment with the anterior compartment, the deep peroneal nerve.

PERONEUS LONGUS TO PERONEUS BREVIS TRANSFER

Transfer of the PL to the PB is a simple and effective transfer to aid in reconstruction of the flexible cavus foot. In this instance, the PL, which typically acts as a plantar flexor of the first ray, is harvested to increase the dorsiflexion and eversion function of the PB. By transferring the PL to the PB, one is able to supplement the PB so that its power is equitable to the tibialis posterior tendon. Moreover, the plantarflexory force on the first metatarsal is reduced. It has been demonstrated in the literature that the PL can switch gait phase in a high percentage of patients.[6,34,51]

The incision is located approximately 4 cm proximal to the base of the fifth metatarsal. The PL is identified as it passes under the cuboid into the peroneal tunnel. The tendon is cut as distally as possible and sutured in a side-to-side manner to the overlying PB tendon with the foot positioned in slight eversion.

PERONEUS LONGUS TRANSFER FOR ADDITIONAL DORSIFLEXION (MODIFIED BRIDLE PROCEDURE)

An additional method for aiding in dorsiflexion is the modified Bridle procedure using the PL tendon. Although not a first-line treatment, it is useful in limited cases. The first incision is made just proximal to the lower third of the lateral leg. As the PL tendon lies superficial to the brevis, it is easily identified. The second incision lies above the lateral edge of the cuboid. The tendon is cut as distal as possible in the plantar peroneal tunnel. It is pulled back through the first incision and rerouted under the extensor retinaculum for fixation in the lateral cuneiform (third incision).[52–55]

POSTERIOR COMPARTMENT TENDON TRANSFERS

Posterior compartment musculotendinous units are the strongest insertions to the foot in the case of cavus foot deformities. Because of this, the posterior compartment is also a main contributor to deforming forces of the foot. Transfer or augmentation of the posterior compartment can and should be considered in 2 instances: drop foot or overpowering of the tibialis posterior tendon in relation to the lateral foot. Augmentation of the tibialis posterior tendon typically results in lengthening to be more equitable in relation to the power of the lateral compartment.

FOOT DROP AND ITS ROLE IN CAVUS

Foot drop in the cavus foot can be a significant contributor to gait dysfunction in the neurologically driven cavus foot, such as seen in CMT. These patients often struggle with ambulation and present with the stereotypical "high steppage gait." Although bracing should be an initial treatment modality, the patient who is not able to comply with bracing may be a candidate for a PT tendon transfer.

TIBIALIS POSTERIOR TENDON TRANSFER VIA INTEROSSEOUS TRANSFER

Transfer of the PT tendon is a critical procedure for the treatment of drop foot for those who are not able to tolerate bracing. Indications include, among others, weak or paralyzed anterior muscle group, CMT, dropfoot, equinovarus deformity, and recurrent clubfoot deformity.[55–60]

The main technique is a 4-incision approach. The first incision is at the insertion at the navicular bone for tendon release. The second posteromedial incision is approximately 7 to 10 cm proximal to the tip of the medial malleolus to free the tibialis posterior muscle belly from the dorsum of the distal tibia. The third incision is anterolateral (approximately 2 cm below the posteromedial incision to alleviate the acute angle of the tendon and to prevent a pulley-effect of the tendon on the tibia) 1 cm lateral to the tibial crest to window the interosseous membrane. Careful dissection must respect the neurovascular bundle lying next to the tibialis posterior muscle belly. The fourth incision is located on the dorsum of the foot for reinsertion of the tendon in the lateral cuneiform. It is fixed after passing beneath the extensor retinaculum with the foot in neutral position with an interference screw.

SPLIT POSTERIOR TIBIAL TENDON LATERAL TRANSFER

Alternatively, a split technique could be used for a more balanced transfer of the tibialis posterior tendon similar to the STATT technique. This technique is useful in the case of spastic but flexible clubfoot deformity. The difference is that one-half of the tendon is left attached to the navicular bone and the other half will be attached to the PB tendon. In addition, the medial incision at the navicular and the posteromedial incision at the lower third of the leg, a third approach is made semicircular around the tip of the lateral malleolus. The peroneal retinaculum is tunneled and a blunt curved Kelly forceps is maneuvered just behind the fibula in close connection to the dorsum of the tibia to catch the armored split tendon. It is then pulled through the lateral wound and fixed in a Pulvertaft technique to the PB tendon.[12,47,61]

AUGMENTATION OF PERONEUS BREVIS WITH FLEXOR DIGITORUM LONGUS TENDON

If the tibialis posterior tendon is strong and the peroneus function is weak with a still flexible midtarsal joint, a transfer of the flexor digitorum longus (FDL) can balance the situation. **Fig. 3** provides a clinical example of an FDL transfer to the PB insertion. The procedure starts with a medial incision between the os naviculare and the base of the first metatarsal. The abductor hallucis is lifted off and the dissection goes further to the master knot of Henry. The tendon of the FDL is harvested in the typical way and armored with a suture 0 or 1. A posteromedial incision is made similar to the PT tendon technique. The third incision follows the steps in the split PT tendon (SPTT) lateral transfer with blunt tunneling behind fibula and tibia. The FDL is then sutured to the distal part of the PB tendon.[62,63]

LENGTHENING OF TENDONS

Tendon augmentation and more specifically tendon lengthening is an important part of pes cavus reconstruction. Balancing of deforming forces through tendon lengthening, in lieu of transfer, allows for appropriate surgical procedure to be used.

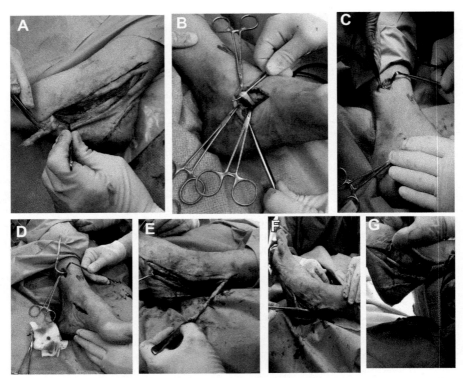

Fig. 3. (*A*) Deteriorated PB in cavus deformity. (*B*) Identification and isolation of FDL before transfer. (*C*) Proximal incision for lateral transfer of FDL to PB tendon. (*D*) Proximal identification and lateral transfer of FDL to PB tendon. (*E*) Lateral transfer of FDL through the peroneal tendon sheath for FDL to PB transfer. (*F*) Transfer of FDL to PB. (*G*) Final repair of FDL to PB transfer.

PLANTAR APONEUROSIS (STEINDLER PROCEDURE)

Release of the plantar aponeurosis together with the short intrinsic muscle origins can have some relaxing effect on the longitudinal arch of the foot. There is still discussion if this will have a beneficial effect on the correction of claw toe deformity in pes cavus or worsen the deformity secondary to the windlass mechanism.[1,64–66]

A 3-cm to 4-cm convex curved medial incision just proximal to the heel pad will expose the medial rim of the plantar aponeurosis. The laminar tendon is cut sharply with scissors from medial to lateral until one can feel the scissors from lateral. The muscular origin of the abductor hallucis and the flexor digitorum brevis and quadratus can be separated from the calcaneus in the next step. The long plantar ligament is left intact to prevent overcorrection. Pushing the foot gently will give the corrective effect. A Steindler procedure is never a stand-alone procedure. It only works if the Achilles tendon as a counterpart is left intact.

ACHILLES TENDON LENGTHENING IN PES CAVUS

If there is a strong equinus deformity, an Achilles tendon lengthening might be considered. One must always keep in mind that correction of an underlying structural (eg, bony) deformity has to be corrected first. Depending on the resistance to dorsiflexion and the degree of plantar flexion one can choose between the following options:

- soft resistance to dorsiflexion → Strayer procedure
- hard resistance with mild shortening → percutaneous Hoke incision
- hard resistance with sever shortening → open Z-plasty of Achilles tendon

Also, in the case of cerebral palsy (CP), one has to rule out pseudo-equinus of the foot in the child because of knee flexion. A tendoachilles lengthening (TAL) in such cases will end up in catastrophic loss of stabilization for gait and verticalization of the calcaneus.

CONSIDERATIONS OF TENDON TRANSFERS DURING RIGID RECONSTRUCTION

To decide whether a tendon transfer is advantageous or not, it is best to stick to the algorithm of correction – stabilization – balancing. The first step is always the correction of the biomechanical axes. Moreover, one has to also consider the levels above the ankle joint (eg, lower and upper leg, knee, hip). In some cases, this surgery has to be done first and then followed by the foot and ankle procedures.

All bony procedures should serve for a plantigrade foot, whether it is via fusion or realignment osteotomies. A tendon transfer on its own can never reduce a malalignment sufficiently unless the axis is not correct due to the immense forces affecting the posture of the foot (or the whole leg, respectively). If surgery has attained appropriate correction, the next step would be to plan the tendon transfer according to the underlying cause for pes cavus, for example, ankle joint stabilization (PL to PB) or supplementing dorsiflexion (PT or PL to lateral cuneiform). Keep in mind that tendon transfers are more efficient than tendon lengthening procedures or tenotomies, even in progressive diseases, due to the lowered risk of recurrence.

There is still an ongoing discussion about whether to do all surgery in one step or to stage the procedures. If staged surgery is chosen, the advantage may be early physical therapy soon after tendon transfer without additional prolonged partial weight bearing, such as with a concomitant arthrodesis. This might serve for less scarring of the transferred tendon and therefore for better mobility. In addition, a staged procedure takes 2 surgeries and the rehabilitation course for the patient is longer, which might be a strain for the patient's compliance.

With single-stage surgery, the correction and balancing are done together. The risk of scarring of the tendon and the breakdown of soft tissue coverage is higher due to prolonged immobilization and can lead to failure of the whole surgery. Moreover, physical therapy must consider partial weight bearing until the osseous procedures have healed.

SPASTICITY

Spasticity can hamper decision making for tendon transfer. Surgery depends very much on the underlying disease of the patient. In CP, surgical procedures can help to enable the patient to be ambulatory with or without bracing. In the first years and up to the age of 7 to 9, conservative treatment often is the treatment of choice. With open physes and an increase of body weight correction, stabilization with an ankle foot orthosis becomes increasingly difficult and surgery might be amenable to the child. As mentioned before, unfortunately, the surgeon has not only to deal with foot deformity, but with deformity and spasticity of the proximal to the foot and ankle as well. A plantigrade posture of the foot needs an unhindered mobility of the hip and knee joints. Therefore, it is essential to develop an overall concept for surgical treatment, including the rehabilitation protocol and socioeconomic factors that may affect the recovery period.[11,44]

It is deleterious to lengthen the Achilles tendon in the case of knee contracture without addressing that as it is "only" a pseudo-equinus position of the foot. This will lead to a pes calcaneus with severe loss of strength resulting in an apropulsive gait and worsening deformity. For treatment of foot deformities in the CP patient, the surgeon has to consider all the techniques (bony corrections and tendon transfers, mild lengthening, and tenotomies) and their combinations to achieve a reasonable result in view of the postoperative capabilities of the disabled patient.

Patients with a cerebral ischemic insult sometimes show spasticity of the lower extremity. Very often the higher activity of the triceps surae and the extrinsic inverters (tibialis anterior [TA], PL) cause a kind of clubfoot deformity. There might also be sensory deficits, such as a lack of proprioception, agnosia, and disturbance of spatial orientation. The main goal of foot surgery is to serve for stability in stance and better control of the foot during swing phase.

Surgery is amenable after 10 to 15 months when an equilibrium has developed after the initial injury. A Steindler procedure might help for the pes equinus as a mild TAL does (Hoke, gastrocnemius recession). To correct alignment, one has to address, after osseous correction has been performed, the function of dorsiflexion and eversion (STATT, PL to PB/lateral cuneiform) to create a balanced foot and ankle. The approach to the patient with posttraumatic brain injury is quite similar. The timing seems to be somewhat delayed (up to 18 months) as there may be some realized improvement in the patient after trauma.

ALGORITHM TO CONSIDER WITH (FLEXIBLE) PES CAVUS RECONSTRUCTION

Establishing a treatment algorithm when considering reconstruction of the pes cavus foot allows for a thorough approach to treating a complex deformity. It is well established in the literature that a possible algorithm for treating pes cavus might be the following:

- Dwyer/Lateral Displacement Calcaneal Osteotomy (LDCO)
- Cole Osteotomy of the Tarsus (OT)
- Dorsiflexory Wedge Osteotomy (DFWO)

If plantigrade posture is accomplished after these osseous procedures, one should look for additional balancing, stabilization, and/or functional improvement with tendon transfer/lengthening/tenotomies. For more functional results, PL transfer or STATT will aid in eversion and dorsiflexion. In the case of loss of anterior and lateral compartment muscle function, one should look for stabilization and reduction of deforming forces (TAL, tibialis posterior transfer). **Box 1** contains a decision-making algorithm to consider when performing a tendon transfer. In addition, one could perform mild lengthening of anterior tibialis to prevent the development of pes cavus, this would be particularly useful in the instance of the CP patient. The overall algorithm for pes cavus surgery should always be correction > stabilization > balancing.[6,34,67]

PEARLS OF TENDON TRANSFER

Tendon transfer can become a time-consuming procedure during surgery, especially when combined with fusions or osteotomies. Therefore, preparation of the site is essential. To split a tendon half way, make a small incision in the middle of the tendon, introduce a Vicryl thread, and cut the tendon by tearing it down with a sawing motion into halves. Armor the stumps of the tendon with a nonabsorbable loop fiber wire. This

---

Box 1
Decision-making algorithm for tendon transfers

ICE with *Triple P*

*I*dentifying the *P*roblem

Choosing the best *P*rocedure

*E*lection of *P*atient

1. Identifying the problem:

What is the etiology of the pes cavus?
- Loss of 1 or 2 motor neuron units
- Bony deformity
- Compartment syndrome
- Hereditary
- Upper vs lower motor neuron dysfunction
- Progressive or stationary (length of duration of deformity, consistent or worsening)

Which structures are involved?
- Osseous deformity with or without arthritis
- Joint contracture
- Joint instability
- Function of muscle compartments:
  - Anterior: tibialis anterior, extensor hallucis longus, extensor digitorum longus, posterior tibial
  - Lateral: peroneus longus, peroneus brevis
  - Posterior superficial: gastroc, soleus
  - Posterior deep: tibialis posterior, flexor hallucis longus, flexor digitorum longus
- Associated deformities proximal to the ankle joint

2. Choosing the best procedure:

Which procedure is suitable?
- Correction of deformity from proximal to distal
- Bony structures/joints in correct alignment and stable, contractures
- Muscle strength of the transferred tendon/muscle unit
- Stable lever arm for the transfer to work on
- In-phase vs non-phasic transfer in relation to the gait cycle
- Effect of deforming forces with weakening of muscle tendon unit (agonist-antagonist relation)
- Intact soft tissue envelope (approach)
- Single vs staged surgical approach
- Rehabilitation protocol (complexity, need for an orthosis, length of rehabilitation)

3. Election of patient:

Do I have the right patient?
- What does the patient want to achieve?
- Age (child, adolescent, adult, elderly)
- Compliance (mentally or physically disabled)
- Single vs staged surgical approach (informed consent of patient!)
- Future course (deterioration of result with time?)
- Alternatives (orthosis, physiotherapy)

- Social context (lack of support structure, time off of work, financial constraints)

---

makes a small solid stump to pull through a soft tissue or bony channel/tunnel and helps the tendon to find its way. Have different long straight and curved clamps available for grasping suture/tendon stump. Temporary transfixation of the joint with K-wires may help to provide for undisturbed tendon transfer and establish the right tension on the construct. Prepare everything for the transfer and then proceed with the definite fixation one after another, especially in the case of more than one transfer.

SUMMARY

Tendon transfer can be a powerful and useful tool in accomplishing a plantigrade foot with reasonable function in the pes cavus patient. It can be used as a stand-alone procedure assuming there is no fixed, structural deformity. Keep in mind the biomechanical axes of the foot and the localization of the tendons to these axes, the surgeon should then be able to choose the right transfer for a successful procedure. The course of the underlying disease must be respected, as well as the compliance and socioeconomic factors of the patient to secure an understanding of the rehabilitation protocol. Structural deformities must be corrected to a plantigrade foot first, whether this is done in the primary surgical setting or in a staged procedure. Careful handling during the procedure and a good concept before starting surgery will save time in theater and achieve better functional results.

CLINICS CARE POINTS

- Tendon transfers are an important adjunctive procedure in the flexible cavus foot at its associated conditions.
- Effective clinical evaluation as well as critical assessment of manual muscle testing is essential before tendon transfer.
- A thorough understanding of the deformity, as well as the antagonistic muscles, allows for precise tendon transfers and limits morbidity of transfer.
- Tendon transfers alone are not a reliable option for transfers in the rigid cavus foot, and alternative osseous procedures must be considered as the primary form of surgical treatment.
- Utilization of a treatment algorithm allows for a stepwise approach to correction of the flexible cavus foot and aids in creating reproducible results.

DISCLOSURE

Dr E. Keeter, Dr J. Wolfe have no disclosures. Dr T.Q. Randt and Dr J. Visser have no conflicts to disclose pertaining to this article.

REFERENCES

1. Wicart P. Cavus foot, from neonates to adolescents. Orthop Traumatol Surg Res 2012;98(7):813–28.
2. Maynou C, Szymanski C, Thiounn A. The adult cavus foot. EFORT Open Rev 2017;2(5):221–9.
3. Samilson RL, Dillin W. Cavus, cavovarus, and calcaneocavus. An update. Clin Orthop Relat Res 1983;177(177):125–32.
4. McCluskey WP, Lovell WW, Cummings RJ. The cavovarus foot deformity. Etiology and management. Clin Orthop Relat Res 1989;247(247):27–37.
5. Levitt RL, Canale ST, Cooke AJ Jr, et al. The role of foot surgery in progressive neuromuscular disorders in children. J Bone Joint Surg Am 1973;55(7):1396–410.
6. Holmes JR, Hansen ST Jr. Foot and ankle manifestations of Charcot-Marie-Tooth disease. Foot Ankle 1993;14(8):476–86.

7. Kaplan JRM, Aiyer A, Cerrato RA, et al. Operative treatment of the cavovarus foot. Foot Ankle Int 2018;39(11):1370–82.
8. Kim BS. Reconstruction of cavus foot: a review. Open Orthop J 2017;11:651–9.
9. van Til JA, Renzenbrink GJ, Dolan JG, et al. The use of the analytic hierarchy process to aid decision making in acquired equinovarus deformity. Arch Phys Med Rehabil 2008;89(3):457–62.
10. Mazaux JM, Debelleix X. The equino-varus foot deformity in patients with hemiplegia. Ann Readapt Med Phys 2004;47(2):87–9.
11. Gasq D, Molinier F, Reina N, et al. Posterior tibial tendon transfer in the spastic brain-damaged adult does not lead to valgus flatfoot. Foot Ankle Surg 2013; 19(3):182–7.
12. Aleksić M, Baščarevic Z, Stevanović V, et al. Modified split tendon transfer of posterior tibialis muscle in the treatment of spastic equinovarus foot deformity: long-term results and comparison with the standard procedure. Int Orthop 2020;44(1): 155–60.
13. Coleman SS, Chesnut WJ. A simple test for hindfoot flexibility in the cavovarus foot. Clin Orthop Relat Res 1977;(123):60–2.
14. Zide JR, Myerson MS. Arthrodesis for the cavus foot: when, where, and how? Foot Ankle Clin 2013;18(4):755–67.
15. Huber M. What is the role of tendon transfer in the cavus foot? Foot Ankle Clin 2013;18(4):689–95.
16. Bohannon RW. Reliability of manual muscle testing: a systematic review. Isokinet Exerc Sci 2018;26(4):245–52.
17. Noakes H, Payne C. The reliability of the manual supination resistance test. J Am Podiatr Med Assoc 2003;93(3):185–9.
18. Allard P, Sirois JP, Thiry PS, et al. Roentgenographic study of cavus foot deformity in Friedreich ataxia patients: preliminary report. Can J Neurol Sci 1982;9(2): 113–7.
19. Eleswarapu AS, Yamini B, Bielski RJ. Evaluating the cavus foot. Pediatr Ann 2016; 45(6):e218–22.
20. Arunakul M, Amendola A, Gao Y, et al. Tripod index: a new radiographic parameter assessing foot alignment. Foot Ankle Int 2013;34(10):1411–20.
21. Perera A, Guha A. Clinical and radiographic evaluation of the cavus foot: surgical implications. Foot Ankle Clin 2013;18(4):619–28.
22. Ritchie GW, Keim HA. A radiographic analysis of major foot deformities. Can Med Assoc J 1964;91(16):840–4.
23. Bouysset M, Tebib JG, Weil G, et al. Deformation of the adult rheumatoid rearfoot. A radiographic study. Clin Rheumatol 1987;6(4):539–44.
24. Burns J, Redmond A, Ouvrier R, et al. Quantification of muscle strength and imbalance in neurogenic pes cavus, compared to health controls, using hand-held dynamometry. Foot Ankle Int 2005;26(7):540–4.
25. Daines SB, Rohr ES, Pace AP, et al. Cadaveric simulation of a pes cavus foot. Foot Ankle Int 2009;30(1):44–50.
26. Mann DC, Hsu JD. Triple arthrodesis in the treatment of fixed cavovarus deformity in adolescent patients with Charcot-Marie-Tooth disease. Foot Ankle 1992; 13(1):1–6.
27. Wapner KL, Hecht PJ, Shea JR, et al. Anatomy of second muscular layer of the foot: considerations for tendon selection in transfer for Achilles and posterior tibial tendon reconstruction. Foot Ankle Int 1994;15(8):420–3.
28. Coughlin MJ, Mann RA, Saltzman CL. Surgery of the foot and ankle. St Louis (MO): Mosby; 1999.

29. Dehne R. Congenital and acquired neurologic disorders. Surgery of the foot and ankle. St Louis (MO): Mosby; 1999. p. 525–57.

30. Fukunaga T, Roy RR, Shellock FG, et al. Specific tension of human plantar flexors and dorsiflexors. J Appl Physiol (1985) 1996;80(1):158–65.

31. Olson SL, Ledoux WR, Ching RP, et al. Muscular imbalances resulting in a clawed hallux. Foot Ankle Int 2003;24(6):477–85.

32. Silver RL, de la Garza J, Rang M. The myth of muscle balance. A study of relative strengths and excursions of normal muscles about the foot and ankle. J Bone Joint Surg Br 1985;67(3):432–7.

33. Aminian A, Sangeorzan BJ. The anatomy of cavus foot deformity. Foot Ankle Clin 2008;13(2):191, 8, v.

34. Ward CM, Dolan LA, Bennett DL, et al. Long-term results of reconstruction for treatment of a flexible cavovarus foot in Charcot-Marie-Tooth disease. J Bone Joint Surg Am 2008;90(12):2631–42.

35. Rosenbaum AJ, Lisella J, Patel N, et al. The cavus foot. Med Clin North Am 2014; 98(2):301–12.

36. Tynan MC, Klenerman L, Helliwell TR, et al. Investigation of muscle imbalance in the leg in symptomatic forefoot pes cavus: a multidisciplinary study. Foot Ankle 1992;13(9):489–501.

37. Dillin W, Samilson RL. Calcaneus deformity in cerebral palsy. Foot Ankle 1983; 4(3):167–70.

38. Benedetti M, Catani F, Ceccarelli F, et al. Gait analysis in pes cavus. Gait Posture 1997;2(5):169.

39. Jahss MH. Evaluation of the cavus foot for orthopedic treatment. Clin Orthop Relat Res 1983;(181):52–63.

40. Younger AS, Hansen ST Jr. Adult cavovarus foot. J Am Acad Orthop Surg 2005; 13(5):302–15.

41. Ryssman DB, Myerson MS. Tendon transfers for the adult flexible cavovarus foot. Foot Ankle Clin 2011;16(3):435–50.

42. Close JR, Todd FN. The phasic activity of the muscles of the lower extremity and the effect of tendon transfer. J Bone Joint Surg Am 1959;41-A(2):189–208.

43. Botte MJ, Santi MD, Prestianni CA, et al. Ischemic contracture of the foot and ankle: principles of management and prevention. Orthopedics 1996;19(3): 235–44.

44. Lawrence SJ, Botte MJ. Management of the adult, spastic, equinovarus foot deformity. Foot Ankle Int 1994;15(6):340–6.

45. Breusch SJ, Wenz W, Döderlein L. Function after correction of a clawed great toe by a modified Robert Jones transfer. J Bone Joint Surg Br 2000;82(2):250–4.

46. Grambart ST. Hibbs tenosuspension. Clin Podiatr Med Surg 2016;33(1):63–9.

47. Vlachou M, Beris A, Dimitriadis D. Split tibialis posterior tendon transfer for correction of spastic equinovarus hindfoot deformity. Acta Orthop Belg 2010; 76(5):651–7.

48. Mindler GT, Kranzl A, Radler C. Normalization of forefoot supination after tibialis anterior tendon transfer for dynamic clubfoot recurrence. J Pediatr Orthop 2020; 40(8):418–24.

49. Limpaphayom N, Chantarasongsuk B, Osateerakun P, et al. The split anterior tibialis tendon transfer procedure for spastic equinovarus foot in children with cerebral palsy: results and factors associated with a failed outcome. Int Orthop 2015;39(8):1593–8.

50. Hosalkar H, Goebel J, Reddy S, et al. Fixation techniques for split anterior tibialis transfer in spastic equinovarus feet. Clin Orthop Relat Res 2008;466(10):2500–6.

51. Hamel J. Corrective procedures and indications for cavovarus foot deformities in children and adolescents. Oper Orthop Traumatol 2017;29(6):473–82.
52. Cohen JC, de Freitas Cabral E. Peroneus longus transfer for drop foot in Hansen disease. Foot Ankle Clin 2012;17(3):425, 36, vi.
53. Vigasio A, Marcoccio I, Patelli A, et al. New tendon transfer for correction of drop-foot in common peroneal nerve palsy. Clin Orthop Relat Res 2008;466(6): 1454–66.
54. Hall G. A review of drop-foot corrective surgery. Lepr Rev 1977;48(3):184–92.
55. Rodriguez RP. The Bridle procedure in the treatment of paralysis of the foot. Foot Ankle 1992;13(2):63–9.
56. Flynn J, Wade A, Bustillo J, et al. Bridle procedure combined with a subtalar implant: a case series and review of the literature. Foot Ankle Spec 2015;8(1): 29–35.
57. Johnson JE, Paxton ES, Lippe J, et al. Outcomes of the bridle procedure for the treatment of foot drop. Foot Ankle Int 2015;36(11):1287–96.
58. Hastings MK, Sinacore DR, Woodburn J, et al. Kinetics and kinematics after the Bridle procedure for treatment of traumatic foot drop. Clin Biomech (Bristol, Avon) 2013;28(5):555–61.
59. Steinau HU, Tofaute A, Huellmann K, et al. Tendon transfers for drop foot correction: long-term results including quality of life assessment, and dynamometric and pedobarographic measurements. Arch Orthop Trauma Surg 2011;131(7): 903–10.
60. Prahinski JR, McHale KA, Temple HT, et al. Bridle transfer for paresis of the anterior and lateral compartment musculature. Foot Ankle Int 1996;17(10):615–9.
61. Liggio FJ, Kruse R. Split tibialis posterior tendon transfer with concomitant distal tibial derotational osteotomy in children with cerebral palsy. J Pediatr Orthop 2001;21(1):95–101.
62. Seybold JD, Campbell JT, Jeng CL, et al. Outcome of lateral transfer of the FHL or FDL for concomitant peroneal tendon tears. Foot Ankle Int 2016;37(6):576–81.
63. Jockel JR, Brodsky JW. Single-stage flexor tendon transfer for the treatment of severe concomitant peroneus longus and brevis tendon tears. Foot Ankle Int 2013;34(5):666–72.
64. Steindler A. Stripping of the os calcis. JBJS 1920;2(1):8–12.
65. Johnson BM, Child B, Hix J, et al. Cavus foot reconstruction in 3 patients with Charcot-Marie-Tooth disease. J Foot Ankle Surg 2009;48(2):116–24.
66. Boffeli TJ, Tabatt JA. Minimally invasive early operative treatment of progressive foot and ankle deformity associated with charcot-marie-tooth disease. J Foot Ankle Surg 2015;54(4):701–8.
67. Chen ZY, Wu ZY, An YH, et al. Soft tissue release combined with joint-sparing osteotomy for treatment of cavovarus foot deformity in older children: analysis of 21 cases. World J Clin Cases 2019;7(20):3208–16.

The Role of Peroneal Tendinopathy and the Cavovarus Foot and Ankle

Harry John Visser, DPM, Blake T. Savage, DPM*,
Jay J. Moradia, DPM, Robert K. Duddy, DPM

KEYWORDS

- Peroneal tendon tears • Cavovarus foot • Peroneal tendon repairs
- Adjunctive operative reconstruction

KEY POINTS

- Evaluation of peroneal tendinopathy requires clinical and radiographic evaluations.
- Weakness and loss of function lead to worsening of the preexisting supinated foot or progressive deformity in the normally aligned foot.
- Evaluation requires diagnosis of the condition, condition of the tendons as well as available muscle strength.
- Residual deformity must be addressed with calcaneal osteotomy, restoration of tendon balance, and stabilization of the subtalar and ankle joints.
- Representative cases describe evaluation and treatment.

INTRODUCTION

Arthur Williams Meyer, a human anatomist, was the first to observe longitudinal tears involving the peroneus brevis tendon noted in a Spanish sailor and an Irish dishwasher.[1] Peroneal tendon tears are often confused with lateral ankle instability. Up to 40% cause delays in definitive diagnosis as a result. Tears of the peroneal tendons have traditionally been considered uncommon.[2–9] However, several investigators have suggested that they are more common than previously recognized.[10–15]

Injuries involving the peroneal tendons may be acute or chronic. Acute peroneal tendon tears occur after a traumatic event. Yet, these injuries often go unappreciated and thus present in a delayed or chronic manner.[16] In this condition, they lack the ability to undergo a gross reparative process.[17] Chronic conditions demonstrate insidious onset of pain. One must then have a high suspicion of existing peroneal pathology. Many investigators suggest a large percentage of peroneal tendon injuries are initially misdiagnosed by a wide variety of health care providers.[11,13,18] One study showed

SSM Health DePaul Hospital, Foot and Ankle Surgery Residency, 12303 DePaul Drive Suite 701, St Louis, MO 63044, USA
* Corresponding author.
E-mail addresses: blaketsavage@gmail.com; tsarhjv@aol.com

Clin Podiatr Med Surg 38 (2021) 445–460
https://doi.org/10.1016/j.cpm.2021.02.006
0891-8422/21/© 2021 Elsevier Inc. All rights reserved.

podiatric.theclinics.com

only 60% of peroneal tendon disorders were accurately diagnosed at the first clinical evaluation.[19] The peroneals act as the main evertors of the foot and play a major role in lateral stability of the ankle.[17] If left untreated, persistent lateral ankle pain and substantial functional disability can occur.[19]

ANATOMY

The peroneal muscles make up the muscle group of the lateral compartment of the lower leg as seen in **Fig. 1**. They are referred to as a group due to their similar actions on the foot but there are 2 different muscles comprising the lateral group: the peroneus brevis and peroneus longus.[20] There is a peroneus tertius muscle located in the anterior compartment with similar actions on the foot in eversion but contributes to dorsiflexion. We are more focused on the 2 muscles of the lateral compartment. The peroneal muscles primarily function as the evertors of the foot, with the longus being the primary evertor, due to its size and strength. Their origin in the lateral compartment of the leg allows pulling the foot laterally when engaged.[21] This motion also has a pronatory effect on the subtalar joint and hindfoot.[22]

In the lateral compartment, the peroneus longus extends from the upper two-thirds of the fibula and fibular head distally and becomes tendinous approximately 4 cm proximal to the fibular tip. The peroneus brevis originates from the distal two-thirds of the fibula and intermuscular septa and extends, on average, 1 to 2 cm more distal than the peroneus longus.[20,21,23] As both of the tendons pass beyond the fibular tip, the brevis tendon is located medially to the longus tendon and, at this point, both tendons share a tunnel to stabilize the tendons as they bend around the distal aspect of the fibula. The tunnel is formed by the superior peroneal retinaculum (SPR), a fibrocartilaginous ridge extending from the fibula, the posterior fibular groove (pulley 1), and fascia from the deep posterior compartment.[21] Any defect of this shared tunnel, especially the SPR, the tendons are at increased risk of subluxation or dislocation.[20,21,23]

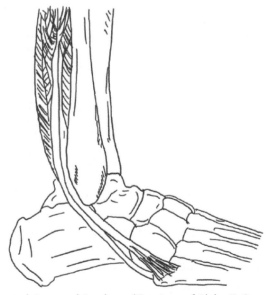

Fig. 1. Peroneal musculature and tendons. (*Courtesy of* Blake T. Savage, DPM, St. Louis, MO.)

The peroneal tendons then separate and continue their own courses once distal to the fibula. They then pass over the calcaneal tubercle with the peroneus brevis passing superior and the peroneus longus coursing inferiorly (pulley 2). The brevis tendon continues its course distally and plantarly toward the base of the fifth metatarsal where it inserts into the styloid process. The peroneus longus also continues distally and plantarly; however, it extends past the cuboid groove (pulley 3) to enter the cuboid tunnel on the plantar aspect of the cuboid and traverses across the plantar aspect of the midfoot and inserts onto the plantar aspects of the base of the first metatarsal and medial cuneiform.[20] The os peroneum is a sesamoid that can be present in the peroneus longus tendon just before the tendon enters the cuboid tunnel and can be a source of pain and tendon pathology.[24,25]

Both peroneal muscles are innervated by the superficial peroneal nerve. Blood supply is provided by the posterior peroneal artery with some minor contributions by the anterior tibial artery.[26] Multiple studies have argued that the peroneal tendons are at high risk of tears and rupture around the lateral malleolus, calcaneal tubercle, and cuboid due to critical zones of avascularity.[20,26] This avascularity was thought to be due to the redirection of the tendons at these points in conjunction with poor arterial blood supply to those very areas. However, a recent study has been published arguing against this notion of avascular zones saying that the blood supply to these areas is adequate.[27] Thus, the peroneal tendons exhibit a 3-pulley system. The peroneus brevis and longus make up pulley 1 at the retrofibular groove and pulley 2 at the calcaneal peroneal tubercle. Pulley 3 involves the peroneus longus only at the cuboid notch. Pathomechanical strain seems to be a major contributing factor.

EXAMINATION

Examination often will note edema, tenderness, and warmth along the course of the tendons in approximately 60% of the cases.[17] The examination involves the tendon pulley points and their connections. Sobel and colleagues[28] described a compression test of the peroneal tendons, as seen in **Fig. 2**. If pain, crepitus, and popping are noted along the posterior edge of the fibula with forced dorsiflexion and eversion, it was considered positive for SPR insufficiency and tendon subluxation. Evaluation of manual muscle strength complicates the diagnosis.[29] Often little or no weakness is noted on manual muscle examination. Ankle stress view radiographs should be performed to rule out ligamentous insufficiency of the lateral collateral ligaments. A

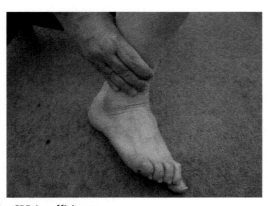

Fig. 2. Sobel test for SPR insufficiency.

Coleman block test may also be needed to assess varus rear foot flexibility. A varus heel should alert the examiner to an underlying neuromuscular disorder, such as Charcot-Marie-Tooth disease.[20]

ZONES OF PERONEAL TENDON INJURY

Brandes and Smith[2] described 3 anatomic zones where peroneal tendon pathology could exist (**Fig. 3**).

Zone A (Pulley 1): Represents tears occurring under the SPR and/or the retrofibular groove (peroneus longus and/or brevis).

Zone B (Pulley 2): Represents tears occurring under the inferior peroneal retinaculum (IPR) in association with the calcaneal peroneal tubercle (peroneus longus and/or brevis).

Zone C (Pulley 3): Involves the cuboid notch and may be associated with an os peroneum (peroneus longus).

Peroneus brevis tears are more common than peroneus longus tears in overall frequency.[30–39] Cadaveric studies note the peroneus brevis is torn between 11% and 37% of the time and the peroneus longus as less frequent.[20] The true incidence is unknown. An MRI study suggested in a retrospective review that 35% of patients with peroneal pathology were asymptomatic.[40] Mechanical and/or local anatomic factors may have a role in peroneal tendon injury.[3,10–12,14,15,28,41–50]

MECHANISMS OF INJURY

Mechanical forms of injury involving the peroneal tendons include the following:

1. Acute inversion (supination, internal rotation) ankle sprains
2. Chronic ankle ligamentous laxity post injury

Acute inversion ankle injuries were the most common precipitating traumatic event involving peroneal tendon injury in 61% of cases.[11] Krause and Brodsky[11] noted 55% of peroneal tendon injury when tears were due to trauma, whereas 45% were unknown in etiology. Another study[17] showed that of 40 patients with peroneus brevis and/or

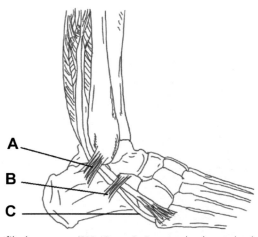

Fig. 3. Zone A: Retrofibular groove/SPR. Zone B: Peroneal calcaneal tuberosity/IPR. Zone C: Cuboid Notch. (*Courtesy of* Blake T. Savage, DPM, St. Louis, MO.)

longus repair, 58% had a history of injury whereas 42% denied injury. Chronic ankle ligamentous laxity in many cases correlates well with peroneal tendon tears.[46–48,50] Sammarco and Diraimondo[50] noted 12 (26%) of 47 patients who required concomitant lateral ankle ligament repair. Symptoms of instability are assessed through stress radiographs evaluating the anterior drawer test (ATFL) and talar tilt (CFL) examinations, as seen in **Fig. 4**. Also, intraoperative inspection of the ligaments and stress examination noticing talar instability should be done.

Functional instability can relate to the peroneal tendons themselves being torn. The peroneal muscles first contract in response to a sudden inversion force and thus provide dynamic stabilization of the lateral ankle complex.[34,51] Delayed action in the torn state to an injury force can thus cause symptoms of ankle instability despite normal stress views. Several sources support this hypothesis.[34–36]

ANATOMIC FACTORS

Peroneal subluxation leading to intrinsic tendon tears include the following conditions involving anatomic pulley 1, the fibular groove:

1. Flat or convex fibular retro-malleolar groove
2. Low-lying peroneus brevis muscle belly encroaching the fibular retro-malleolar groove
3. Accessory peroneal muscles: peroneus quartus or peroneus quintus
4. SPR insufficiency
5. Intrasheath subluxation
6. Peroneal tendon injury at peroneal calcaneal tubercle (pulley 2)
7. Peroneus longus injury at the cuboid notch (pulley 3)
8. Cavus or supinated foot type

Both the peroneus brevis and longus tendons are contained within the fibular retro-malleolar groove. The SPR provides the primary restraint to tendon subluxation.[30] The surface area is increased laterally by the nonosseous fibrocartilaginous ridge.

The retro-malleolar groove evaluated in a cadaveric study by Edwards[52] noted it to be concave in 82%, flat in 11%, and convex in 7%. The flat and concave forms lead to lateral subluxation of the peroneal tendons and strain on the SPR. This leads to tearing of the peroneus brevis in a longitudinal manner over the posterior, lateral fibular ridge.

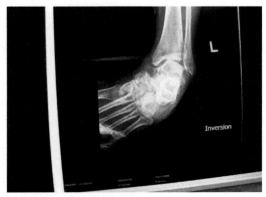

Fig. 4. Inversion stress views noting positive talar tilt due to lateral collateral ligamentous laxity.

The peroneus longus then fills the brevis defect or split and thus the tendon is unable to heal. Demetracopoulos and colleagues,[19] in their intraoperative review, noted only 3 (9%) of 34 patients requiring "groove-deepening" surgical approaches in conjunction with repair. These groove-deepening procedures involve fibular osteotomy, and retro-malleolar core decompression.

The low-lying peroneus brevis muscle belly (**Figs. 5** and **6**) was found to occur in 33% of patients in general.[32,53,54] MRI and cadaveric studies noted presence of the low-lying muscle belly in 10% to 21% of cases.[17] The peroneus quartus was found in 6.6% to 21.7% of cadaveric specimens.[33,55] Van Dijk and colleagues[21] found the quartus or quintus in 10% and 34% of the population, respectively. These conditions lead to overcrowding of the retro-malleolar groove. This causes strain on the SPR and can lead to tendon subluxation. Also, longitudinal compression leading to a split tear can occur. Management involves excision of the muscle tissue to decompress the retro-malleolar groove.

SPR insufficiency can be caused, as already stated, by abnormal groove morphology and crowding with low-lying or accessory muscles. Four authors[12,13,16,56] note injury as a primary cause. Dombek and colleagues[17] noted this condition in 13% of cases with peroneal tendon repairs. Its incompetence as described leads to lateral subluxation and longitudinal tearing along the posterior lateral fibula. Treatment is repair of the SPR in a pants-over-vest manner. Geppert and colleagues[43] noted that the calcaneal attachment of the SPR lays parallel to the CFL. When there is injury and damage to the ATF and CF ligaments, there is associated strain placed on the SPR. This acts to further compound ankle instability with peroneal dislocation. Redfern and Myerson[22] thus preferred in these cases to do a Chrisman-Snook lateral ankle stabilization using the anterior portion of the peroneus brevis rather than an anatomic repair such as a Brostrom.

Intrasheath subluxation concerns a condition in which the peroneus brevis and longus reverse their anatomic positions. This occurs within the peroneal groove and the SPR remains intact. Clinically, there is pain and palpable clicking on ankle circumduction.[20] Raikin and colleagues[57] noted 2 types:

Type A: Peroneus longus is deep to peroneus brevis without a tear.
Type B: Longitudinal split tear of the peroneus brevis. Peroneus longus lies deep and no associated tear of the SPR.

Pulley 2 is where the peroneal tendons cross the lateral calcaneal wall, separated by the peroneal tubercle. The brevis tendon passes above the tubercle and the longus

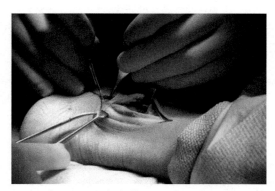

Fig. 5. Low-lying peroneus brevis muscle belly crowding the retro-malleolar groove.

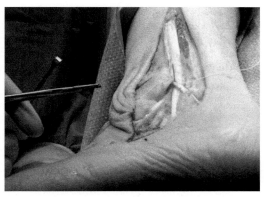

Fig. 6. Chrisman-Snook procedure with peroneal tendon tear and concomitant lateral collateral ligament insufficiency.

below. They are restrained by the IPR. Hyer and colleagues[58] performed a cadaveric study of 114 calcanei and noted 3 main variations of the peroneal tubercle: flat (42.7%), prominent (29.1%), and concave (27.2%). Prominence of the tubercle greater than 5 mm can lead to peroneus longus and brevis impingement, injury (**Fig. 7**), calcaneal varus, and supinated foot types and are often associated with pathology.

Pulley 3 is where the peroneus longus passes under the cuboid to enter a fibroosseous tunnel formed between the long plantar ligament and a groove under the cuboid.[20] The peroneus longus tendon may exhibit a round-shaped sesamoid bone. Sarrafian[32] noted it to be primarily fibro-cartilaginous and osseous in 20%. It can articulate with the lateral calcaneus, calcaneocuboid joint, or inferior cuboid. Sobel and colleagues[25] coined the term os peroneum syndrome. The condition has a spectrum of pathology from acute fracture to peroneus longus tendon entrapment. Surgical management can involve excision with tendon repair, or in cases of extrinsic tendon damage, a transfer of the peroneus longus to the peroneus brevis.

As seen in **Fig. 8**, the varus or supinated foot type has been implicated with associated peroneal tendon tears. Brandes and Smith[2] noted that 82% of patients with peroneal tendon issues exhibited a supinated foot type. Dombek and colleagues[17]

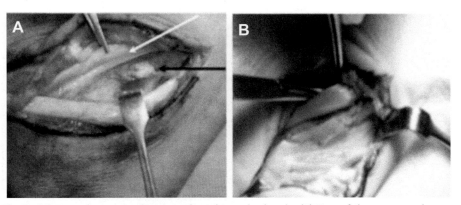

Fig. 7. (*A*) Tear of peroneus brevis at the calcaneal tubercle. (*B*) Tear of the peroneus longus at the calcaneal tubercle.

noted that the cavovarus foot predisposes and contributes to peroneal tendon injury. Their findings noted procurvatum of the ankle architecture and calcaneal position of a mean of 4.1° of varus of their studied patients predisposed to peroneal tendon injury. Grasset and colleagues[59] found 35% of patients had a negative Meary angle on a lateral radiograph and demonstrated a rearfoot varus averaging 4.6° ± 1.5° (range from 3° to 7°).

Redfern and Myerson[22] proposed an algorithm for the intraoperative assessment of the peroneal tendons. They noted that MRIs often did not reflect the extent of the tendon pathology. Demetracopoulos and colleagues,[19] however, found MRI useful in the preoperative planning and visualization of peroneal tendon tears. Redfern and Myerson[22] noted that peroneal tendon pathology was only revealed at the time of surgery. They found that MRI was only accurate in 14 of 23 cases. Eight of 23 peroneus longus tears and 2 of 23 peroneus brevis tears were identified.

Their Algorithm Is as Follows

> *Type I*: Both tendons are intact. Longitudinal split tears were excised and the tendon tubularized. Using Krause and Brodsky's classification,[11] more than 50% of the tendons were found viable (**Fig. 9**).
>
> *Type II*: One tendon was torn involving more than 50% of the tendon diameter. Tenodesis was performed or an allograft could be used (**Fig. 10**).
>
> *Type III*: Represents a condition in which both tendons are torn and unusable with more than 50% of the diameter nonviable or completely ruptured.
>
> *Type IIIa*: Notes no excursion of the proximal muscle. Preoperative MRI presence of fatty infiltration or clinical signs of loss of calf girth could be considered. Options in this case involve a tendon transfer to gain motor power. Satisfactory outcomes have been noted when the flexor digitorum longus (FDL),[16] flexor hallucis longus (FHL)[60] or plantaris[12,13] was used.
>
> *Type IIIb*: Excursion of the proximal muscle. If there is scarring of the tissue bed, a 2-stage allograft with Hunter silicone rod is considered.[11,16,22,61–63] If there is no tissue bed scarring, then a 1-stage allograft or tendon transfer is done.[22]

The peroneal muscles, longus and brevis, are pronators and evertors of the foot.[64] Niemi and colleagues[64] noted eccentric function at midstance and concentric function at heel off. As described, they dynamically augment lateral ankle instability. Injury will offset structural balance of the foot.[65] They account for 63% of eversion strength, with

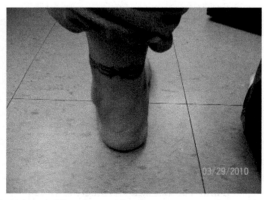

Fig. 8. Supinated foot type with calcaneal heel varus.

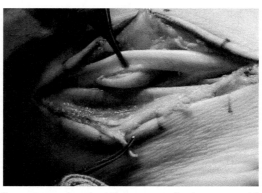

Fig. 9. Split tear of the peroneus brevis at the retro-malleolar groove. More than 50% of the tendon was preserved.

the brevis accounting for 29% and the longus 35%.[23] A tear of the peroneus longus with or without a tear of the peroneus brevis leads to inversion of the rearfoot by an overpowering tibialis posterior muscle tendon.[57,65] As seen, the peroneus longus is approximately 2 times stronger than the peroneus brevis and, therefore, is of greater importance in rearfoot balance.[13,57,65]

Ruptures of both the peroneus longus and brevis tendons are rarely documented.[12,13] Discussion has often been limited to a few case reports.[16,56,66] Treatment of this condition is based on (1) function of the tendon/tendons, (2) mobility and strength of remaining peroneal musculature, (3) scarring of the tissue bed, (4) ankle instability, and (5) heel position.

With loss of function of both peroneal muscles due to tendon injury, their antagonists, tibialis posterior and tibialis anterior, are given a distinct advantage to counterbalance their loss of pull or eversion force. The peroneus brevis, although weaker in comparison, has a distinct representation when torn or ruptured. When in the torn state, it maintains some resistance to the tibialis posterior muscle. Thus, in type I

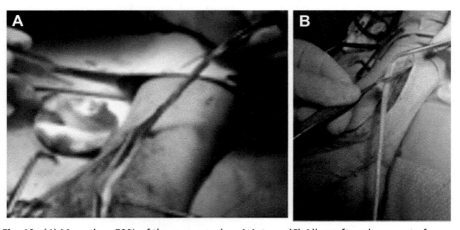

Fig. 10. (*A*) More than 50% of the peroneus brevis is torn. (*B*) Allograft replacement of more than 50% torn peroneus brevis tendon.

and II tears, the foot deformity leads to an adductovarus condition. However, in stage III, the tibialis posterior, and deep flexors (FHL and FDL) then have full mechanical advantage. The result is often an adductocavovarus foot deformity dependent on chronicity, as the more distal insertion of the tibialis posterior tendon manifests itself. Management can include allograft replacement, tendon transfer, and 2-stage Hunter rod exchange in scarred tissue bed, a lateral translational or Dwyer-type calcaneal osteotomy is performed (**Fig. 11**). Calcaneal osteotomy has universally improved position of the rearfoot, but studies have shown a persistent, mild residual deformity.[22] Thus, in cases of peroneal tendon dysfunction, functional lengthening of the tibialis posterior muscle-tendon should be considered along with a plantar fascial release and possible gastrocnemius recession depending on the degree of heel varus. With concomitant ankle instability, a Chrisman-Snook–type stabilization is preferred. This procedure may be necessary when both tendons are ruptured. A Brostrom still can be considered in type I and II conditions of the peroneal tendons. It also must be remembered in cases in which the subtalar joint is fixed or immobile, the tibialis anterior muscle-tendon can be a force creating an adductovarus forefoot deformity. This is centered about the talonavicular (TN) joint or in the case in which the talonavicular joint is fused, the navicular-medial cuneiform joint.

CASE STUDIES
Case 1

A 60-year-old woman presented with a history of having developed pain in her antero-lateral left foot and ankle. Initial medical care failed to make a diagnosis. Subsequently, however, an MRI was performed indicating a tear/rupture of the peroneus brevis tendon at the peroneal tubercle and the peroneus longus at the cuboid notch. Due to her ligamentous laxity as diagnosed by the Beighton examination, dynamic adductovarus was noted to the foot with weight bearing. MRI showed fatty infiltration of the peroneal musculature and calf girth being smaller than the contralateral side. She was diagnosed as an IIIa condition. Intraoperatively, there was no contracture of the peroneal musculature when stimulated. Because the peroneal sheath and tunnel were not fibrosed, an FDL transfer was performed to gain motor power to the lateral foot. The tendon was secured by a Pulvertaft technique to the remaining stump of the peroneus brevis tendon at the fifth metatarsal base. A Dwyer osteotomy with fractional lengthening of the tibialis posterior tendon and plantar fascial release

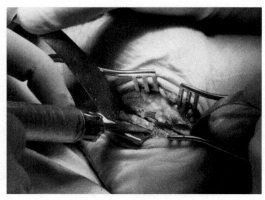

Fig. 11. Dwyer-type posterior body closing wedge calcaneal osteotomy.

were also performed. Postoperative course consisted of 4 weeks in posterior splint and non–weight bearing in boot for another 4 weeks. Active eversion and dorsiflexion exercises began at 4 weeks (**Fig. 12**).

Case 2

Case 2 was a 54-year-old man with a history of rheumatoid arthritis who had a history of 2 prior procedures on the peroneal tendons. The patient's remaining health status and neurovascular function were normal. The patient subsequently had noticed changes in his foot position with the development of a unilateral cavovarus. The MRI noted extensive tendinosis of the peroneus brevis and longus without an associated rupture. There were also no signs of fibrosis or fatty infiltration of the peroneal musculature.

A 2-stage procedure was done, as he was diagnosed with a IIIb condition. Stage 1 involved excision of the stenosed and extensively tendonosed peroneal tendons. A 6-mm silicone Hunter rod was then placed along the anatomic course of the peroneal tendons. Proximally it was incorporated in the remaining portion of the peroneus brevis and longus tendons. Distally, it was secured to the fifth metatarsal base with a suture anchor. At 6 weeks, stage 2 was performed. The Hunter rod was retrieved, and a tibialis anterior tendon allograft was used. It was cut to the proper width to fit the retro-malleolar groove. The proximal and distal ends of the incision were opened. The allograft was then secured to the proximal end of the Hunter rod and the distal end of the rod was mobilized to pull the allograft through the already created peroneal tunnel. The rod had created a mobile sheath and retro-malleolar stability for the gliding function of the allograft. Tensioning occurred with the foot dorsiflexed and everted. A Dwyer calcaneal osteotomy and fractional lengthening of the tibialis posterior tendon were also performed (**Fig. 13**). As stated, the patient remained 6 weeks non–weight bearing with the silicon rod. Once the allograft was placed and the Dwyer and tibialis posterior lengthening procedures were performed, a further 4 weeks of non–weight bearing was ordered. Weight bearing then ensued with active mobilization of the ankle and subtalar joints along with strengthening of the peroneal allograft.

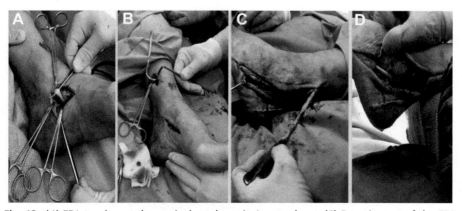

Fig. 12. (*A*) FDL tendon at the navicular tuberosity/master knot. (*B*) Recruitment of the FDL tendon at the proximal ankle 9 cm above the ankle joint. (*C*) FDL tendon passed to lateral compartment posterior to the ankle. Peroneal tendons excised. (*D*) Transfer of the FDL to remaining peroneus brevis stump via Pulvertaft technique.

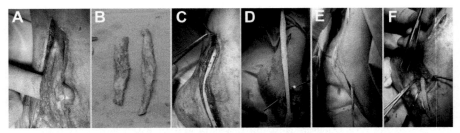

Fig. 13. (*A*) Extensive stenosis and scarring of peroneal tendons at the retro-malleolar groove. (*B*) Extensive peroneal tendinosis. (*C*) Insertion of Hunter silicone rod. (*D*) Tibialis anterior allograft. (*E*) Insertion of allograft with removal of silicone rod. (*F*) Allograft within newly created peroneal tunnel.

Case 3

A 59-year-old man with no significant medical conditions gave a history of feeling a large pop 7 months before the initial evaluation. He had prodromal pain approximately 1 year and after the injury event he had some mild edema but relief of pain. As a ballroom dancing teacher, he noticed weakness and instability of his left ankle. He also noticed changes in the shape of his foot and walking more on the outside of his foot. An MRI showed rupture of both the peroneus brevis and longus tendons without fatty infiltration of the peroneal musculature. Ankle stress views were negative. The peroneus brevis ruptured at the retro-malleolar groove and the longus at the cuboid groove. The patient demonstrated a IIIb condition. The surgical procedure involved a single-stage allograft due to preservation of the tendon sheath and SPR. Excursion of the proximal peroneal musculature was noted intraoperatively. A Dwyer calcaneal osteotomy and fractional lengthening of the tibialis posterior tendon was also performed, as well as a gastrocnemius recession due to its contribution to heel varus (**Fig. 14**). Postoperative course included posterior splint application and non–weight bearing for 4 weeks, followed by weight bearing in a boot. Active mobilization of the peroneal allograft began at 4 weeks.

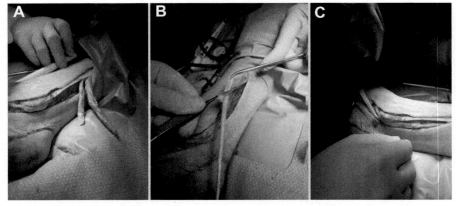

Fig. 14. (*A*) Ruptured peroneal tendons. (*B*) Insertion of a peroneus brevis allograft. (*C*) Securing allograft to proximal peroneus brevis and longus stumps and securing insertion at the fifth metatarsal base.

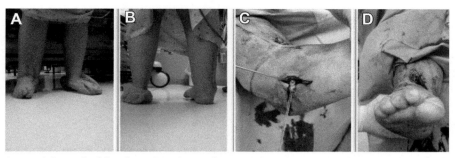

Fig. 15. (A) Residual forefoot elevation and varus. (B) Heel in proper alignment. (C) Transfer of the tibialis anterior tendon to the cuboid with 3-incision approach. (D) Reduction of forefoot with lateral tibialis anterior transfer.

Case 4

A 55-year-old woman with a long history of peroneal tendon tears and a developmental adductovarus deformity presented with a persistent varus forefoot deformity. She had had 2 prior operations on the peroneal tendons. This led to stenosis and dysfunction. As a result, a triple arthrodesis was performed. Postoperatively, a persistent forefoot varus occurred and a revision of the talonavicular fusion was performed. Again, the forefoot varus deformity recurred. She then sought another opinion. On examination, the patient had a residual forefoot varus deformity. The subtalar joint and calcaneal position were in 2° of valgus. The calcaneocuboid joint and talonavicular joint were fused in anatomic position. There was significant elevation of the first metatarsal at the navicular-medial cuneiform joint. The deformity could be reduced manually.

The impression here is that a triple arthrodesis was done to stabilize the cavovarus foot for complete loss of function of the peroneal tendons. This, then, did "neutralize" the tibialis posterior muscle antagonist. However, the tibialis anterior was then without a functioning antagonist. The tibialis anterior was able to pull unopposed at the navicular-medial cuneiform joint and produce a forefoot varus deformity. Thus, the condition was managed with a transfer of the tibialis anterior tendon to the cuboid (**Fig. 15**). This reduced the deformity and returned function. Postoperative course was a bivalved cast with the forefoot in maximal valgus. This was for 4 weeks. At 4 weeks, weight bearing began and active dorsiflexion at the ankle was done.

CLINICS CARE POINTS

- History and physical examination should be focused on diagnosis of the condition, condition of the tendons, and available muscle strength.
- A thorough explanation of the risks and benefits of surgical intervention should be made clear to the patient to improve patient outcomes.

DISCLOSURE

Dr B.T. Savage does not have any disclosures. Dr H.J. Visser, Dr R.K. Duddy, and Dr J.J. Moradia have no conflicts to disclose pertaining to this article.

REFERENCES

1. Meyer AW. Further evidences of attrition in the human body. Am J Anat 1924; 34(1):241–67.
2. Brandes CB, Smith RW. Characterization of patients with primary peroneus longus tendinopathy: a review of twenty-two cases. Foot Ankle Int 2000;21(6):462–8.
3. Dombek MF, Orsini R, Mendicino RW, et al. Peroneus brevis tendon tears. Clin Podiatr Med Surg 2001;18(3):409–27.
4. Minoyama O. Two cases of peroneus brevis tendon tear. Br J Sports Med 2002; 36(1):65–6.
5. Pai V, Lawson D. Rupture of the peroneus longus tendon. J Foot Ankle Surg 1995; 34(5):475–7.
6. Patterson MJ, Cox WK. Peroneus longus tendon rupture as a cause of chronic lateral ankle pain. Clin Orthop Relat Res 1999;365:163–6.
7. Saxena A, Pham B. Longitudinal peroneal tendon tears. J Foot Ankle Surg 1997; 36(3):173–9.
8. Thompson FM, Patterson AH. Rupture of the peroneus longus tendon. Report of three cases. J Bone Joint Surg Am 1989;71(2):293–5.
9. Yao L, Tong DJ, Cracchiolo A, et al. MR findings in peroneal tendonopathy. J Comput Assist Tomogr 1995;19(3):460–4.
10. Alanen J, Orava S, Heinonen OJ, et al. Peroneal tendon injuries. Report of thirty-eight operated cases. Ann Chir Gynaecol 2001;90(1):43–6.
11. Krause JO, Brodsky JW. Peroneus brevis tendon tears: pathophysiology, surgical reconstruction, and clinical results. Foot Ankle Int 1998;19(5):271–9.
12. Sammarco GJ. Peroneal tendon injuries. Orthop Clin North Am 1994;25(1): 135–45.
13. Sammarco GJ. Peroneus longus tendon tears: acute and chronic. Foot Ankle Int 1995;16(5):245–53.
14. Sobel M, Bohne WH, Levy ME. Longitudinal attrition of the peroneus brevis tendon in the fibular groove: an anatomic study. Foot Ankle 1990;11(3):124–8.
15. Sobel M, Dicarlo EF, Bohne WH, et al. Longitudinal splitting of the peroneus brevis tendon: an anatomic and histologic study of cadaveric material. Foot Ankle 1991;12(3):165–70.
16. Borton DC, Lucas P, Jomha NM, et al. Operative reconstruction after transverse rupture of the tendons of both peroneus longus and brevis. J Bone Joint Surg Br 1998;80-B(5):781–4.
17. Dombek MF, Lamm BM, Saltrick K, et al. Peroneal tendon tears: a retrospective review. J Foot Ankle Surg 2003;42(5):250–8.
18. Clarke HD, Kitaoka HB, Ehman RL. Peroneal tendon injuries. Foot Ankle Int 1998; 19(5):280–8.
19. Demetracopoulos CA, Vineyard JC, Kiesau CD, et al. Long-term results of debridement and primary repair of peroneal tendon tears. Foot Ankle Int 2013; 35(3):252–7.
20. Davda K, Malhotra K, O'Donnell P, et al. Peroneal tendon disorders. EFORT Open Rev 2017;2(6):281–92.
21. Dijk PA, Kerkhoffs GM, Chiodo C, et al. Chronic disorders of the peroneal tendons. J Am Acad Orthop Surg 2019;27(16):590–8.
22. Redfern D, Myerson M. The management of concomitant tears of the peroneus longus and brevis tendons. Foot Ankle Int 2004;25(10):695–707.
23. Bahad SR, Kane JM. Peroneal tendon pathology. Orthop Clin North Am 2020; 51(1):121–30.

24. Blitz NM, Nemes KK. Bilateral peroneus longus tendon rupture through a bipartite os peroneum. J Foot Ankle Surg 2007;46(4):270–7.

25. Sobel M, Pavlov H, Geppert MJ, et al. Painful os peroneum syndrome: a spectrum of conditions responsible for plantar lateral foot pain. Foot Ankle Int 1994; 15(3):112–24.

26. Petersen W, Bobka T, Stein V, et al. Blood supply of the peroneal tendons: injection and immunohistochemical studies of cadaver tendons. Acta Orthop Scand 2000;71(2):168–74.

27. Dijk PV, Madirolas X, Carrera A, et al. Peroneal tendons well vascularized: results from a cadaveric study. Arthrosc J Arthrosc Relat Surg 2016;32(6). https://doi.org/10.1016/j.arthro.2016.03.080.

28. Sobel M, Geppert MJ, Olson EJ, et al. The dynamics of peroneus brevis tendon splits: a proposed mechanism, technique of diagnosis, and classification of injury. Foot Ankle 1992;13(7):413–22.

29. Mizel AW, Michelson JD, Wapner KL. Diagnosis and treatment of peroneus brevis. In: Myerson MS, editor. Foot and ankle clinics tendon injury and reconstruction. Philadelphia: Saunders; 1996. p. 343–54.

30. Orthner E, Wagner M. Dislocation of the peroneal tendon. Sportverletz Sportschaden 1989;3:112–5.

31. Athavale SA, Swathi &, Vangara SV. Anatomy of the superior peroneal tunnel. J Bone Joint Surg Am 2011;93(6):564–71.

32. Sarrafian SK. Anatomy of the foot and ankle: descriptive, topographic, functional. Second edition. Philadelphia, PA: Lippincott; 1993.

33. Sobel M, Levy ME, Bohne WH. Congenital variations of the peroneus quartus muscle: an anatomic study. Foot Ankle 1990;11(2):81–9.

34. Konradsen L, Voigt M, Hojsgaard C. Ankle inversion injuries. Am J Sports Med 1997;25(1):54–8.

35. Karlsson J, Andreasson GO. The effect of external ankle support in chronic lateral ankle joint instability. Clin J Sport Med 1992;2(4):291.

36. Palmieri-Smith RM, Hopkins JT, Brown TN. Peroneal activation deficits in persons with functional ankle instability. Am J Sports Med 2009;37(5):982–8.

37. Larsen E, Lund PM. Peroneal muscle function in chronically unstable ankles. Clin Orthop Relat Res 1991;(272):219–26.

38. Dijk CV, Kort N. Tendoscopy of the peroneal tendons. Arthrosc J Arthrosc Relat Surg 1998;14(5):471–8.

39. Oden RR. Tendon injuries about the ankle resulting from skiing. Clin Orthop Relat Res 1987;(216):63–9.

40. O'Neil JT, Pedowitz DI, Kerbel YE, et al. Peroneal tendon abnormalities on routine magnetic resonance imaging of the foot and ankle. Foot Ankle Int 2016;37(7): 743–7.

41. Bonnin M, Tavernier T, Bouysset M. Split lesions of the peroneus brevis tendon in chronic ankle laxity. Am J Sports Med 1997;25(5):699–703.

42. Brage ME, Hansen ST. Traumatic subluxation/dislocation of the peroneal tendons. Foot Ankle 1992;13(7):423–31.

43. Geppert MJ, Sobel M, Bohne WH. Lateral ankle instability as a cause of superior peroneal retinacular laxity: an anatomic and biomechanical study of cadaveric feet. Foot Ankle 1993;14(6):330–4.

44. Harrington KD. Degenerative arthritis of the ankle secondary to long-standing lateral ligament instability. J Bone Joint Surg 1979;61(3):354–61.

45. Rosenberg Z, Feldman F, Singson R, et al. Peroneal tendon injury associated with calcaneal fractures: CT findings. Am J Roentgenol 1987;149(1):125–9.

46. Sobel M, Geppert MJ. Technique tips: repair of concomitant lateral ankle ligament instability and peroneus brevis splits through a posteriorly modified Brostrom gould. Foot Ankle 1992;13(4):224–5.
47. Sobel M, Geppert MJ, Warren RF. Chronic ankle instability as a cause of peroneal tendon injury. Clin Orthop Relat Res 1993;(296):187–91.
48. Sobel M, Warren RF, Brourman S. Lateral ankle instability associated with dislocation of the peroneal tendons treated by the Chrisman-Snook procedure. The Am J Sports Med 1990;18(5):539–43.
49. Tehranzadeh J, Stoll DA, Gabriele OM. Case report 271. Posterior migration of the os peroneum, indicating a tear of the peroneal tendon. Skeletal Radiol 1984; 12(44).
50. Sammarco GJ, Diraimondo CV. Chronic peroneus brevis tendon lesions. Foot Ankle 1989;9(4):163–70.
51. Brunt D, Andersen JC, Huntsman B, et al. Postural responses to lateral perturbation in healthy subjects and ankle sprain patients. Med Sci Sports Exerc 1992;24(2).
52. Edwards ME. The relations of the peroneal tendons to the fibula, calcaneus, and cuboideum. Am J Anat 1928;42(1):213–53.
53. Munn J, Beard DJ, Refshauge KM, et al. Eccentric muscle strength in functional ankle instability. Med Sci Sports Exerc 2003;35(2):245–50.
54. Ebig M, Lephart SM, Burdett RC, et al. The effect of sudden inversion stress on EMG activity of the peroneal and tibialis anterior muscles in the chronically unstable ankle. J Orthop Sports Phys Ther 1997;26(2):73–7.
55. Zammit J, Singh D. The peroneus quartus muscle. J Bone Joint Surg Br 2003; 85-B(8):1134–7.
56. Wind WM, Rohrbacher BJ. Peroneus longus and brevis rupture in a collegiate athlete. Foot Ankle Int 2001;22(2):140–3.
57. Raikin SM, Elias I, Nazarian LN. Intrasheath subluxation of the peroneal tendons. J Bone Joint Surg Am 2008;90(5):992–9.
58. Hyer CF, Dawson JM, Philbin TM, et al. The peroneal tubercle: description, classification, and relevance to peroneus longus tendon pathology. Foot Ankle Int 2005;26(11):947–50.
59. Grasset W, Mercier N, Chaussard C, et al. The surgical treatment of peroneal tendinopathy (excluding subluxations): a series of 17 patients. J Foot Ankle Surg 2012;51(1):13–9.
60. Sobel M, Bohne WHO. In: Master techniques in orthopaedic surgery. New York: Raven; 1994. p. 285–97.
61. Heckman DS, Gluck GS, Parekh SG. Tendon disorders of the foot and ankle, Part 1. Am J Sports Med 2009;37(3):614–25.
62. Squires N, Myerson MS, Gamba C. Surgical treatment of peroneal tendon tears. Foot Ankle Clin 2007;12(4):675–95.
63. Wapner KL, Taras JS, Lin SS, et al. Staged reconstruction for chronic rupture of both peroneal tendons using hunter rod and flexor hallucis longus tendon transfer: a long-term followup study. Foot Ankle Int 2006;27(8):591–7.
64. Niemi WJ, Savidakis J, Dejesus JM. Peroneal subluxation: a comprehensive review of the literature with case presentations. J Foot Ankle Surg 1997;36(2): 141–5.
65. Deluca PA, Banta JV. Pes cavovarus as a late consequence of peroneus longus tendon laceration. J Pediatr Orthop 1985;5(5):582–3.
66. Abraham E, Stirnaman JE. Neglected rupture of the peroneal tendons causing recurrent sprains of the ankle. Case report. J Bone Joint Surg 1979;61(8):1247–8.

The Cavovarus Ankle
Approaches to Ankle Instability and Inframalleolar Deformity

Lawrence A. DiDomenico, DPM[a,b,c,*],
Sharif Abdelfattah, DPM, PGYIII[a,1], David Chan, DPM, PGY III[a,2],
Clay Shumway, DPM, PGY III[a,3]

KEYWORDS

- Cavovarus • Cavus foot and ankle • Deformity • Osteotomy • Arthrodesis
- Reconstruction

KEY POINTS

- It is important to identify the level of the deformity or deformities.
- It is important to get the limb as close to anatomic alignment as possible.
- Many levels and multiple procedures may be involved with this reconstruction.

Pes cavus is a foot and ankle condition that is seen in both children and adults. Pes cavus and cavovarus deformity often are used interchangeably. Cavovarus appears to be the most common manifestation of a cavus foot deformity. As a result of a significant cavovarus foot deformity, the ankle can become impaired. Typically, the ankle is found to be in a pathologic varus position when patients first present. Pes cavus foot and ankle deformities classically are seen with a heighten longitudinal arch of the foot, plantar flexion of the first metatarsal/ray, forefoot valgus, hindfoot varus, and forefoot adduction/metatarsal adducts deformity. Pes cavus frequently is a manifestation of an underlying neurologic process. The cavovarus deformity is a result of an imbalance between antagonist muscles. Particularly of interest, the tibialis posterior and the peroneus longus. There commonly is an imbalance with tibialis anterior and the peroneus brevis, respectively. The primary deforming force can be the peroneus longus, leading to a plantarflexed first ray along with an overpowered tibialis posterior, a weak tibialis anterior, and weak peroneus brevis that pulls the foot into a position of varus. The

[a] East Liverpool City Hospital, East Liverpool, OH, USA; [b] NOMS Ankle and Foot Care Centers; [c] St. Elizabeth Hospital, 8175 Market Street, Youngstown, OH 444512, USA
[1] 2200 N Section Street, Sullivan, IN 47882, USA
[2] 224D Cornwall Street Northwest 102, Leesburg, VA 20176, USA
[3] 256 W Lancaster Avenue #200, Malvern, PA 19355, USA
* Corresponding author.
E-mail address: LD5353@aol.com

Clin Podiatr Med Surg 38 (2021) 461–481
https://doi.org/10.1016/j.cpm.2020.12.015
0891-8422/21/© 2020 Elsevier Inc. All rights reserved.

extensor hallucis longus and extensor digitorum longus then are recruited in order to become ankle dorsiflexors in the absence or weakness of these other forces. As a result of these deforming forces, the lesser digits result in claw toes deformity and potential cock-up deformity of the hallux. In more recent literature, there have been more publications regarding a milder version of cavovarus deformity without an identifiable underlying etiology[1] (**Figs. 1** and **2**).

The key to an effective clinical examination of a cavus foot first and foremost should be assessing the a family history and birth history to assess if there were any developmental delays, premature births, history of club foot, or any history of previously diagnosed neurologic deficits[2] (**Figs. 3** and **4**).

Neurologic conditions largely are observed to be progressive disorders whereas other etiologic factors are not.[3–5] Accuracy in diagnosis of the deformity is an important undertaking because of the implications it has on determining the course of the condition and treatment. In cases of suspected neurologic disorders, electrodiagnostic testing also should be considered as part of the examination to confirm or rule out any motor/sensory neuropathy (**Fig. 5**).

HISTORY

Patients may complain of frequent ankle sprains, arch pain, metatarsal pain, digital pain, and occasionally heel pain. Foot pain is a frequently described symptom, which usually is the result of an imbalance and result of the increased stress on 1 part of the foot secondary to the deformity. Common sites of pain are in the sub–first metatarsal, toes, lateral aspect of the foot along the lateral heel, and the cuboid region. Other complaints may include the ankle, the lateral collateral ligaments, and the peroneal tendons. Often, the shoes wear unevenly and do not fit well and increase the pain secondary to the pressure over existing callus tissue (**Figs. 6–9**).

A family history of similar foot and ankle deformities may indicate a hereditary cause. Care should be taken to obtain a detailed family history. The patient history for the subtle cavus foot is more consistent with long-standing chronic lateral foot and ankle pain. It also may present as ankle instability or peroneal tendon pathology. A good history and physical examination often can establish an underlying diagnosis.

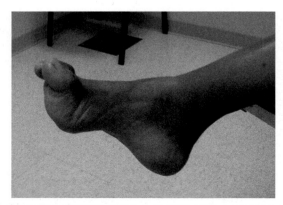

Fig. 1. A medial clinic view demonstrating a patient with a cavovarus deformity and a plantar-flexed first metatarsal from a peroneal longus overdrive with significant plantar flexion of the first ray.

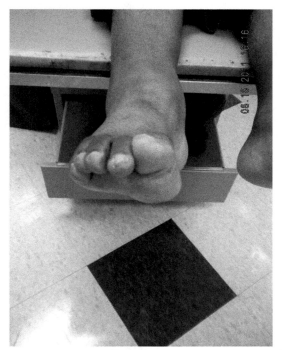

Fig. 2. A forefoot axial clinical view of a patient with a cavovarus deformity demonstrating a forefoot valgus. Note the plantar aspect of the sub–first metatarsal relative to the lesser metatarsals. During weight bearing, the calcaneus compensates and goes into a hind foot varus, which, in turn, stresses the ankle joint.

PHYSICAL EXAMINATION

Patients can present with a wide range of complaints; among them, pain is the main reason for consultation. The patient should be evaluated while ambulating and standing. The lower limb should be evaluated from the hip to the feet.

The physical examination should include muscle strength/weakness and imbalances. Any hypertrophy or muscle wasting should be noted. Weight-bearing posture of the foot typically includes a high-arched foot, metatarsus adductus, clawing of the toes, and callosities beneath the first and fifth metatarsals, the lateral column of the foot, and the lateral aspect of the calcaneus (**Fig. 10**).

Passive and active range of motion should be assessed at the ankle, hindfoot, midfoot, and forefoot.[4] A Silfverskiöld test also is performed by comparing the range of ankle dorsiflexion with the knee in extension and flexion to assess for gastrocnemius or gastrocsoleus complex. A tight posterior muscle group often is a contributing factor for a varus pull on the calcaneus.

Metatarsalgia often is observed with an anterior cavus foot and as a result of a tight posterior muscle group. Hindfoot and ankle pain is seen with a posterior pes cavus. Local tenderness when wearing shoes consisting on the plantar calluses and callosities related to clawed toes are common complaints. Flat-heeled shoes are poorly tolerated and high heels can be more comfortable. Walking is disturbed by cramping and dull aching pain in the calf and foot and ankle. Contraction of the muscle in the

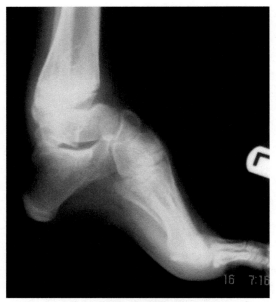

Fig. 3. A preoperative lateral radiograph demonstrating a flat top talus, a posterior rotated fibula following club foot surgery. At the time, the patient had not reached skeletal maturity.

plantar arch is common during prolonged walking. Instability of the ankle leads to repeated sprains and instability secondary to the hindfoot and ankle varus deformity.

Clinical examination is important in the management of pes cavus deformities, especially in subtle cavovarus. The aim is to confirm the presence of rigidity of the

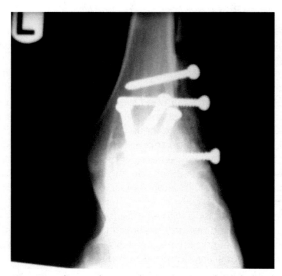

Fig. 4. A postoperative AP radiograph once the patient reached skeletal maturity. An ankle arthrodesis with an anterior rotated and positioned onlay fibular graft.

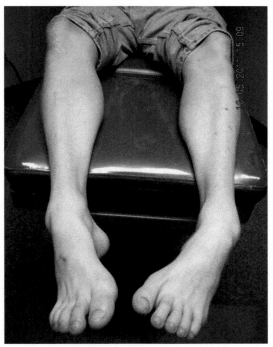

Fig. 5. A clinical view of a CMT patient who experiences weakness and a muscular imbalance of his musculature of both lower extremities. Electrodiagnostic test confirmed a neurologic deficit. Note how the ankle position is more plantar-flexed and inverted.

cavovarus deformity but also to identify any underlying neurologic cause if not known at the time of the examination. An evaluation of the entire lower limb is mandatory. Calf wasting should be noted. The clinical examination of the foot and ankle should begin with the evaluation of the patterns of wear affecting the heels and the soles of the

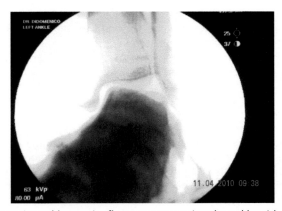

Fig. 6. An intraoperative ankle mortise fluoroscopy stressing the ankle with an inversion stress test demonstrating lateral ankle instability of the cavovarus foot and ankle.

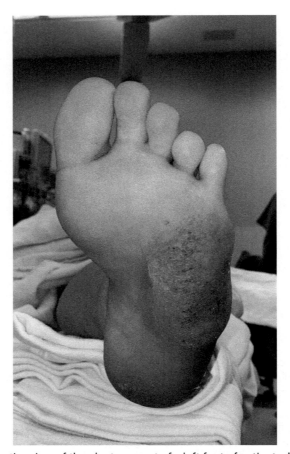

Fig. 7. A preoperative view of the plantar aspect of a left foot of patient who suffers from a cavovarus foot, with a large calcaneal varus, mild metatarsal adductus, and an equinus contracture. These deformities have resulted in an unstable ankle and subsequent peroneal tendon pathology and overload of the lateral column with marked hyperkeratosis.

shoes. It is common to see excessive wear, especially on the lateral side of the sole because of the hindfoot/ankle varus. Much information can be obtained from mere observation of the weight-bearing posture of the foot. Commonly seen are high arch; metatarsus adductus; clawing of the toes; callosity under the first and fifth metatarsal heads, lateral plantar foot, or heel; and prominence or posterior position of the lateral malleolus. In the cavovarus foot, it is not unusual to find marked callosities under the first and fifth metatarsal heads and under the lateral column of the foot.

The function and strength of all muscles in the lower extremity should be evaluated for variations and muscle imbalance. Passive and active range of movement of the ankle, hindfoot, and forefoot should be noted as well as the stability of the given joints. Range of motion of the ankle, subtalar joint, midtarsal joint, and Lisfranc joint can assist in the classification as reducible, semirigid, or rigid. This exam assists in ruling out other pathologies, such as a tarsal coalition or previous posttraumatic arthritis. This helps determined if the pathology is an isolation of a cavovarus foot and ankle alone or a combined deformity.

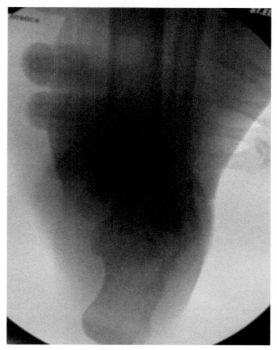

Fig. 8. An intraoperative calcaneal alignment view demonstrating a calcaneal varus deformity. Note the varus calcaneal deformity relative to the tibia; thus, the hindfoot varus had created an unstable ankle joint and peroneal tendon pathology as a result of continuous ankle sprains secondary to the calcaneal varus deformity.

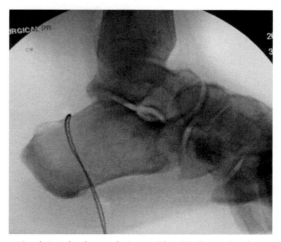

Fig. 9. An intraoperative lateral calcaneal view with a Gigli saw in place to perform a lateral calcaneal displacement osteotomy percutaneously.

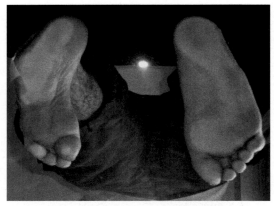

Fig. 10. A weight-bearing view demonstrating a significant cavovarus deformity on this patient's right foot. There is a significant metatarsal adductus deformity and overloading of the lateral column of the right foot.

The soft envelope should be assessed. The consideration for soft tissue healing, especially on the tension side of the deformity, is paramount (**Fig. 11**).

A complete neurologic examination of both the upper and the lower limbs is needed. To detect any muscular imbalance, a full examination of all muscle groups should be performed for power and graded. A lower extremity neurologic examination should be

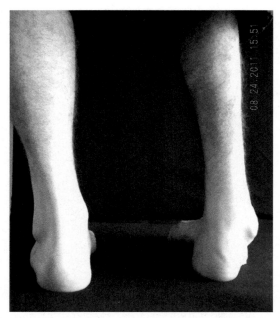

Fig. 11. Muscle imbalance. A posterior view of a patient who suffers from a unilateral muscular imbalance of the right lower extremity. Note the size difference of the muscular soft tissues of the lower extremities, significant calcaneal varus, metatarsal adductus, and lateral foot overload.

performed, and, if there is any concern with the examination, a referral to a physiatrist or a neurologist should be considered.

The foot and ankle surgeon can order electrodiagnostic studies to confirm hereditary motor sensory neuropathies. Unilateral pes cavus should encourage a referral to a physiatrist or a neurologist for work-up of a brain and/or spinal cord injury.

The Coleman block test is a part of the routine physical examination in patients who suffer with a cavovarus foot and ankle. This test should assist the foot and ankle surgeon in comprehending the pathology in more detail. This Coleman block test helps evaluate the flexibility and the rigidity of the cavovarus foot and ankle. The Coleman block test is performed by placing a book or a block of wood under the lateral aspect of the forefoot and heel. This allows the first metatarsal head to hang off the edge of the book, thus relieving the consequence of the plantar-flexed first metatarsal. The hindfoot stays in varus or it reduces to a neutral position. If removing the first metatarsal's deforming force allows the hindfoot to correct from varus to neutral, it should be classified as a nonrigid deformity. If the Coleman block test restores hindfoot alignment, then the deformity is flexible and driven by the forefoot. If the hindfoot varus does not correct and stays in varus, the deformity is rigid and fixed. The surgical decision making can be different for a flexible deformity compared with a rigid deformity.

In the subtle cavus deformity, the presenting complaints or pathology can be seen as fifth metatarsal fracture, stress fracture, peroneal tendon pathology, ankle instability, recurrent sprains, anterior medial impingement at the tibiotalar joint, lateral column pain, Achilles tendon insufficiency/dysfunction, and plantar fasciitis. A thorough assessment is necessary to assess if any of these factors needs to be addressed.[6,7]

The base of the fifth metatarsal should be evaluated in particular for cases of excessive cavovarus deformities associated with a metatarsal adductus deformity. Chronic nonhealing fractures and/or bony hypertrophy secondary can occur at the base of the fifth metatarsal because of the increased stress to this anatomic location (**Fig. 12**).

Examination of the ankle for stability, joint tenderness, peroneal tendinopathy, and ligamentous injuries also should be completed. Pain along the peroneal tendons is not uncommon as well as along the lateral collateral ligaments. Anterior ankle pain can be common due to impingement of a relatively dorsiflexed and mal aligned talus.

A peekaboo heel, first described by Manoli[8] in 1993, is a classic hindfoot varus finding and clinical sign of the subtle cavus foot.[9] This is a clinical condition whereby the heel is visible on the medial side when viewing the patient from the front. Also, the foot and ankle surgeon can see the heel pad easily from the front with the patient standing and both feet pointing ahead. In the normal foot, the heel pad should not be visible when viewed from the front due to the natural valgus alignment of the hindfoot (**Fig. 13**).

Plain radiographs of the foot, ankle, and calcaneus are the initial radiographic examination for the cavus foot and ankle. Recommended views should be done weight bearing and include anteroposterior (AP), medial oblique, and lateral views of the foot and ankle (**Fig. 14**).

A calcaneal axial and or a Colby view is necessary to assess the hindfoot and the hindfoot-leg alignment. A standard evaluation for alignment and degenerative changes should be performed with the radiographic assessment. The anatomic angles and alignment on plains radiographs can help the clinician determine the relative position of the foot and ankle.

The foot and ankle surgeon can view the position of the medial cuneiform and the fifth metatarsal base on a lateral radiograph of the foot in the presence of a cavovarus foot and ankle deformity. A fifth metatarsal base positioned plantarly indicates the foot

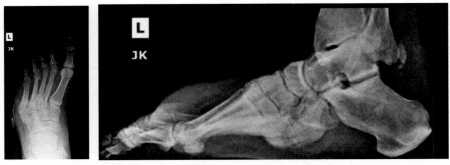

Fig. 12. AP and lateral radiograph of a patient who has a mild cavovarus foot deformity with an increased deformity from the metatarsal adductus. Note the chronic bone hypertrophy of bony callus from the recurring stress fracture to the base of the fifth metatarsal causing an ulceration.

usually is in a cavus position. The Meary line is utilized on a lateral radiograph projection to assess the talus in relation to the first metatarsal position. In a nonpathologic foot, 0° is expected. In a cavus foot deformity, the first metatarsal is plantarflexed relative to the talus alignment, increasing the Meary angle. Mild cavus foot deformities may yield a Meary angle of 5° to 10°. A severe cavus foot deformity may yield a Meary angle greater than 20°. A Hibbs angle also is described and is a measurement between the longitudinal axis of the calcaneus and first metatarsal on a lateral radiographic view. Nonpathologic feet typically are less than 45°, with cavovarus deformities angles often greater than 90°. A talocalcaneal (Kite) angle on the AP radiograph shows a divergent talus and calcaneus in a nonpathologic foot, with angles averaging between 20° and 40°. With the cavovarus deformity, the angle is decreased. The talus and calcaneus tend to be more parallel with a cavovarus foot and ankle. A decreased with the cuboid abduction angle or an increased forefoot adductus commonly is seen with a cavovarus foot and ankle. On a lateral foot view, typically there is a posterior break in the cyma line, or a bullet hole sinus tarsi.

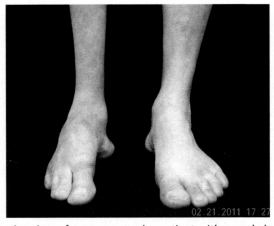

Fig. 13. A preoperative view of a neuromuscular patient with a peekaboo sign.

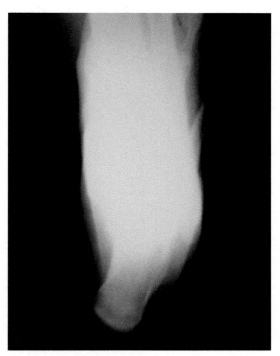

Fig. 14. This is a posterior calcaneal view demonstrating a varus malalignment of the calcaneus relative to the tibia in a patient who is diagnosed with a cavovarus foot and ankle.

An AP ankle radiograph also may show medially localized or with narrowing and osteophyte formation of the tibiotalar joint (**Fig. 15**).

Advance imaging often is utilized in the pes cavus foot and ankle. The advanced imaging can consist of either or both computed tomography and/or magnetic resonance imaging (MRI). These scans also may be performed for evaluation of the osseous structures and evaluation of the joints in the foot and ankle and to assist with surgical planning. MRI classically is utilized for the evaluation of the lateral ligaments, peroneal tendons, and osteochondral lesions as well as other cartilage and bone of the foot and ankle.

A varus ankle deformity can be a result of a more proximal pathology, which can result in a talus and ankle mortise with a varus tilt. The foot and ankle surgeon must assess the ankle joint and the subtalar joint, to determine if subtalar joint is compensating for the ankle varus. If the hindfoot and ankle remain in varus, a correction at the ankle and or subtalar joint may be necessary before reconstructing the more distal midfoot and forefoot deformities.

NONOPERATIVE

Nonoperative and conservative treatment of the cavus foot and ankle depends on the reducibility and severity of the deformity. A flexible deformity often can be managed with nonoperative care. A Coleman block test should be performed to determine if the hindfoot varus is forefoot driven or if it primarily is a hindfoot varus.

Standard nonoperative interventions include activity modification, anti-inflammatory medications, simple accommodative shoes, and custom orthoses. Patients with milder

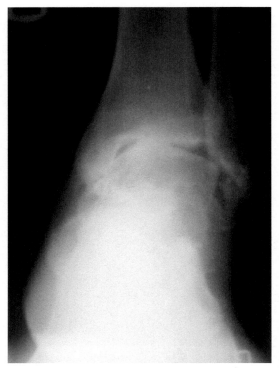

Fig. 15. An ankle view demonstrating a cavovarus foot having long-term secondary effects of the ankle joint. Note the tibial talar mal alignment, the varus position of the talus within the mortise of the ankle and the bone fragments from the long-term sequela of the malaligned cavovarus foot and ankle.

deformities and milder symptoms may be treated successfully using custom orthoses, with the goal being realignment of the hindfoot and to offload the lateral foot. For the flexible cavus foot, lateral hindfoot posting, a recess for the first metatarsal head area, and a heel pad are recommendations to be included with custom orthoses. Attempts may be made to manage more rigid and severe deformities with more restrictive orthoses, such as an ankle foot orthosis.

In addition to bracing and orthotics, the patient may benefit from physical therapy or stretching exercises, along with strengthening of the lateral tendons and ligament. Gastrocnemius stretching programs also are employed to assist and prevent contractures. Strengthening and stretching remain good short-term options.

OPERATIVE

Options for surgical intervention can include 1 or many procedures independently or in combination. Typically, the procedures consist of a posterior muscle lengthening procedure, Steindler stripping, calcaneal osteotomy, dorsiflexion osteotomy of the first ray, midfoot osteotomies, midfoot arthrodeses, in-phase tendon transfer or out-of-phase tendon transfer, tendon lengthening, ankle stabilization procedures, supramalleolar osteotomies, possible ankle replacement, ankle fusion, and tibial talar calcaneal procedures. All of these procedures can be utilized independently or in combination, with the purpose of achieving a plantigrade and balanced foot and ankle. The exact combination of procedures depends greatly on each patient's given deformity and the surgeon's experience and philosophy.

It is the senior author's (L.A.D) experience to initiate surgical reconstruction early if the deformity is progressed or progressing and if there is a muscular imbalance present. The theory is the imbalance only worsens over time, leading to a more progressive deformity and muscular imbalance, resulting in more collateral anatomic injury. It is best to initiate surgical reconstruction prior to the foot and/or ankle becoming unsalvageable.

Posterior Muscle Lengthening

Many patients who experience a cavovarus foot and ankle deformity typically present with an equinus contracture. A Silfverskiöld test should be performed.[10] In most cases, the Silfverskiöld test appears to involve a gastrocnemius contracture. In the scenario that involves an isolated gastrocnemius contracture, the senior author prefers performing an endoscopic gastrocnemius recessing.[11-13] In the scenario of a tight posterior muscle contracture that results in a gastrocnemius-soleus contracture, the senior author prefers performing a percutaneous tendo-Achilles lengthening. These techniques are preferable because most of these surgical reconstructions involve multiple procedures; thus, endoscopic and percutaneous techniques can be more advantageous to the soft tissue envelope.[14]

Calcaneal Osteotomy

Many deformities involving a cavovarus deformity involve a calcaneal varus deformity. In conditions that involve a calcaneal varus deformity, the senior author prefers the percutaneous technique as this minimizes the trauma postoperatively to the soft tissue envelope, because most of these conditions warrant multiple surgical procedures on a relatively small anatomic area.[15-18]

Midfoot Surgery

A large number of patients that have a cavovarus deformity involve a midfoot deformity commonly seen with a metatarsal adductus. This deformity needs to be corrected in all planes. It is essential that the midfoot be corrected because this part of the malalignment contributes to ankle pathology in the cavovarus patient.[19]

SURGICAL CORRECTION FOR ANKLE INSTABILITY AND DEFORMITY

Different surgical techniques have been described, including a combination of soft tissue releases; ligamentous tightening, tendon transfers, osteotomies and arthrodesis, posterior tibial tendon recession, deltoid releases, and lateral ankle stabilization are among the most common procedures employed to correct the soft tissue deformities. Bony deformities may warrant realignment osteotomies of the foot and/or ankle or arthrodesis procedures in the foot and/or ankle. In the scenario of an acute correction, the authors also recommend a prophylactic tarsal tunnel release.

For an ankle to remain balanced and stable, it is mandatory the foot also is balanced and stable; therefore, the surgeon must work through each and every segment of the lower extremity anatomy to ensure that anatomic alignment is restored.

Osteotomies and arthrodesis typically are indicated in severe rigid cavus foot or in degenerative cases. Osseous alignment procedures commonly can consist of a first metatarsal dorsiflexion osteotomy for forefoot-driven cavus or tarsal metatarsal arthrodesis. For hindfoot-driven varus deformities, a lateralizing calcaneal osteotomy commonly is used to realign the pull of the gastrocnemius.[20] Plantar fascia release may be part of the treatment algorithm as well, to allow for further dorsiflexion of the first ray.[1]

Joint-sparing osteotomies are preferred in patients without advanced degenerative disease. Even in those patients in whom arthrodesis is performed, however, balancing of the muscular forces is recommended to avoid fusion failure.[1] Triple arthrodesis remains a surgical option but generally is viewed as a salvage operation because most patients who underwent this procedure as teenagers had significant adjacent joint disease by their 30s.[7]

Surgical treatment of the subtle cavus foot often occurs while the surgeon is addressing other pathologies, such as lateral overload symptoms, stress fractures, and lateral ankle instability.[5]

Joint-sparing surgical procedures along with tendon balancing are recommended in the flexible cavovarus foot. Each segment of the deformity needs to be evaluated and managed individually. There are essential and nonessential joints in the foot, and the essential joints should be preserved as best as possible. For example, in a patient who suffers from Charcot-Marie-Tooth (CMT) disease with significant disease of the peroneal muscles and a drop foot, typically resulting with an unstable lateral ankle.

Posterior Muscle Lengthening

A correction of posterior muscle lengthening should consist of a gastrocnemius recession or a tendo-Achilles lengthening to address the common tight posterior muscle component of the deformity. Performing this posterior muscle release allows the calcaneus to reduce to a neutral or a more neutral anatomic position. The senior author's experience has been that a majority of the tight posterior muscle lengthening warrants a gastrocnemius recession because this appears to involve mostly an isolate gastrocnemius contracture.[11–14]

Calcaneal Osteotomy

In the event that the calcaneus does not completely reduce to a neutral position, a percutaneous calcaneal osteotomy is performed.[15–18]

Steindler Stripping

Next, a Steindler stripping can be performed. This releases the soft tissue contracture of the sagittal plane of the midfoot and releases any adduction of the midfoot and may correcst some forefoot rotation.

Midfoot Osteotomy

Attention then is directed to the midfoot, where a midfoot osteotomy may be needed based on the residual deformity in the sagittal plane or frontal or transverse plane. The midfoot osteotomy can address 1 isolated plane, 2 planes, or all 3 planes with the midfoot osteotomy. This realigns the forefoot to the hindfoot.

Ankle Stabilization

In cases of a long-standing condition, the lateral collateral ankles and the peroneal tendons may be compromised. Patients with lateral ankle instability, who have exhausted conservative measures, such as bracing and physical therapy, may benefit from ligament repair or reconstruction of the ligaments. With regard to reconstruction, there are 2 types: anatomic and nonanatomic. Anatomic reconstruction rebuilds the physiologic orientation of the ligaments. Nonanatomic reconstruction usually involves tendon transfers that are not positioned in the same location as the talofibular ligament and the calcaneofibular ligament. If the peroneal tendons are not compromised, the senior author performs a modified Brostrom-type procedure because the foot below is already balanced and the Brostrom procedure then stabilizes the unstable ankle. If the peroneal tendons are diseased, the recommendation is to split the diseased portion and use this portion of the peroneal tendon as a ligamentous graft as a split peroneal breivs or longus lateral ankle stabilization. Typically, the authors like to fixate this soft tissue with an interference screw for strong soft tissue fixation[21,22] (**Fig. 16**).

Peroneal Tendon Repair

In the event there is a peroneal tendon tear, there should be a direct repair or tendon transfer performed, given the extent of the injury to the tendon or tendons.

Peroneal Longus–Peroneal Brevis Tendon Transfer

In the scenario where a patient has a significant forefoot valgus caused from a peroneal longus overdrive, the patient may or may not present with a sub–first metatarsal ulcer secondary to this pathology. In the event a patient presents with a peroneal longus overdrive, the senior author has had good response to performing a peroneal longus to peroneal brevis tendon transfer. In the case of a patient who suffers from a sub–first metatarsal ulcer, this removes the deforming force. Relative to the cavovarus foot and ankle, this will eliminate some of the deforming force while balancing and strengthening the lateral weaker components of the lateral ankle.[23]

Tendon Transfer to the Anterior Compartment for Repair of a Dropfoot

To address the drop foot, the functioning posterior tibial tendon is split and transferred to the dorsal of the foot. This weakens the overpowering plantar flexion and improves the dorsiflexion of the ankle to approximately 40% to 60% of normal function. The tendon transfer acts as a sling holding the ankle at 90° and it gains approximately 40% to 60% of strength of a nonpathologic ankle[24] (**Figs. 17** and **18**).

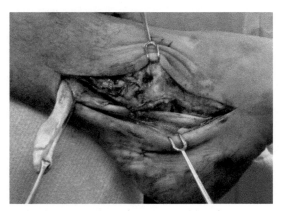

Fig. 16. This is an intraoperative view of a right ankle of a cavovarus deformity with ongoing ankle pain. There was a long-standing complete rupture of the peroneal brevis tendon secondary to chronic stress and malalignment to the soft tissues.

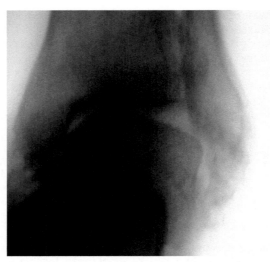

Fig. 17. An intraoperative fluoroscopy view demonstrating secondary osteoarthritis that develops from a pathologic cavovarus foot, causing repetitive damage to the ankle joint.

Posterior Tibial Tendon

In spastic or fixed equinovarus deformities, it may be necessary to lengthen or transfer the posterior tibial tendon in order to adequately reduce the ankle in the mortise. It has been described for use in patients with cerebral palsy and other neuromuscular disorders, including of reducible deformities.[2] Other investigators have described the transfer of the posterior tibial tendon anteriorly and lengthening of the Achilles

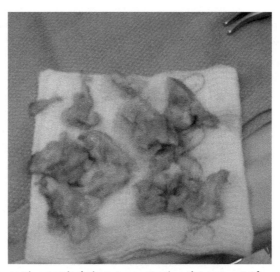

Fig. 18. An intraoperative surgical view remonstrating the amount of secondary cheilus/osteophyte damage to the ankle joint as a result of a significant cavovarus deformity of the foot.

tendon.[7,25] Tibialis posterior tendon recession is not a common procedure; however, in difficult cases of a contractor of the posterior tibial tendon, this can be performed at the location at the aponeurosis.[26] A distal incision of the tendon has been demonstrated to have a higher load to failure and a 48% greater lengthening of the tendon compared with a proximal incision.[20] Another alternative is a Z-lengthening of the tendon. Additionally, the posterior tibial tendon may be transferred through the interosseous membrane and attached to the middle cuneiform as an alternative to a lengthening procedure. This is useful especially when other deformities exist, such as a drop foot.

Tarsal Tunnel Release

The medial structures may cause compression to the posterior tibial nerve related and possible vascular compromise when the ankle and hindfoot are placed into a rectus position moving from a varus position. Prophylactic tarsal tunnel release, especially in the setting of acute corrections for ankle varus deformities, should be considered.

Deltoid Release

A deltoid release may be necessary if there is talar tilt in the ankle mortise and is secondary to deltoid contracture. This appears to occur in cases with long-standing deformities.[27]

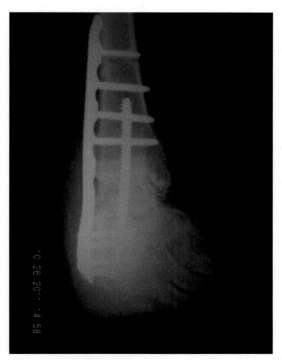

Fig. 19. A postoperative radiograph of a patient who suffered from excessive ankle and subtalar joint deformity as a result of a progressed cavovarus deformity. The fibula was taken down and used for bone grafting of the ankle and subtalar joint in this case. A large fully threaded screw and a femoral locking plate was used for fixation.

Total Ankle Arthroplasty, Ankle Arthrodesis, and Tibial Talar Calcaneal Arthrodesis

The debate for total ankle arthroplasty and ankle arthrodesis continues to be a disputed topic. In the experience of the senior author, if the foot and ankle can be balanced and the patient is an appropriate candidate for an implant arthroplasty, then it is recommended to perform the arthroplasty because it preserves adjacent joints long term in comparison to an ankle arthrodesis. With a properly balanced ankle and foot, both ankle arthrodesis and total ankle replacement are viable options to treat patients' pain and improve function.[27–29] In the senior author's experience, if the foot and ankle deformities are corrected and well aligned, the preoperative pain and function should improve with most patients.

Supramalleolar Osteotomies

Tibial osteotomies may need to be performed to realign the anatomic and mechanical axis. More proximal deformities in the knee and hip as well as limb length discrepancies also should be considered. For deformity above the ankle joint, a biplanar opening or closing wedge or a dome-shaped osteotomy may correct multiplanar deformity. The osteotomy can be combined with an ankle replacement. The osteotomy is made in the metaphysis, leaving sufficient bone distally for fixation. If the fibula requires an osteotomy, it can be performed at the same level laterally or obliquely more proximally. The ankle then is manipulated, rotated, translated, or angulated in any plane until the desired correction is obtained. This osteotomy is particularly useful

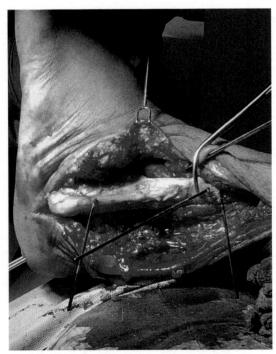

Fig. 20. An intraoperative view of using the fibula as a biologic plate. The lateral aspect of the tibia, talus and calcaneus was resected so the fibula could inlay and serve as a biologic plate.

to correct deformity when the center of rotation of angulation is further away from the ankle joint. In general, a closing wedge osteotomy is more friendly and predictable in comparison to an opening wedge osteotomy. Typically, the medial closing wedge osteotomy heals well and is more predictable because no bone grafting is needed. This osteotomy can be done as a traditional open technique or a percutaneous technique through small incisions.[30]

Subtalar Arthrodesis

Based on the given disease and scenario of each patient, when the disease process is limited to the talar calcaneal joint and it is not possible to realign with the articular structures and preserve the function, then a subtalar joint arthrodesis can be performed. The goal of the subtalar joint arthrodesis is to restore anatomic alignment and to improve function.

Ankle Arthrodesis

Based on the given disease and scenario of each patient, when the disease process is limited to the tibial talar joint and it is not possible to realign with the articular structures and preserve the function, then an ankle arthrodesis can be performed. The goal of the ankle arthrodesis is to restore anatomic alignment and to improve function.

Tibial Talar Calcaneal Arthrodesis

With a deformity that is excessive or advanced and involves both the ankle joint and the subtalar joint, the senior author recommends performing a tibial talar calcaneal arthrodesis. The senior author has utilized a femoral locking plate for added stability.[31] In scenarios with a malalignment and a need of more biologics, the fibula has been used as a biologic plate for fixation of a tibial talar calcaneal arthrodesis[32] (**Fig. 19**).

These procedures may be done in a single-stage or multiple-staged approach, isolated or in combination based on the presentation and given scenario of the extremity. The fibula may be helpful in the use of bone grafting. If a deformity is extremely large, the senior author has used the distal fibula as a cortical cancellous in lay graft. On other occasions, the senior author has used the fibula as a biologic plate for additional fixation and a biological advantage (**Fig. 20**).[31]

SUMMARY

A cavovarus deformity involving the ankle can be a complex problem for the patient and the foot and ankle surgeon. A thorough physical examination and gait assessment are needed. A careful work-up and identification of detailed pathology are required. A comprehensive evaluation of each anatomic segment of the entire lower extremity is needed for a complete balancing of soft tissue and osseous structures. The complex surgical corrections may be staged, allowing the soft tissues to accommodate to the anatomic corrections.

CLINICS CARE POINTS

- Identify the underlying pathology
- Correct the underlying pathology
- Typically, this surgical reconstruction involves multiple procedures and multiple planes of deformity correction

DISCLOSURE

The authors have nothing to disclose.

REFERENCES

1. Manoli A II, Graham B. The subtle cavus foot, "the underpronator". Foot Ankle Int 2005;26:256–63.
2. Burns J, Redmond A, Ouvrier R, et al. Quantification of muscle strength and imbalance in neurogenic pes cavus, compared to health controls, using hand-held dynamometry. Foot Ankle Int 2005;26(7):540–4.
3. Brewerton D, Sandifer P, Sweetnam D. Idiopathic" pes cavus: an investigation into its aetiology. BMJ 1963;2:659–61.
4. Maynou C, Szymanski C, Thiounn A. The adult cavus foot. EFORT Open Rev 2017;2(5):221–9.
5. Eleswarapu AS, Yamini B, Bielski RJ. Evaluating the cavus foot. Pediatr Ann 2016; 45(6):e218–22.
6. Ruda R, Frost HM. Cerebral palsy: spastic varus and forefoot adductus, treated by intramuscular posterior tibial tendon lengthening. Clin Orthop Relat Res 1971; 79:61–70.
7. Lagast J, Mylle J, Fabry G. Posterior tibial tendon transfer in spastic equinovarus. Arch Orthop Trauma Surg 1989;108(2):100–3.
8. Manoli A. The subtle cavus foot, "the underpronator". Graham B Foot Ankle Int 2005;26(3):256–63.
9. Chilvers M, Arthur M II. The subtle cavus foot and association with ankle instability and lateral foot overload. Foot Ankle Clin N Am 2008;13:315–24.
10. Silfverskiold N. Reduction of the uncrossed two joint muscles of the leg to one-joint muscles in spastic conditions. Acta Chir Scand 1923;56:315–30.
11. DiDomenico L, Adams H, Garcahr D. Endoscopic gastrocnemius recession for the treatment of gastrocnemius equinus. J Am Podiatr Med Assoc 2005;95(4): 410–3.
12. Saxsena A, Gollwitzer H, Widtfeldt A, et al. Endoscopic gastrocnemius recession as therapy for gastrocnemius equinus (English and German). Z Orthop Unfall 2007;145(4):499–504.
13. DiDomenico, L.A., Groner, T. W., Szczepanski, J. A., Endoscopic gastrocnemius recession, International Advances in Foot and Ankle Surgery, 2012. DOI: 10. 1007978-0-85729-2_40.
14. Haro AA, DiDomenico LA. Frontal plane-guided percutaneous tendo achilles' lengthening. J Foot Ankle Surg 2007;46(1):55–61.
15. Maffulli N, Easely M. Minimally invasive surgery of the foot and ankle. Springer - Verlag London Limited; 2011. https://doi.org/10.1007/978-1-84996-417-3.
16. Dull JM, DiDomenico LA. Percutaneous displacement calcaneal osteotomy. J Foot Ankle Surg 2004;43(5):336–7.
17. DiDomenico LA, Anain J, Wargo-Dorsey M. Assessment of medial and lateral neurovascular structures after percutaneous posterior calcaneal displacement osteotomy: a cadaver study. J Foot Ankle Surg 2011;50(6):668–71.
18. DiDomenico LA, Butto D. Percutaneous calcaneal displacement osteotomy. In: Scuderi G, Tria A, editors. Minimally Invasive Surgery in Orthopedics. Springer, Cham; 2016. https://doi.org/10.1007/978-3-319-15206-6_79-1.
19. Groner TW, DiDomenico LA. Midfoot osteotomies for the cavus foot. Clin Podiatr Med Surg 2005;22(2):247–64.

20. Altuntas AO, Dagge B, Chin TYP, et al. The effects of intramuscular tenotomy on the lengthening characteristics of tibialis posterior: high versus low intramuscular tenotomy. J children's orthopaedics 2011;5(3):225–30.

21. Baze E, Butto DN, DiDomenico LA. A closer look at the use of interference screws for lateral ankle stabilization. Podiatry Today 2012;25(8).

22. DiDomenico LA, Cross DJ, Giagnacova A. Techniques for utilization of an interference screw for split peroneus brevis tendon transfer in lateral ankle stabilization. J Foot Ankle Surg 2014;53(1):114–6.

23. DiDomenico LA, Abdelfattah SR, Hassan M. Emerging concepts with tendon transfers. Podiatry Today 2018.

24. Ley D, Sadeghi S, DiDomenico LA. A closer look at tendon transfers for non-healing wounds. Podiatry Today 2020.

25. Schneider M, Balon K. Deformity of the foot following anterior transfer of the posterior tibial tendon and lengthening of the Achilles tendon for spastic equinovarus. Clin Orthop Relat Res 1977;(125):113–8.

26. Roukis TS. Tibialis posterior recession. Foot Ankle Surg 2009;48(3):402–4.

27. Roukis TS, Elliott AD. Use of soft-tissue procedures for managing varus and valgus malalignment with total ankle replacement. Clin Podiatr Med Surg 2015; 32(4):517–28.

28. Kim BS, Choi WJ, Kim YS, et al. Total ankle replacement in moderate to severe varus deformity of the ankle. J Bone Joint Surg Br Vol 2009;91(9):1183–90.

29. Schuberth JM, Christensen JC, Seidenstricker CL. Total ankle replacement with severe valgus deformity: technique and surgical strategy. J Foot Ankle Surg 2017;56(3):618–27.

30. Mendicino RW, Catanzariti AR, Reeves CL. Percutaneous supramalleolar osteotomy for distal tibian (near articular) ankle deformities. J Am Podiatr Med Assoc 2005;95(1):72–84.

31. DiDomenico LA, Wargo-Dorsey M. Tibiotalocalcaneal arthrodesis using a femoral locking plate. J Foot Ankle Surg 2012;51(1):128–32.

32. Ley D, Hassan M, DiDomenico LA. Can Biological Fibular Plates Perovied Viable Fixation for Tibiocalcaneal Arthrodesis? Podiatry Today 2020;33(4).

Ankle and Pantalar Arthrodesis

End-Stage Salvage in Cavus Foot

David E. Karges, DO[a],*, Joshua Wolfe, DPM, MHA[b],
Raul Aviles, DPM[c]

KEYWORDS

- Arthrodesis • Cavus • Cavovarus • Foot

KEY POINTS

- Treatment is best individualized to restore ankle, hindfoot, and midfoot alignment when performing arthrodesis to restore a plantigrade foot.
- Ankle, hindfoot, and pantalar arthrodesis is best indicated in the fixed cavovarus foot with advanced arthrosis and chronic pain.
- After successful ankle, hindfoot, or pantalar fusion, the full-length custom orthotic and shoe with the rockerbottom sole modification is necessary to preserve transtarsal motion and diminish secondary arthrosis of the midfoot.

INTRODUCTION

The cavovarus foot is complex and leads to varying degrees of deformity. Very often, the etiologies are not uniform and can range from neuromuscular, idiopathic, to post-traumatic. Severe deformities greatly affect ambulation and quality of life. Less severe forms that are limited to the joints of the foot can in the long term, through progressive compensation, result in more severe forms that affect the ankle joint. For these severe types, bracing, and other methods of nonoperative treatment do not provide a long-term solution.

The ankle or pantalar arthrodesis may be the resulting best long-term surgical limb salvage treatment option.[1] The fusion addresses the deformity and can improve quality of life. For advanced conditions of ankle and hindfoot varus, the goal is to correct the deformity, decrease pain, and possibly provide a brace-free gait, serving as an alternative to below-the-knee amputation.

[a] Department of Orthopaedic Surgery, St. Louis University School of Medicine, 1008 South Spring Avenue, First Floor, Saint Louis, MO 63110, USA; [b] Foot and Ankle Surgery Residency, SSM Health DePaul Hospital, 12303 DePaul Drive, Suite 701, St Louis, MO 63044, USA; [c] Foot and Ankle Surgery Residency, SSM Health DePaul Hospital, 12303 DePaul Drive, Suite 701, Bridgeton, MO 63044, USA
* Corresponding author.
E-mail address: david.karges@health.slu.edu

Clin Podiatr Med Surg 38 (2021) 483–495
https://doi.org/10.1016/j.cpm.2020.12.016
0891-8422/21/© 2021 Elsevier Inc. All rights reserved.

NATURE OF SEVERE CAVUS DEFORMITY

A cavovarus foot typically arises from a muscle force imbalance, often secondary to hereditary sensorimotor neuropathy, but it is also associated with a variety of neurologic insults, developmental abnormalities, and post-traumatic states.[2] The cavus foot is predominantly a sagittal plane deformity; however, any advanced case will present with multiplanar deformity such that understanding the cause and selecting the appropriate treatment is often determined on a case-by-case basis. The vast majority of mature, symptomatic cavus foot conditions are clearly managed best surgically.[3] This correction is most often by way of extra-articular osteotomies and soft tissue balancing.[4] However, severe, recalcitrant, and arthritic deformities of the ankle and subtalar joint are the sequelae of end-stage neurologic, post-traumatic, and congenital conditions. These advanced cases can be effectively managed by ankle and pantalar fusion.[5]

The application of a treatment classification is wise to correlate the etiology and clinical findings with treatment itemizing deformity correction. In the advanced cavus deformity presenting unilaterally, the common causal etiology is trauma and stroke.[6] The patient must be evaluated for upper extremity, spine injury, and a history of lower extremity neuromuscular compartment loss. In addition, cavovarus deformity owing to distal tibial, talar, and calcaneal fracture malalignment must be determined. Any deep posterior compartment injury routinely affects lesser toe function and alignment.

The patient presenting with bilateral cavus foot deformity will likely have a different etiology. These cases may have idiopathic, genetic (Charcot-Marie-Tooth disease) and neurologic (eg, cerebral palsy, post-polio syndrome, spina bifida) causes yet most cases present with only unilateral symptoms of ankle deformity, weakness, and pain warranting surgical care.[7]

DIAGNOSIS AND PRINCIPLES OF CORRECTION

Correction of the cavovarus foot or ankle is a difficult task to accomplish and requires organization of the surgical treatment plan. These patients should be properly counseled on the procedure and its risks. The potential complications arise most often from the multiple soft tissue incisions required with deformity correction and the associated dissections necessary.

The ultimate goal of these procedures is the apical correction of the deformity to obtain a plantigrade, functional foot and ankle on which to ambulate. This factor is particularly important when considering ankle or pantalar arthrodesis as the definitive treatment for this condition. Correction in these advanced cases should be carefully evaluated.

A deformity assessment of the foot and ankle requires preoperative computed tomography scan alignment and degree of any arthrosis. An MRI of the ankle and hindfoot muscle–tendon units should also be included in the surgical treatment plan. The MRI can reveal the status of the peroneus brevis tendon unit, the most powerful, active everter to the foot, which may have undergone significant degeneration over time and the study can provide information concerning a gastrocsoleus contracture in any cavus equinus deformity case.

ANATOMY

The mechanics of normal gait, heel strike to toe-off, is an important understanding to all foot and ankle surgeons. The first phase, in normal gait, involves heel-strike to flatfoot. Initially, the subtalar joint inverts precipitating lateral heel strike. Following, as weight transfers forward, the subtalar joint everts, unlocking the Chopart's joints and the midfoot becomes supple for shock absorption. The tibialis anterior muscle contracts eccentrically, controlling the initiation of foot plantarflexion.

As the body passes over the foot advancing from flat-foot to heel-rise, the gastrocsoleus lever eccentrically contracts to control foot dorsiflexion. The posterior tibialis contracts concentrically returning the subtalar joint to inversion, externally rotating the tibia, and initiating pelvic and contralateral leg motion.

During heel rise to toe-off, the rigid midfoot acts as a lever. The inverted subtalar joint locks Chopart's joint. The talonavicular (T-N) joint while compressed indirectly dorsiflexes the first metatarsal-phalangeal joint, tightening the plantar fascia, and the foot intrinsics contract creating a plantarflexion moment. Along with contracture of both the gastrocsoleus complex and the extrinsic long foot flexors, toe-off is complete while initiation of weight transfer and gait mechanics to the contralateral limb begins.[8]

The cavus foot gait abnormality begins with heel-strike to flat-foot; the inverted subtalar joint is fixed followed by initial strike of the medial first ray rather than the lateral hindfoot. The Chopart's joint is locked yet the foot is rigid, allowing for less shock absorption as body weight advances forward. The primary abnormalities associated with the cavus foot are the flexed first ray and loss of eversion with heel strike creating overload of the lateral foot and ankle, which leads to functional limitation of the foot, lateral column, and forefoot metatarsal pain and eventually ankle instability owing to attenuation of lateral ligaments, capsule, and hypertrophy of the peroneus longus promoting a varus deformity of the foot and ankle.[9]

PREOPERATIVE EVALUATION

The process of diagnosing and assessing appropriate management of a cavus foot patient must start with a detailed interview. The young patient with a cavus foot—those in their 20s to 40s—commonly presents with a minimal or no history of daily symptoms of the foot and ankle, unless there is a history of traumatic injury to the cavus foot. A reason for the initial presentation in the younger patient might merely be lateral hindfoot soreness occurring frequently or a new activity involving exercise or recreation precipitating a lateral metatarsal stress injury or forefoot metatarsalgia. The younger patients commonly believe they have a normal foot, they repetitively load on the foot as needed, have no history of orthotic use, and have never been discriminating of shoe or footwear.

The older patients with cavus—an active 40- to 70-year-old—will routinely present with a daily, painful varus foot and ankle problems that impact work and activities. Many patients describe a crooked ankle and have worn orthotics and may have undergone surgery, such as a soft tissue ankle reconstruction or peroneal tendon evaluation and repair. These patients have commonly been undermanaged and not found relief with brace wear and oral anti-inflammatory medical management. They need further careful evaluation of their chronic foot and ankle pain.

A detailed physical examination should include a gait analysis, Coleman block, Silfverskiöld testing, sensorimotor testing, and a joint motion evaluation.[10] The Coleman block test is especially important for determining whether hindfoot varus is flexible and "forefoot driven." This clinical finding of a flexible hindfoot would preclude the consideration of an ankle or pantalar fusion.

IMAGING

Radiographs are useful in assessing the skeletal posture, screening for the presence and extent of arthritis, and planning osteotomies for treatment. Hindfoot alignment views aid in quantifying hindfoot varus. A computed tomography scan is useful for assessing ankle and subtalar arthrosis, a coalition, and quantitatively determining the precise axial malalignment of the varus ankle and hindfoot. An MRI is frequently used in the setting of the subtle cavus foot, especially for patients presenting with complaints of chronic lateral instability. However, in the advanced end-stage cavus deformity, even when considering the ankle fusion, it is of value to know any degenerative status of the peroneus brevis tendon and the tendo-achilles.[11]

OPERATIVE PLANNING OF THE ANKLE ARTHRODESIS

For noncomplex cavovarus foot deformity management, it is wise to focus on conservative care. The patient's level of pain, gait, and instability, as well as the scale of ankle and hindfoot varus malalignment can generally all be effectively improved by shoe and orthotic modification, custom ankle bracing, and medical management. However, in end-stage varus and cavovarus foot deformity, the abnormality relates to the hindfoot, midfoot, and forefoot.[4] If the deformity presents the hindfoot with fixed subtalar motion, lateral ankle instability, attrition of peroneal tendons, and medial ankle arthrosis, then the midfoot abnormality to this advanced deformity presents with lateral peritalar subluxation, forefoot supination, and digital claw toe deformity.

The cause of the varus abnormality can be a true bone malalignment, chronic ligamentous attenuation, muscle contracture, or imbalance. In most cases, a combination of both bone and soft tissue pathology is responsible for the deformity, which stems from genetic, neurologic, vascular, and traumatic etiologies.[12]

The ankle joint is uncommonly affected by primary osteoarthritis, unlike the hip and knee. Studies evaluating end-stage ankle arthrosis clearly identify trauma as the most common precipitating mechanism. The advanced cavus foot, with no history of trauma, reveals medial tibiotalar degenerative change and often little or no radiographic subtalar arthrosis; however, the varus subtalar rigidity can be severe largely associated to medial hindfoot soft tissue contracture and more distal T-N arthrosis and malalignment.

In these techniques, the patient is positioned supine and a well-padded thigh-high tourniquet applied just distal to the groin crease. I recommend the tourniquet be set at 250 mm Hg and the surgeon should discuss, with the anesthesiologist, keeping the patient systolic blood pressure at less than 120 mm Hg. In addition to the lower extremity preparation, the surgeon must consider incorporating an iliac crest cancellous bone graft for the procedure and this is commonly prepped and performed on the same side as the fusion procedure. In the past 20 years of my ankle and hindfoot fusions requiring iliac crest graft harvesting, I have incorporated a small catheter attached to a pain pump to the cancellous graft defect for the initial 24-hour postoperative period.

In recent years requiring arthrodesis of the ankle and subtalar (S-T) joint, using the retrograde intramedullary nail implant, I have avoided the iliac crest grafting procedure completely by way of application using the Synthes reamer irrigator aspirator system. This system allows the surgeon to effectively harvest cancellous and endosteal cortical bone while performing the standard, preimplant retrograde reaming process. The current reamer diameters now range from 8 mm to 19 mm in sharp end-cutting reamers harvesting bone marrow and morselized bone. The process lends well to retrograde fusion techniques.[13]

ANKLE FUSION INDICATIONS

The main indication for a primary or staged fusion of the cavovarus foot is persistent ankle and hindfoot pain after a lack of response to nonoperative management or extra-articular realignment procedures.

The development of ankle arthritis is a known consequence of a cavovarus foot deformity and an indication to perform an ankle fusion in the recalcitrant and painful ankle.[14] There is literature that supports ankle replacement in the setting of a considerable varus deformity; however, a focus on achieving an aligned, plantigrade foot is important to optimize the outcomes of the patients with an advanced cavovarus foot. One treatment option for the cavovarus foot is total ankle replacement, although it is clearly not a wise long-term treatment option particularly in the younger patient employed as a laborer, owing to the daily demands required of his foot and ankle.[15] Chronic ankle instability is also a risk factor for the development of ankle arthritis, and cavovarus malalignment has been shown to increase medial ankle joint pressures.[16] In addition, both calcaneal osteotomies and supramalleolar osteotomies have demonstrated a change in center of force and ankle joint pressures.

Moderate anteromedial ankle arthritis in the setting of the cavovarus foot treated with lateral ligament reconstruction combined with calcaneal osteotomy and/or first metatarsal osteotomy has been shown, in numerous studies, to provide adequate correction of the deformity and improvement in pain and instability.[5] However, these studies have analyzed only mild to moderate ankle arthritis. More severe ankle arthritis secondary to cavovarus deformity is less amenable to ankle joint–sparing cavovarus reconstruction procedures. Irwin and colleagues[17] in 2010 evaluated the clinical outcome of patients with advanced ankle arthritis and cavovarus deformity. These patients underwent lateral ankle ligament reconstruction and multiple foot realignment procedures for their deformity. They revealed poor American Orthopaedic Foot and Ankle Society scores, worse pain scores, and little patient satisfaction among patients with advanced arthritis. The study found poor ankle–hindfoot scores correlated with advanced ankle arthritis and postoperative residual varus tilting.[18]

The management of ankle fusion is commonly performed using multiple screws, screw and plate fixation, retrograde intramedullary nails, and circular external fixation frame application. Considerations to make when selecting an appropriate implant are the severity of the ankle and hindfoot arthrosis and varus deformity, subtalar stiffness versus instability, existing ankle and hindfoot hardware, and, importantly, the condition of the entire foot and ankle soft tissue envelope.

In the younger patient with advanced ankle arthrosis but clinical evidence of functional nontender subtalar motion, screw fixation of the ankle fusion and possibly a lateralizing calcaneal osteotomy is considered to minimize rigidity of the hindfoot. In the case of both ankle and hindfoot rigidity with arthrosis and varus deformity, either a lateral locked screw plate construct or an intramedullary retrograde fusion of both ankle and S-T joints can be considered. Patients with compromised soft tissues, often from multiple previous ipsilateral procedures and where anticipated surgical approaches are to be minimized, the contemporary designs of circular external fixators, applied correctly, will offer a safe option to performing these fusions.

OPERATIVE TECHNIQUE FOR ANKLE FUSION

The recommendation for cases treated in the supine position is a longitudinal incision beginning 10 to 12 cm in line with the anterior cortical margin of the lateral malleolus. At the distal tip of the lateral malleolus, the incision should extend approximately 3 cm further in line with the axis of the foot. Sharp dissection is advanced down to the anterior portion of the lateral malleolus, after which the dissection is to release the anterior compartment fascia and more distally the lateral retinaculum. The anterolateral ankle syndesmosis and distal tibia are easily palpated and a Hohmann retractor is inserted gently across the malleolus of the distal tibia. A lateral ankle capsulotomy is performed commonly, revealing lateral peritalar subluxation in an advanced cavovarus foot deformity. Another small narrow Hohmann retractor is often inserted next advanced along the talar neck.

A transfibular osteotomy approximately 8 cm above the ankle joint, nicely exposing the ankle joint from a lateral perspective. At this time, a Hohmann retractor is inserted and fixed along the posterolateral distal portion of the ankle joint, externally rotating the lateral malleolus to improve exposure. The ankle joint is now debrided on all surfaces of scar tissue, existing cartilage, and subchondral bone, with all debridement following the contours of the articular plafond and talar dome. When fusing the S-T joint as well, this same preparation technique is necessary. The posterior ankle capsule is carefully excised and the ankle joint is, pinned correcting varus malalignment in no more than 10° of external rotation, neutral dorsiflexion, and approximately 5° to 10° valgus, and then positioned as posteriorly in the ankle joint as possible to diminish the lever arm of the foot.[19] A bone graft is applied in and around the fusion interspace and implant fixation is inserted accordingly. When performing only the fusion of an ankle joint, the initial fixation is a 6.5-mm screw, cannulated or not, inserted percutaneously from the posterior-superior malleolus of the ankle, directed down the axis of talar dome, neck to near the interior subchondral surface of the talar head. I recommend applying a washer with the posterior screw, which acts as a small focal plate. A partially threaded 6.5-mm screw is intuitive to allow of compression of the fusion; however, a well-reduced ankle fusion interface is best controlled by a fully threaded screw. Next, a second 6.5-mm screw, 90° to the posterior screw, is inserted percutaneously from the medial supramalleolar location of the ankle, directed toward the lateral process of the talus. Attention to the excursion of the posterior to anterior screw is critical so as not to block the second medial to lateral screw. At this time, the lateral malleolus is either osteotomized in the sagittal plane and reduced to the lateral surface of the distal tibial and talus and fixed rigidly to the fusion construct with bicortical 3.5-mm interfragmentary screws and washer augmenting the fusion or the lateral malleolus is reduced and plated laterally and two 4-cortical syndesmotic position screws are advanced through the plate and fixed to the distal tibia. In the advance cavovarus ankle fusion, it is also wise to incorporate a lateralizing calcaneal osteotomy at this time. There is likely dynamic S-T varus malalignment, which needs to be corrected. Attention to medial first metatarsal vertical alignment may also require an extension osteotomy.

In the following case, presenting with arthrosis of both the ankle and hindfoot joints. This individual underwent a traumatic injury with a concomitant cavovarus deformity. After initial spanning external fixation and eventual staged ORIF of her injury, she presented later with advanced ankle and hindfoot post-traumatic arthritis. She underwent reconstruction and her case can be seen below through **Figs. 1–7**. The intramedullary retrograde fusion nail is an excellent treatment option in cases such as this.

As described, both the ankle and S-T joints must be carefully prepared; bone grafted and reduced in normal alignment before being provisionally pinned in position and then definitively fused in compression with a self-aligning retrograde fusion nail.

POSTOPERATIVE CARE

Postoperatively a well-padded compressive splint with a posterior mold and bias dressing is applied for a minimum of 24 hours, after which a nonweight-bearing fiberglass cast is applied for 2 weeks followed by a nonweight-bearing removable fracture boot and daily dressing changes with a compressive 4-inch to 6-inch ACE wrap. The fusion(s) are remained absolutely nonweight-bearing for 8 weeks monitored by serial

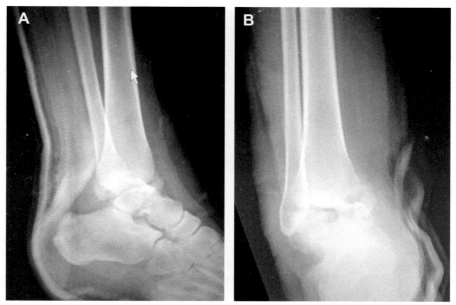

Fig. 1. (*A*, *B*) Lateral and anteroposterior injury radiograph of a closed, displaced, right multifragmentary talar dome and medial malleolar fracture sustained by a 34-year-old woman with a cavovarus deformity.

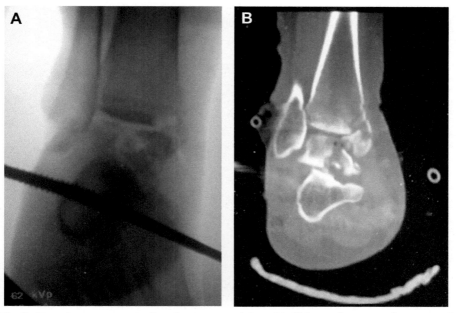

Fig. 2. Staged management of acute cavovarus injury. (*A*, *B*) Immediate spanning external fixator of right ankle with coronal computed tomography image.

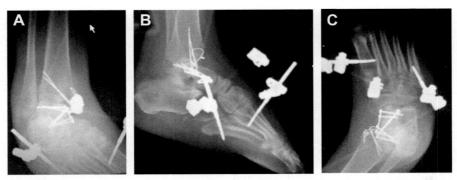

Fig. 3. Definitive management of acute cavovarus injury. (*A–C*) Staged reconstruction of the right talus and medial malleolus of an ankle with a temporary foot and ankle external fixator controlling the cavovarus deformity.

radiographs. After the fusion is confirmed radiographically, gentle and progressive weight bearing initially in the form of a removable fracture boot with daily application of a knee-high 20 to 30 mm Hg compressive stocking to control normal ankle swelling is recommended.

PANTALAR ARTHRODESIS

The most well-regarded indications for the pantalar arthrodesis are chronic pain, cavovarus deformity, and instability, which include the T-N joint. Historically, the pantalar arthrodesis can be performed in either a single-stage or a 2-stage fashion.[20] The procedure involves requiring fusion of the ankle, subtalar, T-N, and calcaneocuboid joints. In the advanced cavovarus case, requiring a pantalar fusion, I prefer the single-stage technique using a direct lateral and dorsomedial exposure.

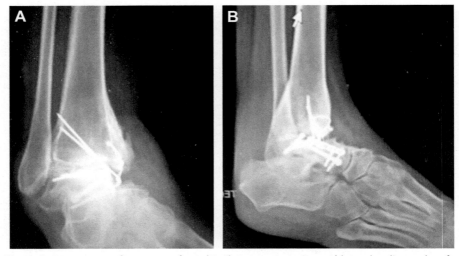

Fig. 4. Late outcome of cavovarus foot. (*A, B*) Anteroposterior and lateral radiographs of a right arthritic ankle and hindfoot of cavovarus deformity at 15 years after injury.

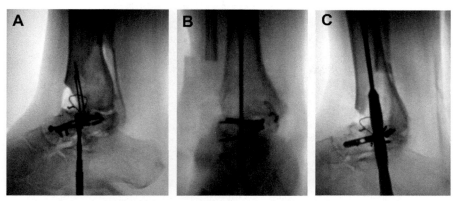

Fig. 5. Surgical technique for cavovarus ankle and hindfoot fusion. (*A–C*) Intraoperative retrograde intramedullary arthrodesis of the right ankle and subtalar joints using a transfibular approach for joint debridement and the correction of a cavovarus deformity.

OPERATIVE TECHNIQUE FOR PANTALAR FUSION

The principles of the ankle and S-T fusions are applied with an isolated lateral longitudinal approach to the ankle and S-T joints for fusion of both access to both joints. The very distal extent of the lateral incision is continued 3 to 5 cm in line with the axis of the foot to expose the calcaneocuboid joint for fusion preparation.

To address T-N fusion, an incision is made either dorsomedially over the T-N joint or strictly along the ankle and T-N joint line. The dorsomedial approach begins from the distal and lateral aspect of the naviculocunieform joint, extending longitudinally to the T-N joint and advancing directly medially over the T-N joint to the anterior margin of the medial malleolus. The primary obstruction to direct view of the T-N joint is the anterior

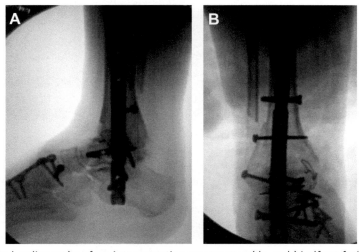

Fig. 6. Final radiographs of an intraoperative cavovarus ankle and hindfoot fusion. (*A*, *B*) Intraoperative lateral and anteroposterior radiographs of the right ankle and hindfoot fusion.

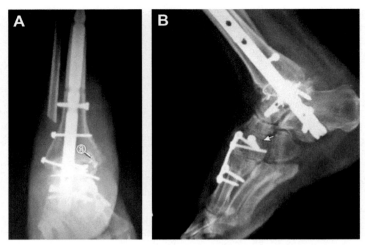

Fig. 7. Ankle and hindfoot fusion complete, cavovarus foot. (*A, B*) Anteroposterior and lateral radiographs of the fused right ankle and hindfoot joints with correction of the cavovarus deformity.

tibial tendon. At the location of the T-N articulation I recommend carefully inserting a full Kessler–type suture, using a #2 nonabsorbable suture inserted into the anterior tibial tendon, on just the proximal side of the T-N joint. Next, approximately 1 cm distal to the nonabsorbable suture, I transect the anterior tibial tendon.[21] This maneuver immediately exposes the entire dorsal T-N capsule, which is excised.

A small lamina spreader is inserted medially or laterally and narrow curved osteotomes are applied, removing all cartilage and subchondral bone. The bone graft is inserted accordingly, and percutaneously an interfragmentary compression screw is inserted medially to posterolaterally, fixing the T-N fusion. A small low-profile dorsal plate can be contoured and laid down, neutralizing forces across the T-N fusion. At the end of the case, after completing all fusion fixation, the tendon is repaired by adding a full Kessler–type nonabsorbable #2 suture into the distal end, with an assistant, both ends of the full Kessler knots are tied down. A continuous 3-0 nylon epitendinous suture is further applied to augment strength to the repair. Attention to avoid any plantarflexion force to the midfoot stressing repair on the knots is necessary.

Laterally, the calcaneocuboid joint is exposed and the articular surfaces are denuded using a thin, narrow flexible osteotome. After insertion of the bone graft, this fusion commonly requires only a single distal to proximal interfragmentary form of screw and washer fixation.

MANAGEMENT

For cavovarus patients with advanced painful arthrosis of the ankle and subtalar joints, arthrodesis is the best common treatment option. However, selective fusion of 1 or all 4 joints in contemporary surgical management is, frankly, uncommon. The goal in realigning joints of the cavus foot is clearly to maintain function while improving patient comfort in gait. Factors to consider when planning an arthrodesis are any existing hardware, the deformity, and the condition of the soft tissues. Uncommonly, an arthrodesis may not be a wise treatment consideration and the options are either nonoperative bracing or a transtibial amputation. Nonoperative care is generally not successful; however, the Intrepid Dynamic Exoskeletal Orthosis, or IDEO brace is a relatively new, effective, custom brace design that should be considered as a nonoperative option. The Intrepid Dynamic Exoskeletal Orthosis brace is a carbon fiber ankle-foot-orthosis exoskeletal brace, designed in the Intrepid military laboratory in San Antonio, Texas, for severely injured recruits as a limb salvage treatment option.[22] The brace fixes the midfoot to the leg, spanning the painful ankle and transferring energy to the limb and off-loading the ankle. The brace is patented and available; however, its high cost and variable availability make it a challenging nonoperative option.

Surgical fusion of the ankle and hindfoot clearly improves the arthritic conditions associated with an advanced cavovarus foot and ankle condition. However, the reality of long-term outcomes is that fusion patients will continue to experience pain and develop secondary midtarsal and transtarsal arthrosis over time owing to the rigidity of the distal limb. It is wise to support the patients' foot with full-length custom orthotics and shoes with rockerbottom sole modifications to minimize stresses on the foot with gait. The patient with recalcitrant pain and soreness after surgical treatment or possibly conditions associated to the cavovarus foot that preclude further ankle and hind-foot reconstruction must be considered and counseled for a transtibial amputation. The prosthetic technology has improved greatly and allows patients the opportunity to be essentially pain free with normal ankle function.

OUTCOME

Management of the advanced cavus foot is challenging and, when this foot undergoes rigid fixation, future surgical treatment options become more limited. Fusions of the tibiotalocalcaneus are reported on more frequently than the pantalar fusion.[5] A well-done ankle fusion will rarely impair a patient's function. The likely reason is that surgeons wish to maintain motion with the patient's foot, particularly in the sagittal plane. Even if the ankle, and S-T joints are fused, the T-N, calcaneocuboid, and transtarsal joints will still allow a small amount of sagittal motion to the foot. However, with ankle, S-T and T-N fusion residual foot motion is largely lost, giving the patient a far more rigid and likely painful foot. In the clinical situation where fusion of the ankle, S-T and T-N joint is performed every attempt to maintain more distal transtarsal motion of the foot must be performed.[23]

Complications associated with ankle, hindfoot, and pantalar fusions have commonly been chronic pain, delayed healing of skin incisions with wound formation of up to 10% in studies. The most notable complication is pseudarthrosis of a joint, found in approximately 12% of patients in reported studies.[24] The need to perform a thorough debridement of joint surfaces is tantamount when performing any fusion and, yet, correcting malalignment as in the cavovarus foot condition is also a primary goal. I performed a retrospective personal study evaluating end-stage ankle and hindfoot arthrodesis incorporating internal fixation and circular Ilizarov external fixation. Sixteen patients were studied with an 87% union rate; 75% of the patients experienced relief of pain. Augmenting the internal fixation with a circular frame construct clearly gave me an opportunity to treat the end-stage deformity patient with greater fixation, particularly with porotic bone.[25]

SUMMARY

The end-stage cavovarus foot deformity has numerous underlying causes precipitating the pathology. In the early stages of a developing cavovarus deformity, it is vital to determine the associated changes that may take place with the patient's foot and ankle over time and counsel the patient about the deformity and apply necessary treatment. In the advanced cavovarus foot condition, there are numerous surgical approaches to treat bone and soft tissue varus overload. Based on the surgeons' experience, it is prudent to individualize any operative plan according to the patients' particular deformity. In severe cavovarus deformities with arthrosis, arthrodesis is necessary to restore function and resolve pain. The most common complication associated with fusion is nonunion and undercorrection of the deformity. Careful operative planning, with attention to soft tissue management and dissection and precise correction of the deformity with fixation all contribute to a successful outcome.

CLINICS CARE POINTS

- The diagnosis of a flexible versus rigid cavovarus deformity associated with arthrosis of the ankle is crucial to determine appropriate treatment.
- A thorough evaluation of the foot and ankle soft tissues plays a significant role in safe surgical care.
- Careful and thorough debridement just deep to the cancellous bone of all fusion surfaces will help to minimize nonunion with compressive fixation.
- Absolute nonweight-bearing of the fusion surfaces for 6 to 8 weeks will help to ensure a successful fusion.

DISCLOSURE

The author has nothing to disclose.

REFERENCES

1. Chien JT, Wu LC. One-stage pantalar arthrodesis for ankle-foot deformity in post-poliomyelitis patients. J Orthop Surg Taiwan 2005;22:28–34.
2. Rosenbaum AJ, Jorden L, Patel N, et al. The cavus foot. Med Clin North Am 2014; 98:301–12.
3. Kai K. Hindfoot issues in the treatment of the cavus foot. Foot Ankle Clin N Am 2008;13:221–7.
4. Kaplan JRM, Aiyer A, Cerrato RA, et al. Operative treatment of the cavovarus foot. Foot Ankle Int 2018;39(11):1370–82.
5. Acosta RA, Uchiba J, Cracchiolo A. The results of primary and staged pantalar arthrodesis and tibiotalocalcaneal arthrodesis in adults patients. Foot Ankle Int 2000;21(3):182–94.
6. Adam W, Ranawat C. Arthrodesis of the hindfoot in rheumatoid arthritis. Orthop Clin North Am 1976;7:827–34.
7. Neumann JA, Nickisch F. Neurologic disorders and cavovarus deformity. Foot Ankle Clin N Am 2019;24:195–203.
8. Gellman H, Leniham M, Halikis M, et al. Selective tarsal arthrodesis and in vitro and analysis of the effect on foot motion. Foot Ankle 1987;8:127–33.
9. Aminian A, Sangeorzan BJ. The anatomy of cavus foot deformity. Foot Ankle Clin 2008;13:191–8.
10. Krahenbuhl N, Weinberg MW. Anatomy and biomechanics of cavovarus deformity. Foot Ankle Clin N Am 2019;24:173–81.
11. Coleman SS, Chesnut WJ. A simple test for hindfoot flexibility in the cavovarus foot. Clin Orthop Relat Res 1977;123:60–2.

12. Recht MP, et al. Magnetic resonance imaging of the foot and ankle. J Am Acad Orthop Surg 2001;9(3):187–99.
13. Myerson MS, Myerson CL. Managing the complex cavus foot deformity. Foot Ankle Clin 2020;25(2):305–17.
14. Herscovici D Jr, Scaduto M. Use of the reamer-irrigator-aspirator technique to obtain autograft for ankle and hindfoot arthrodesis. JBJS Br 2012;94-B(1):47–55.
15. McCluskey WP, Lovell WW, Cummings RJ. The cavovarus foot deformity. Etiology and management. Clin Orthop Relat Res 1989;247:27–37.
16. Fortin PT, Guettler J, Manoli A. Idiopathic cavovarus and lateral ankle instability: recognition and treatment implications relating to ankle arthritis. Foot Ankle Int 2002;39(11):982–94.
17. Irwin TA, Anderson RB, Davis WH, et al. Effect of ankle arthritis on clinical outcome of lateral ankle ligament reconstruction in cavovarus feet. Foot Ankle Int 2010;31(11):941–8.
18. Zide JR, Myerson WS. Arthrodesis for the cavus foot: when, where, and how? Foot Ankle Clin 2013;18:755–67.
19. King HA, Watkins TB, Samuelson KM. Analysis of foot position in ankle arthrodesis and its influence on gait. Foot Ankle Int 1980;1(1):44–9.
20. Provelengios S, Papivasiliou KA, Krykos MJ, et al. Role of the pantalar arthrodesis in the treatment of paralytic foot deformities. JBJS Am 2009;91:575–83.
21. Kessler I. The "grasping technique for tendon repair. Hand 1973;5(3):253–5.
22. Bedigrew KM, Patzowski JC, Wilken JM, et al. Can an integrated orthotic and rehabilitation program stop pain and improve function after lower extremity trauma. Clin Orthop Relat Res 2014;472:3017–25.
23. AlSayel F, Valderrabano V. Arthrodesis of a varus ankle. Foot Ankle Clin 2019; 24(2):265–80.
24. Thevendran G, Shah K, Pinney SJ, et al. Perceived risk factors for nonunion following foot and ankle arthrodesis. J Orthop Surg 2017;25(1):1–6.
25. Crawford B, Watson JT, Jackman J, et al. Case reports and series end-stage hindfoot arthrosis: outcomes of tibiocalcaneal fusion using internal and Ilizarov fixation. J Foot Ankle Surg 2014;53(5):1–6.

Consideration for Total Ankle Replacement in the Varus Ankle and Cavovarus Foot Type

Jordan Tacktill, DPM, FACFAS[a,b], Zachary Rasor, DPM, AACFAS[b],
Benjamin Savasky, DPM, AACFAS[b], Charles M. Zelen, DPM, FACFAS[b,*]

KEYWORDS

• Varus • Total ankle • Cavus

KEY POINTS

- Total ankle replacement is an excellent surgery to allow the patients to ambulate more normally without the pitfalls of a fusion.
- Total Ankle Replacement in the varus ankle is possible when performed in an appropriate manner and with the most appropriate implant.
- Complex total ankle replacement should be left to the foot and ankle surgeon that performs this procedure on a regular basis due to complexity.

Varus malalignment of the ankle joint commonly is categorized as intraarticular and extraarticular.[1] The extraarticular, incongruent joint originates from ligamentous and other soft tissue imbalance, including constriction of the deltoid ligament and also abnormal morphology of the tibia or talus. In distinction to the extraarticular incongruent joint, the intraarticular congruent varus deformity stems from erosive change occurring within the ankle joint and degradation of the medial tibial plafond.[2] The erosive changes can be seen with any degree of varus and often are associated with injury, predisposing a patient to end-stage arthritic malformation of the ankle joint.

Clinical and radiographic evaluations of patients with both varus ankle and cavovarus feet predetermine the designated procedures. The Coleman block test differentiates patients from a rigid osseous deformity requiring arthrodesis of joints, compared with a reducible deformity to a neutral angulation, which is treated with soft tissue balancing and ancillary osseous realignment procedure.[3] The Coleman block test

[a] Kaiser Permanente Midatlantic, Washington Hospital Center Residency, 1221 Mercantile Ln, Upper Marlboro, MD 20774, USA; [b] Professional Education and Research Institute, 222 Walnut Avenue, Roanoke, VA 24016, USA
* Corresponding author.
E-mail address: Cmzelen@periedu.com

Clin Podiatr Med Surg 38 (2021) 497–504
https://doi.org/10.1016/j.cpm.2021.03.003
0891-8422/21/© 2021 Elsevier Inc. All rights reserved.

should be performed to find out if the deformity is forefoot or rearfoot driven. If the rearfoot is moved back into slight valgus with the lateral aspect of the foot on the block, the deformity is considered reducible and forefoot driven.[3] The anterior drawer and talar tilt tests must be performed because there could be ankle instability due to lateral ankle overload. The ankle joint should be palpated for pain as anterior medial impingement of the talus and tibia could illicit discomfort. Silfverskiöld test should be performed and findings should dictate whether a tendo-Achilles lengthening or a gastrocnemius recession is appropriate.[4]

Advanced imaging, such as computer-aided topography or computed tomography scan with 3-dimensional reconstructions, illustrate bony contour and alignment challenges. Radiographs should be taken and are crucial for surgical planning (osteotomy, rearfoot fusions, ankle arthroplasty, ankle arthrodesis, or combination) and help to objectively quantify the amount of correction needed. At minimum, 3 weight-bearing views are needed: lateral ankle, frontal ankle, and dorsoplantar foot. On the lateral view, the talar–first metatarsal angle (Meary angle), calcaneal inclination angle, lateral talocalcaneal angle (Kite angle), first metatarsal calcaneal angle (Hibb angle), cyma line, and ankle joint congruity should be examined. On the frontal view, metatarsal overlap and talar tilt could be seen while ankle joint congruity should be examined (ankle stress views may be taken). On the dorsoplantar plane, talar-navicular congruency, Kite angle, and cyma line are examined. With a cavus foot type, there is an increase in Meary angle, Hibb angle, and calcaneal inclination angle, a decrease in Kite angle, and percentage of talar head uncoverage by the navicular, a posterior break in the cyma line. On lateral view, the apex of deformity is noted where the first metatarsal axis intersects with the axis of the talus.

The cavus foot type and the varus ankle do have inherent challenges with ankle joint replacement surgery. These are due to angular deformity of the joints and the potential for uneven ankle implant device wear following implantation. Considering that, and knowing varus deformity and the cavus foot type can be a more rigid deformity, the decreased range of motion of surrounding joints may offer more predictable outcomes. As noted by Daniels,[5] a varus ankle of less than 10° is suitable for ankle replacement. An incongruency of greater than 10° of varus deformity is unsuitable for ankle replacement and requires either an ankle arthrodesis or an adjunct procedure.[5] Adjunct procedures for total ankle replacement fitment and longevity can include soft tissue balancing. These soft tissue balance procedures consist of medial ankle contracture release, including the deltoid ligament and lengthening of the posterior tibial tendon with conjoined lateral ankle stabilization and augmentation of the lateral ligaments. Additionally, tendon transfers, including partial posterior tibial tendon transfer to the peroneus brevis or augmenting the peroneus brevis by transferring the peroneus longus to the peroneus brevis, are options for balancing the ankle joint. More rigid and higher angle deformities of the foot and ankle can be corrected with osseous procedures, including tibial lengthening medial wedge, supramalleolar osteotomies of the tibia, and Dwyer calcaneal wedge resection with dorsiflexory wedge osteotomy of the first ray. Osteoarthritis often is observed at the subtalar and talonavicular joints, adding to the rigidity of the deformity. This requires wedge osteotomies with joint arthrodesis involving the arthritic joints.

Varus ankles have been researched thoroughly with regard to ankle replacement surgery to regain anatomic alignment and resolve the arthritic condition. Kim and colleagues[6] performed soft tissue balancing on severe varus total ankle arthroplasty patients with success. Soft tissue balancing consisting of medial ankle contracture release and plication of the lateral ankle soft tissue was performed, in addition to a peroneus longus to peroneus brevis tendon transfer and modified Broström procedure.[6]

The lateral soft tissue procedures were utilized if residual angular deformity of the talus was visualized on intraoperative fluoroscopic examination in the anterior-posterior plane. Kim reported a 87% patient satisfaction rating following the procedures, which is consistent with the patient satisfaction of total ankle replacement in neutral ankles.[6]

Adjunct osseous procedures for varus hindfoot deformities and cavus foot types also include isolated subtalar joint arthrodesis, a talonavicular and subtalar joint double arthrodesis, and a triple arthrodesis consisting of fusion of the talonavicular, subtalar, and calcaneocuboid joints. These procedures aide in distal alignment of the hindfoot and, therefore, reduce unwanted stress and strain on the ankle implant and increase its longevity.[7] After following 288 total ankle replacement surgery patients for a mean of 39.5 months, Kim and colleagues[7] discovered patients did show significant improvement when scored with the American Orthopaedic Foot and Ankle Society Score system. As noted by the investigators, the angular deformity must be addressed prior to or during the total ankle arthroplasty to obtain optimal results and increase the survivorship of the implant.

In attempt to decrease the medialization of the ankle and correct the mechanical axis to a neutral position, Colin and colleagues[8] performed supramalleolar osteotomies of the tibia on 52 of 104 patients. Colin and colleagues[8] research revealed that although the realignment of the ankle does reduce pain, realignment of the ankle while performing a total ankle arthroplasty gained more function and a greater reduction in pain. The supramalleolar osteotomy alone does not address the degraded cartilaginous articular surface, and the ankle replacement group was found to have superior outcomes when related to osteoarthritis or posttraumatic osteoarthritis of the ankle joint. Colin and colleagues[8] hypothesized that the supramalleolar osteotomies would correct the ankle joint malalignment in 3 planes, including the talar tilt angle, sagittal talocalcaneal angle, and the talo–first metatarsal angle, but, as a result of radiographic evaluation in preoperative and postoperative evaluation, the supramalleolar osteotomy did not fully correct the talar tilt geometry. Although the osteotomy did improve the overall geometry of the ankle, the functional outcome the total ankle replacement demonstrated superior results.[8]

Preoperative radiographic evaluation of ankle joint angular deformities measuring greater than 14° of varus has been deemed a contraindication for total ankle replacement surgery. A study performed in 2013 concluded that of 104 patients who underwent total ankle arthroplasty, those with varus malalignment showed statistically similar outcomes to patients with a rectus ankle when adjunctive procedures, such as deltoid release and lateral ankle stabilization, were performed. This study followed patients for 2 years postoperatively and, although this is a relatively short length of follow-up, the results are a testament to the statistical significance of angular ankle deformity correction with adjunct procedures and joint replacement surgery.[9]

After conducting 10 total ankle arthroplasties on 8 patients with cavovarus feet and combining the ankle replacement with calcaneal and metatarsal osteotomies, Hong-Geun and colleagues[10] found a statistical significance in patient satisfaction with reduction of the hindfoot deformity and returning the foot and ankle to a neutral position. The reduction of the deformity avoids asymmetric edge loading and subsequent subluxation or dislocation of the ankle joint and eventual implant failure. Additional procedures performed in this study to correct the varus alignment of the foot and ankle included deltoid ligament release, Broström lateral ankle stabilization, peroneus longus to peroneus brevis transfer, lateral calcaneal slide osteotomy, and first metatarsal dorsiflexory wedge osteotomy. Of the patients enrolled in this study, more than half were recorded as very satisfied with the outcome of the surgery, whereas some were satisfied and minimal unsatisfied.[10]

With medial impaction for the tibial plafond and incongruency of the lateral ligament structures in a varus ankle, the necessity for realignment and neutralization is crucial for proper procedural implantation of the total ankle replacement and permanence of the prosthetic device. A 2011 study by Shock and colleagues[11] observed 26 patients with a varus ankle angulation suffering from osteoarthritis and posttraumatic osteoarthritis for up to 37 months. This study incorporated ancillary procedures similar to from other studies, discussed previously, but supplemented lateral gutter resection to allow rotation of the talus. As noted by the investigators in this study and other studies of similar nature, a varus ankle deformity of great than 15° with result in 6.52-times great medial edge load on the implant polymer spacer and therefore led to premature failure of the implant and ultimately revisional surgery.[11]

Ryssman and Myerson[2] formed an algorithmic approach to correcting varus angular deformities of the ankle beginning with intratibial deformity correction, including opening medial distal tibial wedge osteotomies and lateral closing wedge osteotomies of the tibia and fibula as well as talar dome osteotomies. Although realignment of the mechanical axis has been beneficial in relieving some pain, as discussed previously, the erosive changes to the articular surface remain; thus, ankle replacement surgery is ideal for not only retaining motion and function but also eliminating the complications of the formerly pathologic joint surface. Intra-articular deformity rectification is achieved by altering the talar dome via resection to remove the deformity while taking care to remove as little bone of the talus as necessary. Extra-articular correction relieves the constricted medial ankle deltoid ligament and stabilizes the lateral ankle ligaments to provide stability and a congruent ankle joint and may be accompanied by a tibial medial malleolar osteotomy and a thicker polymer spacer. If the varus deformity is distal to the ankle joint, then standard cavovarus foot reconstruction techniques can be completed to achieve neutral alignment.[2]

As the varus deformity increases beyond 14°, the statistical evidence concludes increased edge loading and decreased survivorship of the implant. Coetzee[12] discovered 50% failure rates when greater than 20° varus deformity was seen in the patients during preoperative radiographic evaluation. An additional study published in 2013 directly reviewed patient outcomes with varus angular deformities over 10°. This study of 33 patients, over a 6-year period, concluded, after an American Orthopaedic Foot and Ankle Society Score questionnaire was completed by the patients, that no statistical difference was seen in the varus group compared with the neutral group, showing both had similar outcomes. A complication rate of 19% was encountered in the varus ankle group, with 36% requiring subsequent surgery, and a complication rate of 14% was seen in the neutral group, with a subsequent surgery rate of 17%.[13]

Atves and Miller[14] stressed the importance of balancing the varus ankle to protect the ankle replacement device, including soft tissue procedures to gain the neutral mechanical alignment position. In concurrence with the previous studies, Atves and Miller[14] described the release of the medial ligament structures with subsequent lateral ankle stabilization, possible peroneus longus to peroneus brevis transfer, and lengthening of the posterior tibial tendon. Osseous correction included a medial malleolar osteotomy, lateral displacement calcaneal osteotomy, and first ray dorsiflexory wedge osteotomy, further reiterating the importance to balance the foot and ankle to a neutral and plantar-grade position and, therefore, reducing edge loading and overall wear of the ankle implant.[14]

A study of 131 patients enrolled for total ankle arthroplasty with varus ankle alignments of greater than 10°, published in 2012, defined the type of ankle varus deformity. The definition of the incongruent varus ankle with regard to this study was that which featured a gap of the talocrural angle of greater than 10°. Congruent ankle distinction showed no gaping with increased varus angulation. Supramalleolar osteotomies and ligament balancing of the medial and lateral ankle achieved a rectus ankle for implantation of the ankle replacement. The researchers proposed that neutral alignment can be attained in 80% of patients who require supramalleolar and hindfoot osteotomies in congruent ankles and in all patients with incongruent ankle varus who required associated soft tissue corrective procedures. Postoperative revision surgery was seen in 40% of patients as a result of edge loading in both congruent and incongruent ankle varus patients. The investigators concluded that varus ankle alignments of greater than 10° to 15° were noted to have greater complication rates following initial surgery, and ankle arthrodesis should be considered for those patients if neutral mechanical alignment cannot be accomplished.[15,16]

Two cases clearly illustrate that the varus total ankle almost always will fail and require revision with ancillary procedures to the address the varus. In the first case (**Fig. 1**), a very active sprinkler mechanic underwent a total ankle with heel osteotomy

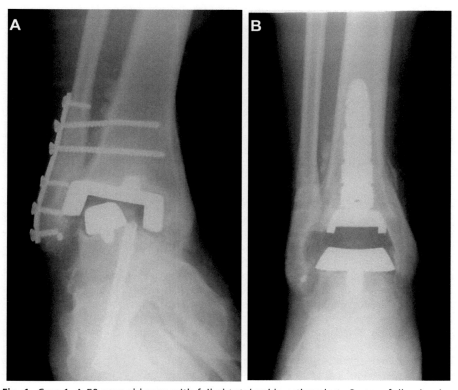

Fig. 1. Case 1. A 50-year-old man with failed total ankle arthroplasty 2 years following implantation. Although the varus deformity was corrected with heel osteotomy and subtalar fusion as well as soft tissue construction at the lateral ankle, injury to his ankle while doing sprinkler maintenance led to failure of the soft tissue reconstruction and a recurrence of the varus deformity. Revision total ankle arthroplasty surgery and extensive soft tissue balancing were performed, leading to a successful revision (A) Varus total ankle after work injury leading to loss of soft tissue stability and recurrent varus led to fast failure of the implant (B) Revision to more stable total ankle and revisional lateral ankle reconstruction led to long-term satisfactory result.

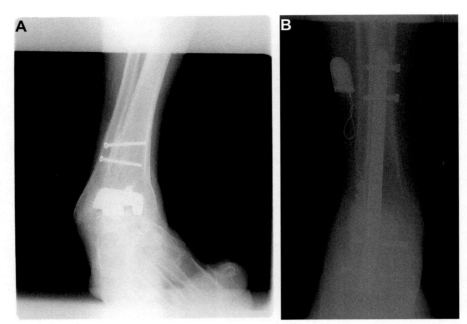

Fig. 2. Case 2. A 70-year-old man with failed total ankle arthroplasty almost immediately after placement, due to the extensive varus angular deformity related to Charcot-Marie-Tooth disease with peripheral neuropathy. Tibiotalocalcaneal arthrodesis was performed. In subsequent evaluation, the patient was full weight bearing without pain. (*A*) Total ankle in severe varus due to Charcot Marie Tooth disease. (*B*) Satisfactory fusion with femoral head graft and intermedullary nail.

and lateral ligament reconstruction. Despite initial satisfactory result, after a work injury twisting his ankle and losing stability, the ankle returned to a varus position and the implant failed. Revision with more stable ankle replacement and extensive lateral ankle reconstruction was needed to salvage this patient's arthroplasty. In the second case (**Fig. 2**), a total ankle was placed into a patient with a progressive neuromuscular deformity (Charcot-Marie-Tooth disease) and almost immediately after surgery went into varus. There is no indication for total ankle in this type of varus/cavus foot due to the progressive nature of this deformity and the ensuing neuropathy; therefore, this was revised to a fusion with femoral head block and intermedullary nail.

In conclusion, ankle varus alignment is a complicated deformity and does present a challenge for surgeons to successfully treat with ankle arthroplasty surgery. The current research does show some success with varus angulation of less than 10°, but the postoperative complication rates do increase as the degree of preoperative deformity increases. Common postoperative pathology includes edge loading and residual deformity following corrective surgery. The consensus of the research agrees that ligamentous and soft tissue balancing typically combined with adjacent bony osteotomies or arthrodesis is recommended to attain a neutral mechanical alignment. Total ankle arthroplasty is a reasonable surgical option for nonprogressive varus ankle and cavus foot deformities when appropriate adjunct procedures are performed either prior to or during the arthroplasty surgery. Total ankle arthroplasty is contraindicated in the presence of progressive cavus foot and ankle deformities. This class of deformity is treated more properly with arthrodesis procedures in patients looking for curative surgical options. The surgeon must conduct a thorough history with detailed neurologic, musculoskeletal, and radiologic examinations during the preoperative encounters. As described in recent literature, patient satisfaction scores and complication rates after total ankle arthroplasty in those with mildly noncongruent ankles are similar to those of rectus ankles.

CLINICS CARE POINTS

- Total Ankle Replacements are one of the most complex procedures a foot and ankle surgeon can perform. More complex replacements should be left to the surgeon who performs the procedure on a more regular basis.
- Total Ankle Replacement is a need procedure as it is far more functional then a fusion with a greater patient satisfaction.
- There are a large number of replacement options and all should be considered to allow your patient to get the best results and appropriately correct deformity.

DISCLOSURE

The authors have nothing to disclose.

REFERENCES

1. Piazza S, Ricci G, Caldarazzo Ienco E, et al. Pes cavus and hereditary neuropathies: when a relationship should be suspected. J Orthop Traumatol 2010;11(4): 195–201.
2. Ryssman D, Myerson MS. Surgical strategies: the management of varus ankle deformity with joint replacement. Foot Ankle Int 2011;32(2):217–24.
3. Coleman SS, Chesnut WJ. A simple test for hindfoot flexibility in the cavovarus foot. Clin Orthop Relat Res 1977;123:60–2.
4. Barouk P, Barouk LS. Clinical diagnosis of gastrocnemius tightness. Foot Ankle Clin 2014;19:659–67.
5. Daniels TR. Surgical technique for total ankle arthroplasty in ankles with preoperative coronal plane varus deformity of 10° or greater. JBJS Essent Surg Tech 2013;3(4):e22.
6. Kim BS, Choi WJ, Kim YS, et al. Total ankle replacement in moderate to severe varus deformity of the ankle. J Bone Joint Surg Br 2009;9:1183–90.
7. Kim BS, Knupp M, Zwicky L, et al. Total ankle replacement in association with hindfoot fusion. J Bone Joint Surg Br 2010;92-B(11):1540–7.
8. Fabrice C, Bolliger L, Lang TH, et al. Effect of supramalleolar osteotomy and total ankle replacement on talar position in the varus osteoarthritic ankle: a comparative study. Foot Ankle Int 2014;35(5):445–52.
9. Queen RM, Adams SB, Viens NA, et al. Differences in outcomes following total ankle replacement in patients with neutral alignment compared with tibiotalar joint malalignment. J Bone Joint Surg Am 2013;95(21):1927–34.
10. Hong-Geun J, Jeon S-H, Kim T-H, et al. Total ankle arthroplasty with combined calcaneal and metatarsal osteotomies for treatment of ankle osteoarthritis with accompanying cavovarus deformities: early results. Foot Ankle Int 2013;34(1): 140–7.
11. Shock RP, Christensen JC, Schuberth JM. Total ankle replacement in the varus ankle. J Foot Ankle Surg 2011;50(1):5–10.

12. Coetzee JC. Surgical strategies: lateral ligament reconstruction as part of the management of varus ankle deformity with ankle replacement. Foot Ankle Int 2010;31(3):267–74.
13. Trajkovski T, Pinsker E, Cadden A, et al. Outcomes of ankle arthroplasty with preoperative coronal-plane varus deformity of 10° or greater. J Bone Joint Surg Am 2013;95(15):1382–8.
14. Atves JN, Miller JR. Pertinent pearls on rebalancing procedures with total ankle replacement. Podiatry Today 2019;32(5):38-45.
15. Kouyoumdjian P, Asencio G. Total ankle arthroplasty and coronal plane deformities. Orthop Trauma Surg Res 2012;98(1):75–84.
16. Smith R, Wood PLR. Arthrodesis of the ankle in the presence of a large deformity in the coronal plane. J Bone Joint Surg Br 2007;89-B(5):615–9.

Moving?

Make sure your subscription moves with you!

To notify us of your new address, find your **Clinics Account Number** (located on your mailing label above your name), and contact customer service at:

Email: journalscustomerservice-usa@elsevier.com

800-654-2452 (subscribers in the U.S. & Canada)
314-447-8871 (subscribers outside of the U.S. & Canada)

Fax number: 314-447-8029

Elsevier Health Sciences Division
Subscription Customer Service
3251 Riverport Lane
Maryland Heights, MO 63043

*To ensure uninterrupted delivery of your subscription, please notify us at least 4 weeks in advance of move.

USA
2023